T0138221

Community Health Equity

Community Health Equity

A Chicago Reader

EDITED BY FERNANDO DE MAIO,
RAJ C. SHAH, MD, JOHN MAZZEO,
AND DAVID A. ANSELL, MD

THE UNIVERSITY OF CHICAGO PRESS   CHICAGO AND LONDON

The University of Chicago Press, Chicago 60637
The University of Chicago Press, Ltd., London
© 2019 by The University of Chicago
All rights reserved. No part of this book may be used or reproduced in any manner whatsoever without written permission, except in the case of brief quotations in critical articles and reviews. For more information, contact the University of Chicago Press, 1427 E. 60th St., Chicago, IL 60637.
Published 2019
Printed in the United States of America

28 27 26 25 24 23 22 21 20 19   1 2 3 4 5

ISBN-13: 978-0-226-61459-5 (cloth)
ISBN-13: 978-0-226-61462-5 (paper)
ISBN-13: 978-0-226-61476-2 (e-book)
DOI: https://doi.org/10.7208/chicago/9780226614762.001.0001

Library of Congress Cataloging-in-Publication Data

Names: De Maio, Fernando, 1976– editor. | Shah, Raj C., editor. | Mazzeo, John (Medical anthropologist), editor. | Ansell, David A., editor.
Title: Community health equity : a Chicago reader / edited by Fernando De Maio, Raj C. Shah, MD, John Mazzeo, and David A. Ansell, MD.
Description: Chicago ; London : The University of Chicago Press, 2019. | Includes bibliographical references and index.
Identifiers: LCCN 2018042357 | ISBN 9780226614595 (cloth : alk. paper) | ISBN 9780226614625 (pbk. : alk. paper) | ISBN 9780226614762 (e-book)
Subjects: LCSH: Minorities—Medical care—Illinois—Chicago. | Medical care—Illinois—Chicago—Social aspects.
Classification: LCC RA448.C4 C65 2019 | DDC 362.1089/00977311—dc23
LC record available at https://lccn.loc.gov/2018042357

♾ This paper meets the requirements of ANSI/NISO Z39.48-1992 (Permanence of Paper).

Contents

Foreword

Today, in American health circles, health equity is the in thing. All manner of organizations claim to be addressing health disparities or health equity. Government and philanthropic organizations issue requests for proposals to attempt to reduce or eliminate health disparities. The call for the elimination of health disparities (still a peculiar American formulation) and the achievement of health equity graces our national health goals and appears in many strategic plans of our local public health departments.

This collection of readings gets back to basics.

It pulls together work over a wide range of disciplines, but all anchored in the nation's heartland—Chicago. Chicago is an apt lens through which we can study the changes in health inequities and what we can do to achieve equity.

The Chicago region was a trading center for a variety of Native American tribes, including the Illinois, Miami, and Potawatomi. Their lands were stolen, and most were forced west. Later—to meet the needs of industry and especially during the 1950s and 1960s as part of the federal government's relocation program—thousands of Native Americans came to Chicago. Former slaves fleeing the terrorism that destroyed the promise of emancipation fled to Chicago. The numbers of blacks exploded in later decades as part of the Great Migration. Chinese, Mexicans, Irish, Italians, and Russians are just some of the people from throughout the world who joined the city to work in the factories and build the railroads. Japanese Americans were relocated to Chicago after the American concentration camps began to be closed. The difficult economic realities of Puerto Rico forced many to come to the city seeking jobs. It is here in Chicago that the Haymarket demonstrations in 1886 called for an eight-hour workday. It would take another half century to win the eight-hour day in law and profoundly improve the health of the American people. The Haymarket police riots set the tone for community–police relations. The 1937 Republic Steel Massacre—where striking workers were killed by police—echoes today in the sixteen shots that brought down a black teenage boy. Chicago is a labor town, and the Coalition of Black Trade Unionists was born here. Today, the Chicago Teacher's Union fights for the preservation of public education, and health care unions struggle to preserve institutions that serve the poor.

As Chicago grew, the white men in charge made sure it became one of the most segregated cities in the nation. Racism—the bedrock of these United States—is nurtured and protected in Chicago. Careful hierarchies designed to protect white supremacy were erected and maintained. New European immigrants came and occupied lower rungs until they were assimilated and became white. Native Americans remain invisible, but they are still here, still alive. People of color from Asia and Latin America and Africa face the racist structures of the city. The very bottom rung is reserved for the sons and daughters of former slaves. The health status of the people discussed in this volume cannot be understood without understanding American racism—Chicago style.

Chicago represents a location where workers from all over the world engage in a power struggle with the captains of finance and industry. It is a city built on racism and its ideological foundation of white supremacy. Women faced oppression as workers. In Chicago, women had to fight for the basic right to vote, to raise families, to obtain basic dignity and human rights for their children. They are the glue. It is not an accident that Ida B. Wells kept her name after marrying and was a leading suffragette and a warrior in the antilynching movement. Today, Chicago remains a city where women still earn less than men and women of color die in greater numbers.

Chicago considers power and politics a local sport. A legendary big city machine has dominated local electoral politics. The First Congressional District of Illinois is the longest-held black district in the nation, dating from Oscar DePriest's election as a Republican (the party of Lincoln) in 1929 through today's congressman, Bobby Rush, who learned leadership as a member of the Black Panther Party. Former congressmen from the First District include the labor leader Charles Hayes and Chicago's first black mayor, Harold Washington. Washington's coalition and election helped pave the way for the first black president, Barack

Obama. However, Chicago's real political power resides in its neighborhoods; organizing is in its blood. Through its mosques and synagogues,
its churches, block clubs, and ethnic organizations, people fight to define the questions. These struggles for social justice outline the research
questions to be described and explored. It is people's struggles that produced much of the work cataloged in this book.

Class, race, and gender are the three fundamental hierarchies around
which power and resources are structured in the United States. Health
inequities are not defined only by differences between those on the top
and those on the bottom. Inequities are preventable injustices that occur
along a gradient. The working poor suffer more than those with union
jobs, who suffer more than the middle class. Indeed, even our rich have
poorer health than their peers in OECD nations.

It is for this reason that *Community Health Equity: A Chicago Reader*
holds lessons for us all. Each article in the collection represents the intersection of the exploration of a problem and a struggle for basic justice
to solve that problem. The book contains no recipes or certain solutions. It illuminates a process that explores the structural origins—the
root causes of health inequities—as well as efforts to reduce pain and
suffering.

Health and well-being are basic human rights desired by all people.
This *Reader* is one small tool that can help us find a way to create a city,
a region, and a planet that are sustainable and at peace and where social
justice is the law of the land.

Linda Rae Murray, MD, MPH, FACP

Acknowledgments

A lot of people helped us in the preparation of this book. We benefited from the thoughtful suggestions of many colleagues at the
Center for Community Health Equity, including Doug Bruce, Brittney
Lange-Maia, Stephen Rothschild, and Dan Schober. We are particularly
grateful to Jana Hirschtick, Maggie Nava, and Noam Ostrander, who discussed the book at the 2016 Health Disparities and Social Justice conference. James Bloyd, Jaime Dircksen, Bijou Hunt, Linda Rae Murray,
and Pat O'Campo all gave thoughtful comments on the proposal or early
drafts. Linda Levendusky from DePaul's Social Science Research Center offered helpful copyediting notes.

We were fortunate to have had the assistance of excellent research
assistants and interns who helped in many aspects of the work, from
early literature reviews to image processing to final referencing and
proofreading: Kerianne Burke, Peter Contos, Camille DeMarco, Kinga
Guziak, Celie Joblin, Amber Miller, LaShawn Murray, and Rosio Pa-
tino. Funding from a DePaul University Academic Initiatives Grant and
several Undergraduate Research Assistant Grants from the College of
Liberal Arts and Social Sciences facilitated this project.

This book is the result of a truly collaborative effort by four colleagues
who share a passion for health equity work and who wanted to better
understand the history of this work in Chicago. We worked together over
several years on this project, and, along the way, each of us drew on the
support of our own networks.

Fernando De Maio. I am most grateful for the support of my family, including my parents, Susana and Domingo, as well as my brother,
Pablo. Fate had it that we would all live in different countries, but that

has never hindered our connection and the support that I know I can count on from them. I owe a particularly important thanks to Cecilia De Maio, *que siempre estuvo a mi lado*. My daughters, Lucy and Joy, are everything and inspire me with their kindness and curiosity. Lastly, I want to acknowledge the support of good colleagues in the Department of Sociology at DePaul University, including Black Hawk Hancock and Deena Weinstein (who reminded me to listen to the Ramones and turn the volume up).

Raj C. Shah. I acknowledge my parents, Chandravadan and Vanitaben Shah, who left the only lives they knew in Tanzania to provide a better life for their children. I acknowledge my sister, Rakhee Stonestreet, and my diverse friends from Bolingbrook, Illinois, who shaped my early life experiences, which involved appreciating multiple viewpoints and cultures. I am grateful for the mentoring provided by professional colleagues, patients, and community leaders in Chicago who have nurtured my academic growth and interests. Most importantly, I am forever grateful to my wife, Falguni R. Vasa, for supporting my curiosity about how things work, and to my children, Ashini and Arjun Shah, for developing as leaders to make the society they will inherit a better place for all.

John Mazzeo. I acknowledge my outstanding colleagues in the Master of Public Health Program at DePaul University, whose work to prepare the next generation of the public health workforce places into action the spirit of this volume. I am grateful for my wife, Ruth, who provides insightful perspective and constant encouragement. I am particularly thankful for my three energetic boys, Ethan, Gavin, and Jacob, whose early determination to make the world a better place makes me a very proud father.

David A. Ansell. I am grateful for the love and support of my wife, Dr. Paula Grabler, my two children, Jonah and Leah Ansell, their spouses, and my grandson, Rafael. I am also grateful for my many friends and colleagues at Rush University Medical Center and across the United States who have provided me guidance and insight.

As a group, we are humbled by the creativity and sophistication of the authors of the publications collected in this book. As a group, we are also grateful for the support of this project by the University of Chicago Press and, in particular, to Tim Mennel and Rachel Kelly Unger for their work shepherding the book through the process of publication.

We sincerely hope that this book will serve as an inspiration to our students, colleagues, and community partners. All of us have the potential to contribute to making Chicago a fairer and more equal city, one in which all its residents can thrive and live out their full potential. May we work together so that a future edition of this book tells a story of that achievement.

Introduction

You must always remember that the sociology, the history, the economics, the graphs, the charts, the regressions all land, with great violence, upon the body. — Ta-Nehisi Coates

This *Reader* tells the story of a divided city, a metropolis whose unequal distribution of power and resources limits the capacity of its residents to live long and healthy lives. We present a rich collection of documents and research studies, taking a historical and interdisciplinary perspective. At their best, these documents challenge the status quo—identifying inequalities (which were previously hidden), highlighting historical patterns (often neglected), and exerting all of us to think critically about the fundamental causes of health inequities in Chicago. As we will see, these documents also show us important weaknesses in our collective efforts; in particular, they remind us that it is not enough simply to collect data and write reports—simply to *describe* the problem (when we already know it exists) would be unethical.[1] Rather, the documents in this *Reader* are a testament to a powerful idea: deliberate action based on data can change seemingly intractable problems.

In Chicago, the latest evidence indicates that life expectancy varies by as much as sixteen years between the worst-off and the best-off communities.[2,3] Similarly, we know that infant mortality varies from a low of 2.2 deaths per 1,000 live births to more than 17—meaning that, while affluent communities like Lincoln Park have infant mortality rates that are on par with those in Japan and Sweden, African American communities such as West Garfield Park, Auburn Gresham, and Roseland are more similar to so-called Third World countries. One's zip code should not predict one's life expectancy, but it does.

The numbers are clear: Chicago suffers from profound health inequities. But why? Is this the result of poor lifestyle choices? After all, we know what it takes to be healthy: eat the right foods, get sufficient exercise, don't smoke, and follow medical advice as needed. In the United States, many of us think nothing else matters because we consider health a personal issue, a personal responsibility. Yet that is not the whole story. While each of us has some degree of control over our health, our capacity to make healthy choices is constrained not just by our own resources but by the characteristics of the places where we live. Our health is shaped by society, not just by our own individual choices and behaviors. In Chicago—a large and highly segregated city—we can see powerful evidence of what are called *the social determinants of health*.[4,5]

In today's Chicago, sixteen-year-old black males have a 50% chance of surviving to age sixty-five—a statistic many people attribute to violence and homicide. While those things do account for a significant proportion of those deaths, more than half of the burden is due to premature heart disease and cancer, which in turn are linked to stress caused by social and economic inequities.[6] Social, economic, and racial inequities can be considered a form of violence called *structural violence*, and they are every bit as deadly as gun violence when it comes to health. We are dealing, in other words, with a burden of largely preventable and treatable conditions made worse by social conditions.[7] This reality shatters the idea that health is solely a personal responsibility when, instead, it is more appropriately seen as a public issue, one shaped by economics, politics, the legal system, and the education system as well as by the health system.[8] Together, those forces are often known as *social structure*.

Chicago is the focus of our book, and, while it is one of the largest and most unequal cities in the United States, it is of course not the only city grappling with health inequities. In the past decade, the concept of health equity has received increasing attention both nationwide and around the world. It features in academic research in a wide range of disciplines and is invoked in the mission statements and strategic plans of numerous hospitals and medical centers. Its importance is clear.

Over time, the research community has explored different ways of defining *health equity*. Perhaps the most powerful definition comes from the Centers for Disease Control, which argues that "health equity is achieved when every person has the opportunity to attain his or her full health potential." Similarly, *Healthy People 2020*—an agenda-setting report published by the US Department of Health and Human Services—defines *health equity* as the "attainment of the highest level of health for all people. Achieving health equity requires valuing everyone equally with focused and ongoing societal efforts to address avoidable inequalities, historical and contemporary injustices, and the elimination of health and health care disparities."[9] Recently, the Commission on the Social Determinants of Health of the World Health Organization (WHO) concluded: "Reducing health inequalities is . . . an ethical imperative. Social injustice is killing people on a grand scale."[10] The WHO commission took an openly progressive political stance, emphasizing: "It does not have to be this way and it is not right that it should be like this. Where systematic differences in health are judged to be avoidable by reasonable action they are, quite simply, unfair. Putting right these inequities—the huge and remediable differences in health between and within countries—is a matter of social justice."[10] Health equity has become a concern for us all.

We believe that, with its rich history of inquiry and activism, Chicago is a particularly fitting case study in the long campaign for health equity. Today, health equity has become the central plank in the city's public health plan, Healthy Chicago 2.0,[3] but studies of the city and its characteristics have a long pedigree. One early example is C. T. Bushnell's 1901 map linking child mortality and factors that would now be called *social determinants of health*: overcrowding, lack of sanitation, and economic distress (see figure 1).[11]

One hundred sixteen years later, we have better data and better maps, but the fundamental problem is the same. If anything, the association between place and health that Bushnell's map illuminated geographically is even more pronounced.

The same is true of residential segregation, which remains a key driver of social inequity in Chicago.[12] The structural roots of residential segregation in Chicago were laid in the 1930s, with the infamous "redlining" of nonwhite neighborhoods by the Federal Home Owners' Loan Corporation. Residents of red areas—nearly all of whom were nonwhite—were effectively denied access to Federal Housing Administration–backed mortgages.[12-14] Coates's assessment of redlining is poignant: "Redlining destroyed the possibility of investment wherever black people lived."[13] This and other discriminatory practices (from restrictive covenants to

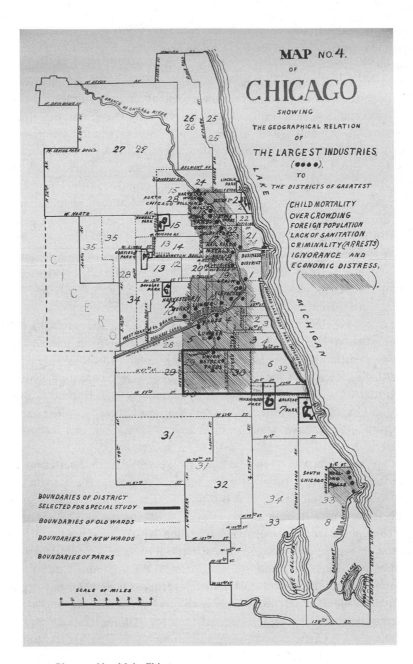

FIGURE 1. Place and health in Chicago, 1901

Source: Bushnell CT. Some social aspects of the Chicago Stock Yards: Chapter II. The Stock Yard community at Chicago. *American Journal of Sociology*. 1901;7(3):289–330.

physical violence) excluded black people from the real estate market—a policy that has affected families across generations.[15] This historical injustice is one of many that continue to affect people today, constraining our collective capacity to achieve health equity across the city.

Redlining is only one example of *structural violence*, which Paul Farmer defined as "social arrangements that put individuals and populations in harm's way. The arrangements are structural because they are embedded in the political and economic organization of our social world; they are violent because they cause injury to people."[16] Above all, this book is a record of the impact structural violence exacts on health.

Structural violence manifests in many ways, including through socioeconomic divisions, gender inequality, ageism, sex discrimination, and—as the record of Chicago illustrates—racism. We argue that *structural* racism—and not biology—explains many of the patterns that will be depicted in this book. By *structural racism*, we mean "the totality of ways in which societies foster racial discrimination through mutually reinforcing systems of housing, education, employment, earnings, benefits, credit, media, health care, and criminal justice. These patterns and practices in turn reinforce discriminatory beliefs, values, and distribution of resources."[17] Used similarly by Camara Jones, *structural racism* is "normative, sometimes legalized, and often manifests as inherited disadvantage. It is structural, having been codified in our institutions of custom, practice, and law, so there need not be an identifiable perpetrator. Indeed, institutionalized racism is often evident as inaction in the face of need."[18]

By reflecting on the contours of health equity research in Chicago, we can take stock of what we know, what we have tried, and what has been debated. Taking a wide and historical view of health equity in Chicago will remind us of, among other things, the importance of social structure, the frustrating permanence of structural violence, and the ongoing burden of racism in our society. Taken together, these documents teach us about the importance (and limits) of research. On the one hand, research can identify inequalities—this is often by disaggregating averages, which can hide differences between groups, or by describing historical trends and geographic differences. Examples in this *Reader* teach us about the importance of local (community-level) data and show historical echoes (e.g., as we will see later in the book, findings from analyses of white-black differences in mortality from tuberculosis in the 1920s

are not dissimilar from the same analyses of mortality from breast cancer in the first decade of the twenty-first century). On the other hand,
research has often been rooted in *description*—identifying the scope of
problems, testing hypotheses about correlation, association, and sometimes causality, but then falling short of naming the fundamental causes
of our health problems. Thus, structural violence is an *unnamed* source
of health inequities in the documents in this *Reader*, despite evidence
pointing to the health-damaging consequences of structural racism seen
in many of these documents.

About This *Reader*

A careful review of decades' worth of articles, reports, and other documents about health equity in Chicago preceded the assembly of
this book. We chose documents primarily for what they taught us—
sometimes in their presentation of new data or the use of a new research
method. Sometimes this involved the creation of a new quantitative measure (e.g., measures of community vitality or collective efficacy); other
times the document involved the application of qualitative techniques to
gather data on peoples' lived experiences (personal narratives that are
often missing in quantitative research). But we were also drawn to documents that seemed to have a lasting importance—those that we wanted
our students and colleagues to read and discuss with us. Our collection is certainly not a meta-analysis or a systematic review, so by design
it cannot wholly represent the literature—there are thousands of published papers and reports on health equity in Chicago, far too many to
include or even cite. Nevertheless, we believe that it tells an important
story about Chicago, its history, and our attempts to make it healthier
and fairer.

The book is divided into five parts to mirror the most important elements of the Healthy People 2020 definition of *health equity*. Part 1, "A
Divided City," illustrates historical and contemporary injustices. Part 2,
"The Health Gap," focuses on Chicago's problems in achieving the highest level of health for all people and documents contemporary patterns
of avoidable inequalities. Part 3, "Separate and Unequal Health Care,"
and part 4, "Communities Matter," reflect on two fundamental drivers of
community health: access to the health care system and the social condi-

tions of communities themselves. Part 5, "Taking Action," engages with ongoing societal efforts to address avoidable inequalities at the level of health care access or community.

A Divided City

Cities are divided. Why? Are they intentionally designed that way according to some master urban plan about how cities should be structured? Is their evolution based on choices favored by the many? Is the evolution of a city characterized by some of both? Chicago as a city is a dynamic and multilayered construct. It had a unique opportunity to redefine itself as it reemerged from the ashes of the Great Chicago Fire of 1871 and as waves of immigrants poured in from elsewhere in the United States and abroad. As stated in Daniel Burnham's 1909 Plan of Chicago: "The people of Chicago have ceased to be impressed by rapid growth or the great size of the city. What they insist [on] asking now is, How are we living?"[19] How *are* we living? That question remains current a century later. Excerpts from Sampson's *Great American City* provide a glimpse at the effects of the interplay between time and space have left on Chicago's lived environment and deep-rooted patterns of segregation. The other documents in this part—published between 1927 and 2012—reflect critical aspects of the city's social divisions. In different ways, they express the importance of the social determinants of health, and they document with startling detail the value of community-level data in a city as divided as Chicago.

The Health Gap

Part 2 examines a rich collection of studies describing health inequities in Chicago, often with a focus on race/racism. While we highlight a wide range of conditions—cancer, birth weight, AIDS, breast cancer, and hypertension—our emphasis is not on the conditions but on how these health outcomes reflect social inequalities. Most of these studies are quantitative in design, reflecting the strengths of epidemiology and population health research. Not only are these studies important for their descriptive insight (they tell us about the scope of the problem); they also begin to illuminate how these health gaps came to be. They are not natural but, rather, a reflection of the social, structural, and political determinants of health. Nor are they static—health gaps change over time and vary from community to community.

Separate and Unequal Health Care

Health equity requires the elimination of unjust health care disparities, an issue of profound importance in Chicago. Our selection of articles here starts with a 1954 pamphlet from the Committee to End Discrimination in Chicago Medical Institutions analyzing the distribution of Negro births and deaths in Chicago hospitals. Its scathing critique of racism in health care directly asked: "What color are your germs?" This part also quotes the Black Panthers, who ran a community clinic in the city. Other selections document the work of the Uptown People's Health Center, quantify the harm of patient dumping at Cook County Hospital in the 1980s, and investigate trauma deserts in the poorest parts of the city in 2015. Altogether, these documents reveal how structural violence is manifest within the health care system and also give a glimpse of the change that is possible through concerted social action.

Communities Matter

This part explores the literature on how community characteristics affect the health of residents—either increasing the risk of disease or protecting health. Here, readers will begin to see how structural violence is linked to community characteristics, through concepts such as collective efficacy, structural disadvantage, social capital, and community vitality. The studies selected raise methodological challenges about how to measure community characteristics and how to link them to individual health. Again, we did not restrict our choice of studies by disease categories. Readers will find a wide range of topics—from smoking cessation to life expectancy, from pregnancy outcomes to heart disease, and from childhood asthma to gun violence.

Taking Action

The final part features Chicago's historical and contemporary efforts to address avoidable inequalities and nurture health equity through two key structural targets: health care systems and communities themselves. In this part, readers will discover successful initiatives to reduce the gap in mortality between blacks and whites with breast cancer. They will also explore the youth-led movement that pushed for the opening of an adult trauma center on the South Side. We conclude with the public health metrics of Healthy Chicago 2.0—quantitative targets for improving health in the city's most disadvantaged communities. We also explore a tension in the literature between problem-focused and solution-focused research, raising the question of how to change to help make Chicago a healthier and more equitable city.

What Must Be Done?

In total, this collection documents more than a century of work on health equity. While the history of Chicago's profound inequality can overwhelm, this work testifies to the relentless efforts of many people from many communities determined to achieve something better, more humane and just. Public health research shows that history matters. Our health is not just the product of our individual behaviors, and disease is in many ways the embodiment of structural violence, generations in the making.[20]

All our solutions are interrelated. We cannot address inequities in diabetes and diabetes-related hospitalizations without first addressing food security. We cannot address the obesity epidemic without recognizing the place of neighborhood safety. Nor can we reduce preventable and avoidable morbidities without considering the social determinants of health—ranging from poverty and economic inequality to racism and gender inequality—as well as political processes that disenfranchise and marginalize whole communities.

While, by design, this *Reader* looks back into the literature—our concern is with the present and the future. Thus, we urge readers to approach this book with a critical perspective, questioning what must be done to make a difference. Whether college students, medical students, or established professionals, they will, we hope, be inspired to join this struggle. What can we do together so that someday the story will be different and we can say that everyone in Chicago really has the opportunity to attain his or her full health potential? The readings that follow offer lessons for taking up that critical task.

References

1. Muntaner C, Sridharan S, Solar O, Benach J. Against unjust global distribution of power and money: The report of the WHO Commission on Social Determinants of Health: Global inequality and the future of public health policy. *Journal of Public Health Policy*. 2009;30(2):163–175.

2. Hunt BR, Tran G, Whitman S. Life expectancy varies in local communities in Chicago: Racial and spatial disparities and correlates. *Journal of Racial and Ethnic Health Disparities*. 2015;2(4):425–433.

3. Dircksen JC, Prachand NG. *Healthy Chicago 2.0: Partnering to improve health equity*. City of Chicago; 2016.

4. De Maio F, Mazzeo J, Ritchie D. Social determinants of health: A view on theory and measurement. *Rhode Island Medical Journal*. 2013;96(7):15–19.

5. De Maio F, Shah RC, Schipper K, Gurdiel R, Ansell D. Racial/ethnic minority segregation and low birth weight: A comparative study of Chicago and Toronto community-level indicators. *Critical Public Health*. 2017;27(5):541–553.

6. Geronimus AT, Bound J, Colen CG. Excess black mortality in the United States and in selected black and white high-poverty areas, 1980–2000. *American Journal of Public Health*. 2011;101(4):720–729.

7. Ansell D. *The death gap*. Chicago: University of Chicago Press; 2017.

8. De Maio F. *Health and social theory*. Basingstoke: Palgrave Macmillan; 2010.

9. Office of Disease Prevention and Health Promotion. *Healthy People 2020*. Washington, DC: US Department of Health and Human Services; 2010.

10. WHO. *Closing the gap in a generation: Health equity through action on the social determinants of health*. Geneva: World Health Organization; 2008.

11. Bushnell CT. Some social aspects of the Chicago Stock Yards: Chapter II: The Stock Yard community at Chicago. *American Journal of Sociology*. 1901;7(3):289–330.

12. Satter B. *Family properties: Race, real estate, and the exploitation of black urban families*. New York: Metropolitan; 2009.

13. Coates T. The case for reparations. *Atlantic*. June 2014.

14. Massey DS. American apartheid: Segregation and the making of the underclass. *American Journal of Sociology*. 1990;96(2):329–357.

15. Sampson RJ. *Great American city: Chicago and the enduring neighborhood effect*. Chicago: University of Chicago Press; 2012.

16. Farmer PE, Nizeye B, Stulac S, Keshavjee S. Structural violence and clinical medicine. *PLoS Medicine*. 2006;3(10):e449.

17. Bailey ZD, Krieger N, Agenor M, Graves J, Linos N, Bassett MT. Structural racism and health inequities in the USA: Evidence and interventions. *Lancet*. 2017;389(10077):1453–1463.

18. Jones CP. Levels of racism: A theoretic framework and a gardener's tale. *American Journal of Public Health*. 2000;90(8):1212–1215.

19. Smith C. *The plan of Chicago: Daniel Burnham and the remaking of the American city*. Chicago: University of Chicago Press; 2006.

20. Krieger N. Public health, embodied history, and social justice: Looking forward. *International Journal of Health Services*. 2015;45(4):587–600.

PART I

A Divided City

Health equity means that everyone should have a fair opportunity to live a long, healthy life. It implies that health should not be compromised or disadvantaged because of one's race, ethnicity, gender, income, sexual orientation, neighborhood, or other social characteristics. Applying an equity lens on health outcomes requires the researcher and the public health practitioner to ask, Who is not thriving? This part of the *Reader* presents studies that highlight the great neighborhood divides between black and white residents of Chicago and their consequences for health (acknowledging that inequities exist between other racialized groups as well). Ranging from the early twentieth century to the early twenty-first, these readings remind us that, while time has passed, the structural nature of health inequity has not.

This part of the *Reader* opens with an article by H. L. Harris, originally written in response to a 1926 *Chicago Tribune* article proclaiming, "This is World's Healthiest City" (see figure 2). In one of the first empirical assessments of health inequities in Chicago, Harris provided a striking rebuke to that claim. From a certain perspective, the claim that Chicago was the world's healthiest city was true. The ranking of world cities with populations of over 1 million inhabitants showed that Chicago's death rate (11.5 per 1,000 population) was lower than those of Berlin, New York, Vienna, and other cities. Yet Harris argued that this claim was supported only by aggregated data; it was correct only if we ignored the differences in death rates between whites and blacks in Chicago. Looking at death rates for whites and blacks revealed profound differences, with black death rates in Chicago closer to those of residents of Bombay than other American cities. Harris's analysis is a powerful

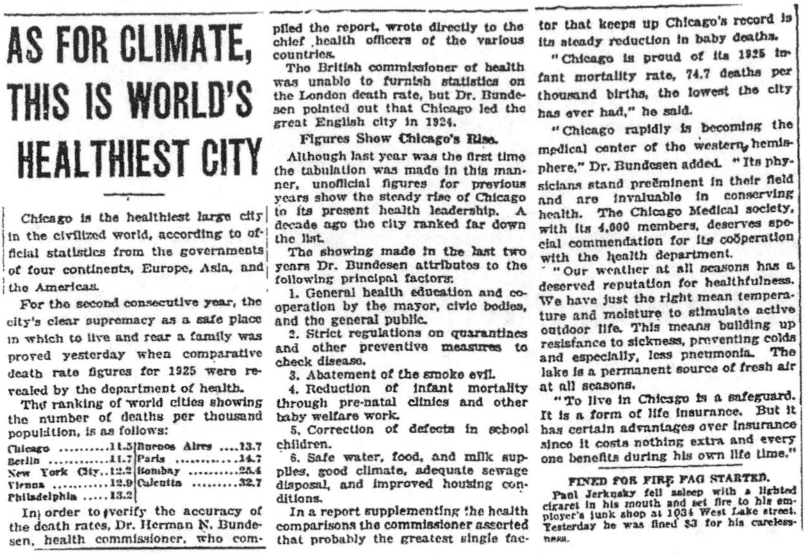

AS FOR CLIMATE, THIS IS WORLD'S HEALTHIEST CITY

Chicago is the healthiest large city in the civilized world, according to official statistics from the governments of four continents, Europe, Asia, and the Americas.

For the second consecutive year, the city's clear supremacy as a safe place in which to live and rear a family was proved yesterday when comparative death rate figures for 1925 were revealed by the department of health.

The ranking of world cities showing the number of deaths per thousand population, is as follows:

Chicago 11.5	Buenos Aires 13.7
Berlin 11.7	Paris 14.7
New York City...12.2	Bombay 25.4
Vienna 12.9	Calcutta 32.7
Philadelphia 13.2	

In order to verify the accuracy of the death rates, Dr. Herman N. Bundesen, health commissioner, who com-

piled the report, wrote directly to the chief health officers of the various countries.

The British commissioner of health was unable to furnish statistics on the London death rate, but Dr. Bundesen pointed out that Chicago led the great English city in 1924.

Figures Show Chicago's Rise.

Although last year was the first time the tabulation was made in this manner, unofficial figures for previous years show the steady rise of Chicago to its present health leadership. A decade ago the city ranked far down the list.

The showing made in the last two years Dr. Bundesen attributes to the following principal factors:

1. General health education and coöperation by the mayor, civic bodies, and the general public.
2. Strict regulations on quarantines and other preventive measures to check disease.
3. Abatement of the smoke evil.
4. Reduction of infant mortality through pre-natal clinics and other baby welfare work.
5. Correction of defects in school children.
6. Safe water, food, and milk supplies, good climate, adequate sewage disposal, and improved housing conditions.

In a report supplementing the health comparisons the commissioner asserted that probably the greatest single fac-

tor that keeps up Chicago's record is its steady reduction in baby deaths.

"Chicago is proud of its 1925 infant mortality rate, 74.7 deaths per thousand births, the lowest the city has ever had," he said.

"Chicago rapidly is becoming the medical center of the western hemisphere," Dr. Bundesen added. "Its physicians stand preëminent in their field and are invaluable in conserving health. The Chicago Medical society, with its 4,000 members, deserves special commendation for its coöperation with the health department.

"Our weather at all seasons has a deserved reputation for healthfulness. We have just the right mean temperature and moisture to stimulate active outdoor life. This means building up resistance to sickness, preventing colds and especially, less pneumonia. The lake is a permanent source of fresh air at all seasons.

"To live in Chicago is a safeguard. It is a form of life insurance. But it has certain advantages over insurance since it costs nothing extra and every one benefits during his own life time."

FINED FOR FIRE FAG STARTED.

Paul Jerkusky fell asleep with a lighted cigaret in his mouth and set fire to his employer's junk shop at 1034 West Lake street. Yesterday he was fined $3 for his carelessness.

FIGURE 2. "World's healthiest city"
Source: *Chicago Tribune*. June 27, 1926.

example of the potential for research to identify and expose otherwise hidden inequities.

There are three observations that one can make about this relatively simple analysis and the discussion of it provided by Harris. The first is that inequities can be hidden within aggregated data. Simply reporting an average rate can hide the differences within that average, glossing over the differences that exist in that place.[1,2] The second is that the belief that a rising tide of health improvements will raise the health of everyone is, ultimately, incorrect. History has shown that those marginalized in society benefit last and least from technological improvements that have the potential to improve health.[3,4] The third is that the public health improvements touted as being responsible for the life span improvement in the first decades of the twentieth century were likely disproportionately extended to the population with the most economic resources, political power, and access to health care—a fact that is as true in 2018 as it was in 1926.

Harris's work foreshadows many of the studies in this *Reader*. For example, Harris emphasized the importance of local data, something that the Sinai Urban Health Institute brought to the forefront of health eq-

uity work in Chicago starting in the 1990s, exemplified by the work of
Ami Shah et al. in part 2 of this *Reader*. Harris's analysis of the trajectories of tuberculosis death rates for whites and blacks is not at all dissimilar from more contemporary analyses of breast cancer mortality also
shown in part 2 of this *Reader* by Steve Whitman et al. In addition, his
observation of racial segregation in Chicago hospitals is echoed in the
work of the Committee to End Discrimination in Chicago Medical Institutions in the 1950s and the Medical Committee for Human Rights in
the 1960s, discussed in part 3 of this book. In assembling this *Reader*, we
have been struck by the relevance of Harris's work—many of the issues
he identified ninety years ago remain salient in our city today.

Part 1 highlights contributions from the classic Chicago school of sociology. Robert Faris and H. Warren Dunham apply the concentric zone
model of the city developed by Robert Park and Ernest Burgess to the
study of mental disorders, examining the geographic distribution of economic wealth and social characteristics, arguing: "The characteristics of
the populations in these zones appear to be produced by the nature of
the life within the zones rather than the reverse." Their work is among
the earliest and clearest expressions of what we now call *the social determinants of health*. The community issues that Faris and Dunham discuss remain critical today—from the breakdown of social cohesion to the
problematic nature of acculturation to the fundamental social causes of
mental disorder. Faris and Dunham "reveal that the nature of the social
life and conditions in certain areas of the city is in *some way a cause* of
high rates of mental disorder" (emphasis added).

In *Black Metropolis: A Study of Negro Life in a Northern City*,
St. Claire Drake and Horace Cayton offered a powerful assessment of
residential segregation. After documenting the perspectives of community members, Drake and Cayton lay out the health effects of residential
segregation—emphasizing that the black tuberculosis rate was five times
higher than the white rate and that the black "venereal disease" rate was
as much as twenty-five times higher than the white. Perhaps most poignantly, in their analysis of white versus black death rates for tuberculosis, Chicago fared much worse than other major cities in the United
States.

We then turn to Abraham's ethnography of the Banes family in North
Lawndale—*Mama Might Be Better Off Dead*. It is here where the divisions in Chicago became most striking, in an account written *fifty years*
after Drake and Cayton's work: "The medical and technological might

of the [Illinois Medical District] contrasts dramatically with the area around it. Just past the research buildings and acres of parking lots lie some of the sickest, most medically underserved neighborhoods in the city." Beyond the epidemiological indicators that quantify health inequities in Chicago, Abraham's qualitative work gives us insight into a world that few health professionals or academics can truly understand. The plight of the Banes family remains representative of a large proportion of the city's population today.

Part I of this *Reader* concludes with a selection from urban sociology— Robert Sampson's *Great American City*. This selection features a walk down Michigan Avenue, starting at Chicago's Magnificent Mile, a glittering high-priced shopping area bustling with tourists and wealthy residents. Sampson describes the changing landscape of the city as he walks south on Michigan Avenue, leaving high-end shops for single-room occupancy hotels, transitioning from areas of "concentrated advantage" to communities of "concentrated disadvantage" and economic hardship. He observes: "There are vast disparities in the contemporary city on a number of dimensions that are anything but randomly distributed in space." Tracing the lineage of his work to *Black Metropolis*, Sampson notes that many of the disadvantaged communities identified by Drake and Cayton in 1945 continue to be disadvantaged today; while some specific communities may change, "the broader pattern of concentration is robust." In other words, the structural inequality in Chicago communities is deeply embedded in society, affecting populations over generations, and directly causing profound and preventable morbidity and premature mortality.

Together, these selections describe a divided city, a metropolis with deep-rooted and man-made segregation. They illustrate the historical presence of structural violence and how it has worked in Chicago. As you read these texts, we encourage you to consider the following: What are the key elements of social division in these analyses? How do race, class, gender, *and* place intersect in these cases? To what extent do these selections reflect *your experience* of Chicago? How has your life been influenced by your city's social divisions?

References

1. Asada Y. *Health inequality: Morality and measurement.* Toronto: University of Toronto Press; 2007.

2. De Maio FG, Linetzky B, Virgolini M. An average/deprivation/inequality

(ADI) analysis of chronic disease outcomes and risk factors in Argentina. *Population Health Metrics.* 2009;7(8). https://pophealthmetrics.biomedcentral.com/articles/10.1186/1478-7954-7-8.

3. Farmer P. *Pathologies of power: Health, human rights, and the new war on the poor.* Berkeley: University of California Press; 2003.

4. Bartley M. *Health inequality: An introduction to theories, concepts and methods.* Cambridge: Polity; 2004.

CHAPTER ONE

Negro Mortality Rates in Chicago

H. L. Harris Jr.

A recent bulletin by the Health Commissioner of the City of Chicago cites figures showing that for 1925 Chicago had the lowest death-rate of any city of a million or more population, and calls attention to the major factors underlying this enviable record.[1]

Only a few days after the publication of this article, however, the Commissioner of Health said to the members of the Negro Health Committee of Chicago that the Negro citizens of Chicago had a death-rate more than twice that of the whites and an infant mortality-rate of 118 for Negroes as compared to 71 for whites. He further stated that Negroes have a still-birth rate more than twice as great as that of whites, a death-rate from tuberculosis and syphilis nearly six times as great, and a death-rate from pneumonia more than three times that of the whites. The Commissioner stated that although approximately $2,000,000 has been spent each year by the municipal tuberculosis sanitarium in the fight against tuberculosis in Chicago, the Negro death-rate from tuberculosis for the past twelve years shows no appreciable decline but, on the contrary, has increased so rapidly for the past three years that deaths among this group, which comprises only one-twentieth of the city's population, have raised the total rate for the city.

In giving the causes for the favorable health record for the city at large, a Chicago newspaper, quoting from the Commissioner of Health, lists the following.[2] (1) General health education and cooperation by the mayor,

Originally published in *Social Service Review* 1, no. 1 (March 1927): 58–77.

civic bodies and the great general public. (2) Strict regulations on quarantines and other preventive measures to check disease. (3) Abatement
of the smoke evil. (4) Reduction of infant mortality through prenatal
clinics and other baby welfare work. (5) Correction of defects in school
children. (6) Safe water, food and milk supplies, good climate, adequate
sewage disposal, and improved housing conditions. The newspaper article added: "Chicago is the healthiest large city in the civilized world, and
has proved for the second consecutive year the city's clear supremacy as
a safe place in which to live and rear a family."

With the statement of the Health Commissioner appears a chart comparing death-rates in all cities of over 1,000,000 population in the world
for which data were available for 1925. This chart is reproduced as figure 1.1 with a modification in order to show the separate rates for the Negro and white population in Chicago.

The striking fact brought out by this chart is the close agreement between the Negro death-rate in Chicago and that of the most unhealthy
cities in the world. Although the death-rate for the entire city of Chicago
is lower than that of any of these large cities, we must go down the list to
Bombay, with the second highest death-rate in the group, to find a rate
higher than that of the Chicago Negroes. Would the Negro, then, be as

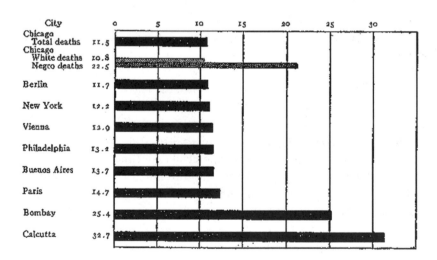

FIGURE I.I. Death-rates in cities of over 1,000,000 population for which data are available,
1925

Note: Number of deaths per 1,000 population. Data not available for London and Osaka.

well off in Bombay as in Chicago? The following editorial from the *Chicago Whip* of January 23, 1926, shows the attitude of this organ of public opinion concerning Chicago as a safe place for Negroes to live:

> Health statistics indicate that the death-rate on the South Side, Chicago's throbbing center of black people, is higher than any other section of the city. This fact, adduced from vital statistics, sent broadcast without mention of any of the causes which contribute, appeals to our enemies and is bruited about to our detriment and confounds us on all sides. No mention is made of the equally true fact that, in proportion to population, the South Side has less of those agencies which combat disease, pestilence, and death than any other section of the city.
>
> Aside from congested housing conditions, there is a woeful, almost criminal, lack of hospital facilities, free clinics, and dispensaries. Recreational provisions for the growing youth are almost nil. The absence of infant welfare stations, sufficient in number and convenient of location, account for [the] telling toll taken by the "grim reaper" among the infants of the race. Public baths are conspicuous by their absence. Playgrounds are just beginning to make their appearance. Perhaps later there will be swimming pools.
>
> If the Department of Health of Chicago recognizes one fact, it ought to be interested in the other. If there is a cause, there is a cure. If it is not the duty of the city to make all parts of the city a healthy place in which to live, it is certainly the duty of a community to see that it gets all that the city has to give for the protection of health. If we desire to be more healthy, conserve our numbers, and make our tribe increase, then we must make our wants known. We can at least let the city know that we recognize the danger and ask that proper safeguards be given us. If the demand is made with the solid backing of the whole community, it cannot be ignored.

The *Chicago Whip* denies neither the fact that Chicago is the healthiest large city in the world, nor the reasons for its supremacy, but does indicate that the same forces and agencies which have caused the improvement of the general health of the city have not been used among Negroes, and argues that they should be used in order that Chicago may become a healthier city. Chicago has not as yet achieved the healthy conditions of some of the smaller cities in the United States. Is Chicago held back in the struggle for public health by conditions in a few sections of the city? Let us examine the facts.

The United States Census Bureau estimates the population of Chicago for 1925 as 2,964,875, of which 160,000 are Negroes. The Negro plays a prominent part of the development of Chicago. The first settler . . . was a Negro, Jean Baptiste Pointe du Sable, a native of Santo Domingo. In the whole history of the development of Chicago, the Negro has occupied a considerable place, and since the curtailing of European immigration, has played an increasingly important role in supplying the unskilled labor necessary to the efficient working of the steel and packing industries, two of the most important sources of Chicago's prosperity. Chicago is becoming increasingly well known as a convention city, and the large number of Negroes, male and female, who are occupied in the various avenues of domestic service play no inconsiderable part in maintaining the city's reputation as an agreeable hostess. The Negro is represented in every publication showing the various phases of Chicago's life, from Dun and Bradstreet to *Who's Who.*

There are very few areas in Chicago in which a few Negroes do not live. The larger proportion, however, live in the Second and Third wards. The accompanying maps (figures 1.2 and 1.3) indicate the proportion of Negroes in the total population of certain areas in Chicago and the ward boundaries of the city. In parts of the Second and Third wards more than 80 per cent of the population are Negroes.

We may think of the Second and Third wards as comprising in 1925 a homogeneous city with a population of 124,000 and a voting strength of 61,212.[3] How does this city compare in essential particulars with metropolitan Chicago?

Figure 1.4, reproduced from the annual report of the Department of Health for the city of Chicago, presents a comparison between these two wards and other wards in Chicago.

A glance at this chart shows that the death-rates from all causes were much higher in the Second and Third wards than in any other wards in the city. The death-rate for Chicago as a whole in 1925 was 11.5 per thousand. In the Second Ward the rate was 19.5, and in the Third Ward, 18.2 per thousand.

The fact that the only other rate above 15 per thousand is to be found in the Twenty-seventh Ward, an area on the near West Side well known as one of the most densely populated and unhealthful regions of the city, makes the higher death-rate of the Negro wards even more significant.

Comparative mortality rates compiled by the Chicago Department

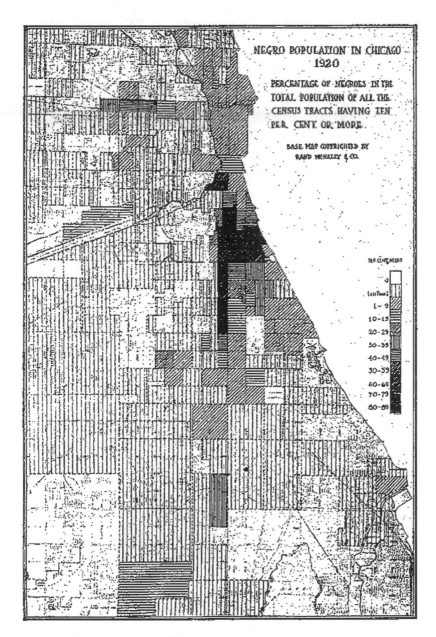

FIGURE 1.2. Negro population in Chicago, 1920

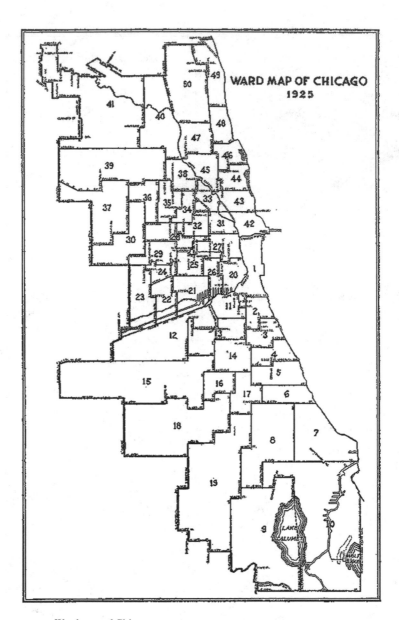

FIGURE 1.3. Ward map of Chicago, 1925

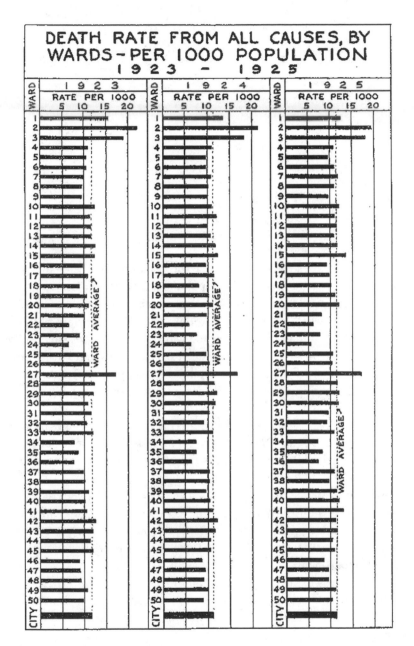

FIGURE I.4. Death-rate from all causes, by wards, per 1,000 population, 1923–1925

Source: Annual Report for 1923, 1924, and 1925: 778.

TABLE 1.1 **Death-rate per 100,000 population from specified causes for the white and Negro population of Chicago in 1925**

Cause of death	Total	White	Negro
Tuberculosis	83.2	65.7	382.5
Pneumonia	102.7	91.2	301.8
Alcoholism	9.2	9.2	8.7
Scarlet fever	4.3	4.3	5.6
Measles	3.9	3.8	5.6
Nephritis	103.2	100.0	367.5
Cancer	107.6	108.5	91.2
Heart disease	210.6	201.8	367.5
Diphtheria	8.0	8.1	7.5
Puerperal causes	10.1	9.4	21.8
All causes	1,146.0	1,082.0	2,248.0

Note: Compiled from records in the Health Department.

of Health and presented in table 1.1 show also wide discrepancies in the rates for the white and Negro populations for certain diseases.

The Negro rates for diseases such as tuberculosis, heart disease, and pneumonia, in which care and sanitation play a very important part, are very much higher than the rates for the whites. On the other hand, there is close agreement in the rates of cancer, which strikes and kills regardless of care, and in the rates for diphtheria, whose deadly nature and rapid spread have caused its almost universal diagnosis and early and adequate treatment.

Moreover, the Negro infant mortality rate was 118.6 per 1,000 births in 1925, while the death-rate for the white infants was only 71.4 per 1,000. Of course, the unduly high rate for Negroes may be partly explained by a failure to report all births.

While the total death-rate has fallen from 23.19 to 11.46 per thousand population in the fifty years since the organization of the Health Department, the Negro rate shows considerably less improvement. It now stands 22.5, nearly as high as the total rate before the organization of the Health Department.

The progress made in the reduction of the white death-rate from tuberculosis between 1912 and 1925, as shown in table 1.2 and figure 1.5, is a marked contrast to the history of the Negro death-rate from the same disease.

The Negro rate for deaths from pulmonary tuberculosis, to be sure, did decline considerably between 1918 and 1921, but more slowly than that of the white population. Moreover, after 1921, while the white rate continued to decline, the Negro rate increased rapidly, from that year up to 1925 (see figure 1.5). During this period a rapid migration from southern rural areas to northern city conditions must undoubtedly explain in part the increasing death-rate. In 1912 the Negro death-rate from pulmonary tuberculosis was three and one-half times as great as the white rate; in 1925 the Negro rate was more than six times that of the white population.

Figure 1.6 indicates an even more unfavorable history of deaths from other forms of tuberculosis.

While the rate for such deaths among white persons has declined almost steadily since 1912, the rate of Negro persons shows fluctuations about a trend that is practically stationary. No real advance has been made since 1912.

The high death-rate in the Negro wards, comparable, however, to the rate of the most congested area inhabited by white persons, suggests that environmental conditions may affect decidedly the health of Negro citizens. It is impossible in a brief article to set forth all the necessary facts to show the lack of facilities proved to be of benefit in promoting the public health. It is certain, however, that if for any part of the community there is insufficient attention given to the matter of [the] spread of disease, if there are insufficient facilities for promoting the public health,

TABLE 1.2 **Death-rates from tuberculosis per 100,000 population for white and Negro population of Chicago in 1925**

Year	Pulmonary			All other forms	
	White	Negro		White	Negro
1912	124	430		22	58
1913	133	341		23	52
1914	134	334		21	56
1915	145	313		23	49
1916	122	292		19	38
1917	120	331		19	47
1918	119	344		19	77
1919	96	309		15	64
1920	76	258		12	62
1921	63	230		10	63
1922	59	232		9	48
1923	60	258		9	50
1924	59	300		10	62
1925	58	366		7	52

Note: Compiled from Grace L. Robey, "A Statistical Study of Tuberculosis for the City of Chicago" (1926), an unpublished master's thesis in the University of Chicago Library.

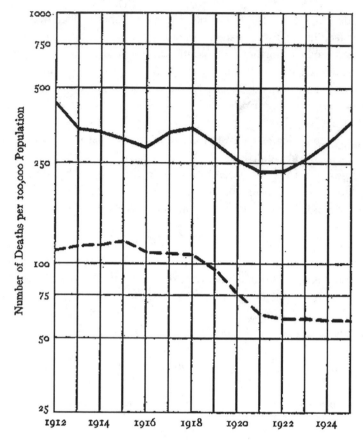

FIGURE I.5. Death-rates from pulmonary tuberculosis per 100,000 population for the white and Negro population of Chicago, 1912–1925
Note: Solid line, Negro death-rate; broken line, white death-rate.

such as hospitals, dispensaries, infant welfare stations, parks, and play-grounds, we may expect an unfavorable record of sickness and death. What conditions exist with regard to these facilities in the Second and Third wards?

[. . .]

[. . .] Although ten hospitals are located within the Second and Third wards, only two of these, Wilson and Provident hospitals, admit Negroes without restriction. These are both small hospitals, with sixty and fifty beds, respectively. The others either admit no Negro patients or admit them only in emergency cases. Among the ninety-five hospitals throughout the city, more than one-third have some restrictions on the admission of Negro patients.

[...]

Insanitary housing conditions also may be in part responsible for the high Negro death-rate. In a recent report on housing conditions by the Department of Public Welfare of the City of Chicago the following statement is made:

"An almost complete cessation in the building of dwellings in Chicago extended over the greater part of the period when Negro migration was heaviest. As the most recent comers into the tenement districts of the city, Negroes and Mexicans have found shelter in the most used, most outworn and derelict housing which the city keeps."[4]

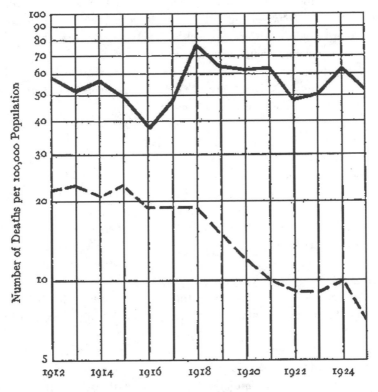

FIGURE 1.6. Death-rates from other forms of tuberculosis per 100,000 population for the white and Negro population of Chicago, 1912–1925
Note: Solid line, Negro death-rate; broken line, white death-rate.

This investigation found that "contrary to popular current opinion, the overcrowding among Negro households was of relatively infrequent occurrence, though instances were not lacking; as, for example, of eleven persons in three rooms and a closet; of thirteen in five or six rooms; or of ten in four rooms."

The degree of deterioration, however, and lack of conveniences for comfort and health could hardly be surpassed in these Negro dwelling houses. "About 1 per cent of the 1,526 homes visited could unhesitatingly be condemned as dwelling places on the lack of conveniences alone." Eleven per cent of the toilets provided in Negro houses were used by ten or more persons. One-third of all families visited had no toilets within their apartments, but were dependent upon toilets in public halls, on porches, in basements, in yards, or under the sidewalk. "The great bulk of tenants (85 per cent) were living in 'cold water' flats with nothing but stove heat. Many bathtubs were not used because there was nothing but a cold water tap in them. Hall, porch, and basement toilets outside apartments in these unheated flats were sometimes useless for long periods in cold weather because frozen."

In spite of such housing conditions the Negro tenants are paying comparatively high rents. "As a group, Negroes are paying much more for shelter than any other class in the community."

Outdoor recreation also is a recognized prerequisite of health. Urban life with its crowded living conditions and lack of yard space forces the city dweller to seek his fresh-air exercise in public parks and playgrounds. As the Playground and Recreation Association of America points out, "public playgrounds and recreation centers are providing a strong ally to the new science of illness prevention." To keep well, the individual must balance work and rest with sufficient outdoor play of a type adapted to his needs; at least a portion of the prevalent nervous disorders are ascribable to a lack of the mental relaxation gained from real recreation.

This need of her citizens for outdoor space is one which the city of Chicago has met admirably in her excellent system of parks. In the city as a whole, the average population to each acre of park area is 507.4. Yet within ward boundaries the population per acre of park space is very much greater in the case of the Second and Third wards.

Table 1.3 compares population per acre of park area for the city and these two wards.

Of the 15.1 acres in the Second Ward, 3.8 acres in Groveland Park

TABLE 1.3 **Population per acre of park area for the city compared to Second and Third Wards**

Area	Estimated population for 1925	Acres of public park space	Average population per acre of public park space
Chicago	2,964,875	5,912,260.0	507.4
Second Ward	60,611	15.1	4,019.2
Third Ward	63,298	9.6	6,559.3

Note: *The Chicago Daily News Almanac and Yearbook* (1926), 894, 905.

and 3.8 acres in Woodlawn Park are not open to the public, since these are private parks. This leaves but 7.5 acres of parks and playgrounds in the Second Ward, or an average population to each acre of park space of 8,059.9. Thus the average resident of the Second Ward has, within ward boundaries, about one-fifteenth the park and playground space available to the average resident of Chicago. However, two of the city's largest parks, Jackson Park and Washington Park, are at no great distance from these two wards.

Nearly three years ago the South Park Commissioners went on record as promising that a portion of a bond issue would be used to establish a recreation park in this area. To date, January, 1927, nothing has been done, and the prospects of immediate accomplishment seem remote.

The public schools also may be made an active agency for the promotion of public health. The report of the Children's Committee of the Illinois Department of Public Welfare already referred to calls attention to the fact that in schools attended largely by Negroes "there is reason to believe that the general equipment is less ample than that generally provided for white children."[5] Equipment for manual training and household arts, gymnasiums, baths, penny lunches, anemic [*sic*] divisions, and special instructors for speech defects are either limited or entirely absent from the schools of the Second and Third wards. The parent-teacher associations fail to function. The parents should be aroused to their responsibilities; the teachers should be sure that their attitudes invite co-operation.

At the Forestville School, in the Third Ward, beginning at about 7:30 in the morning and continuing until about noon, large numbers of children are to be seen buying breakfasts of ice cream, pickles, and "hot dogs" at the shops in the neighborhood. It would seem that a properly supervised school lunchroom would add much to the efficiency of this school and to the health of the neighborhood.

TABLE 1.4 **Death-rates of five northern and six southern cities, 1925**

Cities	Estimated population			Deaths per 1,000 population		
	Total	White	Negro	Total	White	Negro
Northern						
Chicago	2,995,239	2,832,239	160,000	11.5	10.8	22.5
Cleveland	936,485	886,485	50,000	10.4	9.6	23.5
Detroit	1,291,724	1,209,893	81,831	10.1	10.0	19.4
New York	5,877,354	5,709,469	159,305	12.2	11.8	25.7
Philadelphia	1,979,364	1,815,666	163,698	13.2	12.4	21.9
Southern						
Baltimore	796,296	678,365	117,931	14.6	12.8	24.9
Birmingham	205,670	124,962	80,708	17.0	12.6	23.8
Louisville	305,939	265,357	40,582	13.9	12.2	24.9
New Orleans	433,000	320,000	113,000	18.3	14.5	29.1
Richmond	186,404	131,130	55,274	14.7	11.9	21.1
Washington	497,906	378,261	119,645	14.1	11.4	22.7

Note: Compiled from data furnished by the Departments of Health of the cities listed.

The Negro death-rate in Chicago is more than twice as high as the death-rate of the city's white population. In the preceding pages an effort has been made to call attention to environmental factors possibly contributory. It is, of course, true that a higher death-rate for Negroes as compared with white persons is to be found in other large cities both in the North and in the South. Table 1.4 lists the death-rates for important cities in the North and South. It may be seen from this table that in every case the death-rate for the Negroes is considerably higher than that of the white population.

One essential feature of any program for lowering the Negro death-rate is undoubtedly an active public opinion. No effort to decrease the death and sickness rates for Negroes in Chicago can be successful in the face of an opposed or apathetic public opinion. The Negro must realize that it is his problem, and that to its solution he must bring every force within him and every factor subject to his control. His home, his church, his lodge, his business organization must take a positive stand and an active interest. The white man must realize that disease knows no boundary lines, and that disease germs cannot be segregated and kept out of restricted neighborhoods. Chicago must realize that it spends, through loss to time in industry, through retardation in school, through decreased property values, many times the amount necessary to bring the Negro death-rate down to the city's average.

The fear of the Negro that knowledge of his illness or of the illness in his home will cause him to lose his job must be combated. He must be taught to recognize its early stages and secure professional treatment for it. The fear of the white man that aid extended the Negro will develop a large parasitic growth must be given scientific examination.

In the case of civic organizations, timidity, rather than opposition, seems to be the rule. In many cases the fiction of public disapproval of a program is created in the mind of the official who voices that disapproval. Public opinion is shaped from above, downward; if the social forum, pulpit, press and enlightened family circle unite in a demand that the health of the Negro be given the aid of the things proved to be of value in promoting public health, then parks, playgrounds, schools, hospitals, day nurseries, infant welfare stations, and other agents of health will be provided.

Unless these agencies and activities are available to the average inhabitant of the Negro districts, it is premature to expect a worth-while improvement from the Negroes' own efforts. The efforts of Negro and white leaders must be combined under a common leadership; it must be recognized that the problem is a municipal, and not merely a Negro, concern. The press, pulpit, and the forum must think of the Negro as a part of Chicago and must make a place for him in every purely civic program.

References

1. *Chicago's Health*, weekly bulletin edited by Herman N. Bundesen, M.D., Commissioner, Chicago Department of Health; June 29, 1926.

2. *Chicago Tribune*, Sunday, June 27, 1926.

3. *Chicago Daily News Almanac*. 1926:814, 894.

4. Hughes EA. *Living conditions for small wage-earners in Chicago*. Chicago: City of Chicago, Department of Public Welfare; [1925]:7.

5. Illinois Department of Public Welfare. Children's Committee. *Report of the Sub-Committee on Colored Children*. December 1920:132–133.

CHAPTER TWO

Selections from *Mental Disorders in Urban Areas: An Ecological Study of Schizophrenia and Other Psychoses*

Robert E. L. Faris and H. Warren Dunham

Natural Areas of the City

A relationship between urbanism and social disorganization has long been recognized and demonstrated. Crude rural-urban comparisons of rates of dependency, crime, divorce and desertion, suicide, and vice have shown these problems to be more severe in the cities, especially the large rapidly expanding industrial cities. But as the study of urban sociology advanced, even more striking comparisons between the different sections of a city were discovered. Some parts were found to be as stable and peaceful as any well-organized rural neighborhood, while other parts were found to be in the extreme stages of social disorganization. Extreme disorganization is confined to certain areas and is not characteristic of all sections of the city.

Out of the interaction of the social and economic forces that cause city growth a pattern is formed in these large expanding American cities which is the same for all cities, with local variations due to topographical and other differences. This pattern is not planned or intended, and to a certain extent resists control by planning. The understanding of this or-

Originally published as chapters 1, 2, and 11 of Robert E. L. Faris and H. Warren Dunham, *Mental Disorders in Urban Areas: An Ecological Study of Schizophrenia and Other Psychoses* (Chicago: University of Chicago Press, 1939).

der is necessary to the understanding of the social disorganization that characterizes urban life.

The Natural Areas Depicted as Circular Zones

The most striking characteristic of this urban pattern, as described by Professor Burgess,[1] may be represented by a system of concentric zones, shown in figure 2.1. Zone 1, at the center, is the central business district. The space is occupied by stores, business offices, places of amusement,

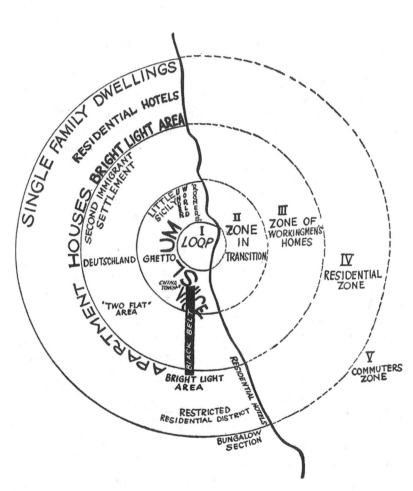

FIGURE 2.1. Natural areas and urban zones

Source: From Park RE, Burgess EW. *The City*. Chicago: University of Chicago Press; 1925.

light industry, and other business establishments. There are few residents in this area, except for transients inhabiting the large hotels, and the homeless men of the "hobohemia" section which is usually located on the fringe of the business district.

Zone II is called the zone in transition. This designation refers to the fact that the expanding industrial region encroaches on the inner edge. Land values are high because of the expectation of sale for industrial purposes, and since residential buildings are not expected to occupy the land permanently, they are not kept in an improved state. Therefore, residential buildings are in a deteriorated state, and rents are low. These slums are inhabited largely by unskilled laborers and their families. All the settlements of foreign populations as well as the rooming-house areas are located in this zone.

Zone III, the zone of workingmen's homes, is inhabited by a somewhat more stable population with a higher percentage of skilled laborers and fewer foreign-born and unskilled. It is intermediate in many respects between the slum areas and the residential areas. In it is located the "Deutschlands," or second immigrant settlement colonies, representing the second generation of those families who have migrated from Zone II.

Zones IV and V, the apartment-house and commuters' zones, are inhabited principally by upper-middle-class families. A high percentage own their homes and reside for long periods at the same address. In these areas stability is the rule and social disorganization exceptional or absent.

The characteristics of the populations in these zones appear to be produced by the nature of the life within the zones rather than the reverse. This is shown by the striking fact that the zones retain all their characteristics as different populations flow through them. The large part of the population migration into the city consists of the influx of unskilled labor into the second zone, the zone in transition. These new arrivals displace the populations already there, forcing them to move farther out into the next zone. In general, the flow of population in the city is of this character, from the inner zones toward the outer ones. Each zone, however, retains its character whether its inhabitants be native-born white, foreign-born, or Negro. Also each racial or national group changes its character as it moves from one zone to the next.

Within this system of zones, there is further sifting and sorting of economic and social institutions and of populations. In the competition for land values at the center of the city, each type of business finds the place in which it can survive. The finding of the place is not infrequently by trial and error, those locating in the wrong place failing. There emerge from this competition financial sections, retail department store sections, theater sections, sections for physicians' and dentists' offices, for specialized shops, for light industry, for warehouses, etc.

Similarly, there are specialized regions for homeless men, for rooming-houses, for apartment hotels, and for single homes. The location of each of these is determined ecologically, and the characteristics also result from the interaction of unplanned forces. They maintain their characteristics in spite of the flow of various racial and national groups through them and invariably impress their effects on each of these groups. These have been called "natural areas" by Professor Park,[2] because they result from the interaction of natural forces and are not the results of human intentions.

Fortunately, the city of Chicago has been studied somewhat more intensively than most other cities of its size. Certain of these areas are significant in relation to social disorganization. It is possible to define and describe these areas with certain kinds of objective data. The major divisions of the city can be seen in figure 2.2. Extending outward from the central business district are the principal industrial and railroad properties. The rooming-house sections extend along three arms radiating from the center to the north, west, and south. The slum areas are roughly defined by the regions containing over 50 per cent foreign-born and native-born of foreign parentage and over 50 per cent Negro. Beyond these areas is the residential section. In the Lake Calumet section at the southeastern corner of the city is another industrial region inhabited by a foreign-born population.

Too small to be shown on this map are the areas of homeless men— the "hobohemia" areas.[3] These are located on three radial streets and are just outside the central business district. Their inhabitants are the most unstable in the city. The mobility and anonymity of their existence produces a lack of sociability and in many cases deterioration of personality. Although spending their time in the most crowded parts of the city, these homeless men are actually extremely isolated. For the most part they represent persons unable to obtain an economic foothold in society, and so they maintain themselves by occasional labor, by petty thievery, by begging, and by receiving charity. As they have no opportunity for normal married life, their sexual activities are limited to relations with the lowest type of prostitutes and to homosexuals. The rate of venereal

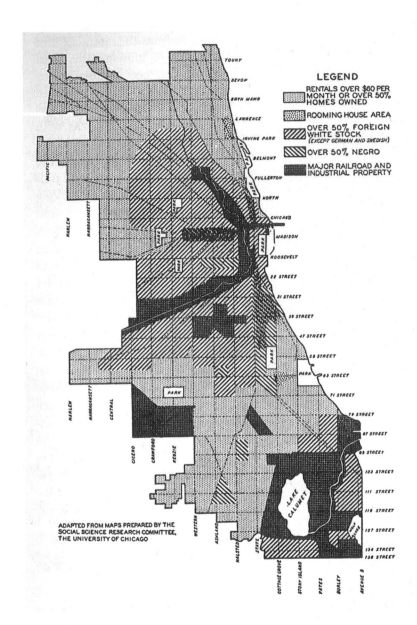

ADAPTED FROM MAPS PREPARED BY THE
SOCIAL SCIENCE RESEARCH COMMITTEE,
THE UNIVERSITY OF CHICAGO

FIGURE 2.2. Types of cultural and economic areas

infection is high among these men. Chronic alcoholism is also a common characteristic of the members of this group. Their lives are without goal or plan, and they drift aimlessly and alone, always farther from the conventional and normal ways of living.

Another area of importance is the rooming-house area. This is usually located along main arteries of transportation and a little farther from the center of the city. In Chicago there are several rooming-house sections, the three largest consisting of arms radiating to the north, west, and south, just beyond the hobohemia areas, each extending for something over two miles in length and from a half-mile to over a mile in width. The populations of these areas are principally young, unmarried white-collar workers who are employed in the central business district during the day and live in low-priced rented rooms within walking distance or a short ride from their work.[4] Within the area the population is constantly shifting, turning over entirely about once each four months. Anonymity and isolation also characterize the social relations in this area; no one knows his neighbors, and no one cares what they might think or say. Consequently the social control of primary group relations is absent, and the result is a breakdown of standards of personal behavior and a drifting into unconventionality and into dissipations and excesses of various sorts. The rates of venereal diseases and of alcoholism are high in this area, and the suicide rate is higher than for any other area of the city.[5]

The foreign-born slum areas occupy a large zone surrounding the central business and industrial area. Within this zone there are a number of segregated ethnic communities, such as the Italian, Polish, Jewish, Russian, and Mexican districts. The newly arrived immigrants of any nationality settle in these communities with their fellow countrymen. In these groups the language, customs, and many institutions of their former culture are at least partly preserved. In some of the most successfully isolated of these, such as the Russian-Jewish "ghetto," the Old-World cultures are preserved almost intact. Where this is the case, there may be a very successful social control and little social disorganization, especially in the first generation. But as soon as the isolation of these first-settlement communities begins to break down, the disorganization is severe. Extreme poverty is the rule; high rates of juvenile delinquency, family disorganization, and alcoholism reflect the various stresses in the lives of these populations.

Two distinct types of disorganizing factors can be seen in the foreign-born slum areas. The first is the isolation of the older generation, the foreign-born who speak English with difficulty or not at all and who are never quite able to become assimilated to the point of establishing intimate friendships with anyone other than their native countrymen. Within the segregated ethnic communities these persons are well adapted to their surroundings, but as soon as they move away or are deserted by their neighbors, they suffer from social isolation.[6] The second type of disorganizing factor operates among the members of the second and third generations. The very high delinquency rate among the second-generation children has been shown by Shaw.[7] This disorganization can be shown to develop from the nature of the child's social situation. Also growing out of the peculiar social situation of the second generation is the mental conflict of the person who is in process of transition between two cultures—the culture of his ancestors and the culture of the new world in which he lives. As he attends American schools and plays with children of other than his own nationality, the child soon finds himself separated from the world of his parents. He loses respect for their customs and traditions and in many cases becomes ashamed of his own nationality, while at the same time he often fails to gain complete acceptance into the American group of his own generation. This is particularly true if he is distinguished by color or by features which betray his racial or national origin. This person is then a "man without a culture," for though he participates to some extent in two cultures, he rejects the one and is not entirely accepted by the other.[8]

The Negro areas are, in general, similar in character to the foreign-born slum areas. The principal Negro district in Chicago extends for several miles southward from the business district. Two smaller Negro districts are located on the Near West Side, as well as one on the Near North Side. In the larger area of the South Side, the social disorganization is extreme only at the part nearest the business district.[9] In the parts farther to the south live the Negroes who have resided longer in the city and who have become more successful economically. These communities have much the same character as the nearby apartment-house areas inhabited by native-born whites.

For some miles along the Lake Front in Chicago a long strip of apartment-hotel districts has grown up. These districts occupy a very pleasant and favorable location and attract residents who are able to pay high rentals. The rates of various indices of social disorganization are in general low in these sections.

The outlying residential districts of middle-class and upper-middle-class native-born white population live in apartments, two-flat homes, and single homes. In these districts, and especially the single home areas in which there is a large percentage of homes owned by the inhabitants, the population is stable, and there is little or no social disorganization in comparison with those areas near the center of the city.

[. . .]

Urban Distribution of Insanity Rates

All cases of mental disorder in Chicago that are cared for in public institutions are first brought to the Cook County Psychopathic Hospital, where they are held for a week or more for examination and a tentative diagnosis. The number of new cases brought here average over 3,000 each year. Some are judged not insane; some cases are mild enough to be allowed to live at home or with relatives. Those needing hospital care are committed to one of several state institutions in the vicinity of Chicago.

Distribution of Insanity Rates for the Psychopathic Hospital

The distribution of the rates for 7,069 first admissions to this hospital for the two years of 1930–31 are shown in figure 2.3. The total number of cases in each of the sixty-eight communities[a] was divided by the 1930 adult population of the community. The adult population was used because of the very small number of persons under twenty-one years among these cases. The resulting rates range from a low of 110 per 100,000 adult population in Community 39, a high-class residential area, to a high of 1,757 in Community 32, the central business district. The distribution, as shown in figure 2.3, shows a very definite pattern. The highest rates are clustered about the center of the city, and the rates are progressively lower at greater distances from the center. The slight rise of the rates in the Lake Calumet region reflects the deteriorated condition of that region, which, although less severe, is similar to that of the areas surrounding the central part of the city.

Distribution of Rates for State Hospitals

Figure 2.4 shows the distribution of 28,763 cases, a much larger number, and presents the average rates for the more detailed 120 subcom-

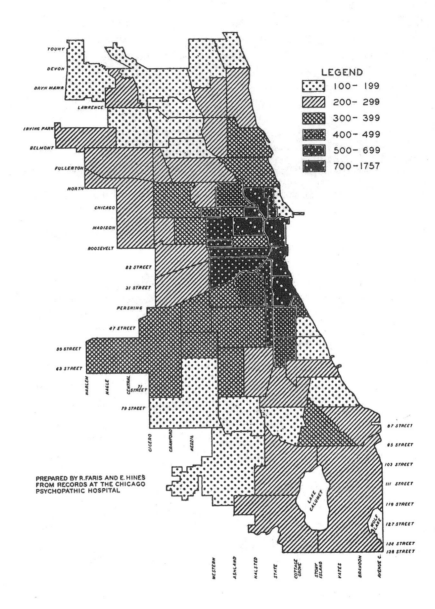

PREPARED BY R. FARIS AND E. HINES
FROM RECORDS AT THE CHICAGO
PSYCHOPATHIC HOSPITAL

LEGEND

⠿	100 - 199
▨	200 - 299
▓	300 - 399
▣	400 - 499
■	500 - 699
■	700 - 1757

FIGURE 2.3. Insanity rates in Chicago, 1930–1931, per 100,000 adult population

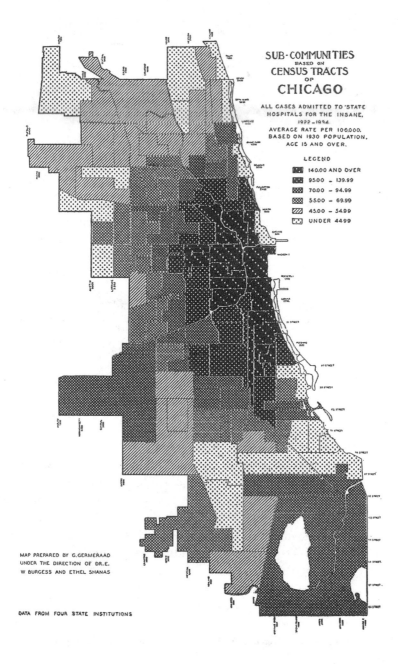

FIGURE 2.4. All cases admitted to state hospitals for the insane, 1922–1934, average rate per 100,000. Based on 1930 population, age 15 and over.

TABLE 2.1 **Percentage of all cases of mental disorder admitted to state hospitals and percentage of the population in each fourth of the 120 subcommunities grouped on the basis of the magnitude of the rates**

Quartile grouping	Percentage of cases in each quartile	Percentage of population in each quartile
Fourth or upper	45.6	23.1
Third	24.7	26.0
Second	16.7	24.4
First	13.0	26.5
Total	100.0	100.0

munities. The cases used are from four state institutions,[b] and consist of all those committed to those institutions from Chicago during the years 1922–34. The distribution resembles closely that shown in the preceding map.

The heavy concentration of high rates in and around the central business district represents a real concentration of cases, as can be seen in table 2.1.

This table shows that the high-rate communities in the two upper quartiles have 70 per cent of the cases but only 49 per cent of the population. It is significant to note that while each quartile contains approximately the same percentage of population, the percentage of cases within each quartile shows significant variations and decreases consistently from the upper quartile to the lowest or first quartile.

The state hospital records do not include all psychotic persons in the city of Chicago. Because of the possibility that these cases may represent a selection of the poorer classes in the population, it seemed necessary to compare the distribution of private hospital cases with those from state hospitals. It is an obvious possibility that the concentration of high rates of mental disorder in the central parts of the city might mean no real concentration at all, but merely a concentration of those patients whose families are too poor to maintain them in private institutions.

Hypotheses and Interpretations of Distributions

The establishment of the fact that there are great differences in the patterns of rates for different psychoses in the natural areas of the city is in itself a complicated task. The interpretation of the meaning of these facts is a separate problem; different methods of study are necessary for this part of the research. The distributions of certain psychoses can be fairly successfully explained; others are more difficult, and explanations can only be suggested.

It is necessary before discussing the meaning of the configuration of rates for the different psychoses to examine certain possible flaws in the method. It may be possible that insanity is not concentrated, and that it appears to be so only because of some statistical illusion. Several possible explanations for the appearance of concentration are discussed below.

An obvious possibility is that the concentration of cases in certain areas of the city may be due to chance. This suggestion has been made by Professor Frank Alexander Ross,[10] with reference to the computation of rates based on data for a single year. Using a formula to test the chance variation of a rate, he tested whether each rate was significantly different from the rate in an adjacent community. In some cases he found differences were not significant and in other cases they were. By combining two communities and computing a rate he was able to show more definitely that the concentration of rates could not be due to chance alone. The logic of this procedure has been questioned by Charles C. Peters, who pointed out the fact that many rates combined into a pattern greatly increased the statistical significance of the pattern itself, and that the possibility that chance variation alone could produce such a pattern is too small to be considered.[11] Since this preliminary study was made, much larger numbers have been used, further decreasing the possibility that the patterns could be due to chance. It was therefore considered necessary to use the formula for testing chance variation only once—in the study of foreign-born rates of schizophrenia. In those maps which show a clear pattern of distribution, the conclusions are drawn from the pattern and not from differences between adjacent communities. It seems permissible to dismiss the possibility that these patterns are due to chance variation.

A second possibility is that the patterns of rate distribution represent only a concentration of cases of mental disorder which have been institutionalized because of poverty. If the actual incidence of mental disorder is equal in all parts of the city and if those in the higher-income classes are more frequently cared for at home or sent out of the state, the hospitalized cases would show a bias toward the lower-income classes and therefore toward the slum section of the city. An attempt is made to minimize this bias by including in the rates all the cases from the regional private hospitals as well as from public hospitals. Because of the small number of patients in the private hospitals, the rates were only slightly affected by the addition of these cases. No way has been found to estimate the amount of bias in the rates caused by the practice of caring for some patients in the homes. It is possible that there is an income selection in such cases. But it appears unlikely that such an effect dominates the patterns of distribution, because of the fact that different psychoses show different patterns of distribution. If a poverty concentration were the only, or the principal, factor in producing these patterns, they should be reasonably similar for all psychoses.

Another possibility is that the apparent concentration of cases is due to a statistical error or failure to adjust the rates for transiency. That is, if the cases from an area taken during the period of a year are divided by the population taken as of a single day, the rate may be regarded as too high if the population during the year had turned over enough to make a significantly larger population than was present on the one census enumeration day. Professor Ross made this point in the discussion previously mentioned.[10] No satisfactory method was found to make a direct adjustment for this criticism. It is known, however, that in the hobo and rooming-house areas, which show very high rates for several types of mental disorder, the population is transient enough to turn over, perhaps two or three times or more. Ross made the suggestion that in such cases the rate be reduced to one-half or one-third. To justify this, however, it would be necessary to know where the excess population was the rest of the year and what the chances of hospitalization were wherever the people were. Only if it is true that the other cities and towns in which this transient population spends a part of the year do not take their quota in their hospitals should the rate be adjusted. It seems significant, here, to point out that if the rates in the hobohemia communities for all types of mental disorders were divided by three, the resulting rates would still be two of the highest in the distribution of the rates. These considerations appear to be important in the statistical criticism presented by the factor of mobility.

An interpretation frequently made of the concentration in the center of the city of insanity rates, and the schizophrenia rates particularly, is that persons who are mentally abnormal fail in their economic life and consequently drift down into the slum areas because they are not able to compete satisfactorily with others. Such a process is, of course, possible, although the explanation does not appear to be valid in the case of the manic-depressive patterns. Many of the cases of schizophrenia consist of persons who were born in and have always lived in deteriorated areas.[c] These did not drift into the high-rate areas. There are also cases that are hospitalized from high-income areas, persons who developed a mental disorder before their failure had caused them to drift to the slums. It is a question whether this drift process, which undoubtedly contributes something to the apparent concentration of rates, is anything more than an insignificant factor in causing the concentration.[d] No decisive material on this point was obtained in this study. Some relevant findings should be stated, however.

One method of testing this drift hypothesis is the comparison of the distribution of young and old cases. For this purpose the paranoid and catatonic types of schizophrenia were selected because of the radical difference in both the pattern of the rates and the age distribution. Since those who are first committed at an advanced age have had a longer time in which to fail in their economic life and consequently to drift toward the slums, the distribution of the older cases should show a sharper concentration than the younger cases. Figures 2.5 and 2.6 show the concentration of the paranoid schizophrenia cases between the ages of fifteen and twenty-nine years and between the ages of thirty and sixty-four years, respectively. The younger cases, mostly too young to have had much time to drift, are concentrated in the central areas in much the same pattern as the older cases.[e] Table 2.2 shows the measurement of concentration of these cases. Both show roughly the same degree of concentration.

[...]

A possible interpretation of the concentration of rates in the central areas might be that this measures the racial tendency to mental disorders of the foreign-born populations that inhabit these areas. [However,] rates for foreign-born cases divided by foreign-born populations are distributed similarly to the rates for all cases. Likewise, rates for Negroes show a variation, being high in the central disorganized areas not populated primarily by members of their own race and low in the actual Negro areas. Some factors other than being foreign-born or Negro are necessary to explain these patterns that are the same no matter which race or nationality inhabits the area. Furthermore, not all psychoses are concentrated in foreign-born areas. Although the correlation of several psychoses with percentages of foreign-born and Negro population is high or medium, such as catatonic schizophrenia (0.86), epilepsy (0.53), and alcoholic psychoses (0.48), others such as paranoid schizophrenia

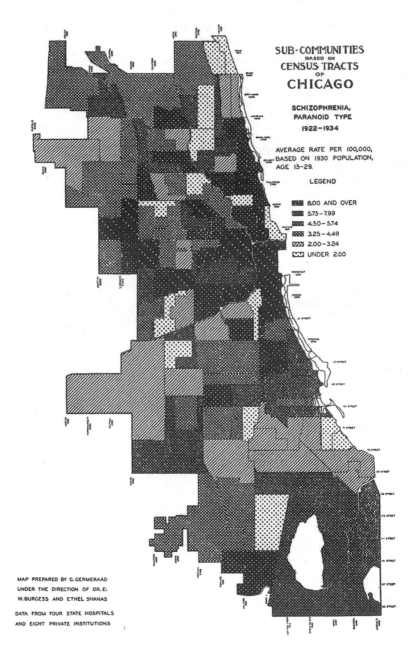

SUB-COMMUNITIES
BASED ON
CENSUS TRACTS
OF
CHICAGO

SCHIZOPHRENIA,
PARANOID TYPE
1922-1934

AVERAGE RATE PER 100,000,
BASED ON 1930 POPULATION,
AGE 15-29.

LEGEND

- 8.00 AND OVER
- 5.75 – 7.99
- 4.50 – 5.74
- 3.25 – 4.49
- 2.00 – 3.24
- UNDER 2.00

MAP PREPARED BY G. GERMERAAD
UNDER THE DIRECTION OF DR. E.
W. BURGESS AND ETHEL SHANAS

DATA FROM FOUR STATE HOSPITALS
AND EIGHT PRIVATE INSTITUTIONS

FIGURE 2.5. Schizophrenia, paranoid type, 1922–1934, average rate per 100,000. Based on 1930 population, age 15–29.

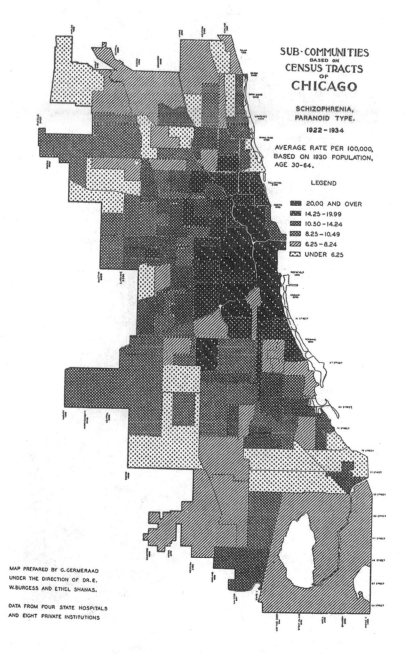

FIGURE 2.6. Schizophrenia, paranoid type, 1922–1934, average rate per 100,000. Based on 1930 population, age 30–64.

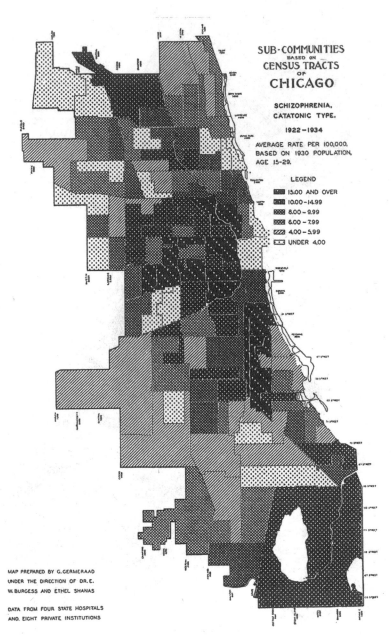

FIGURE 2.7. Schizophrenia, catatonic type, 1922–1934, average rate per 100,000. Based on 1930 population, age 15–29.

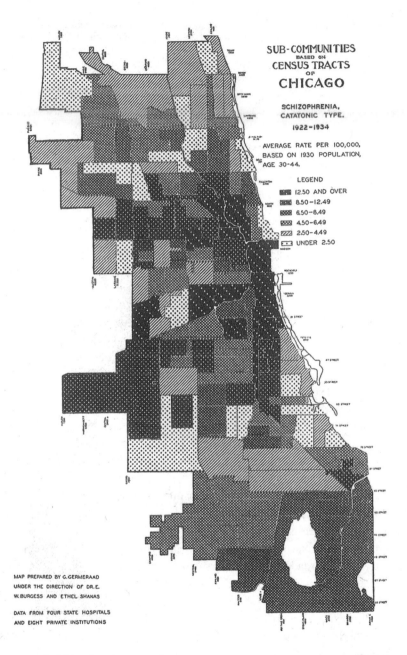

FIGURE 2.8. Schizophrenia, catatonic type, 1922–1934, average rate per 100,000. Based on 1930 population, age 30–44.

TABLE 2.2 **Percentage of paranoid schizophrenic cases, 15–29 years, and 30–64 years, and
the percentage of the population in each one-fourth of the 120 subcommunities
grouped on the basis of the magnitude of the rates**

Quartile grouping	Percentage of cases in each quartile		Percentage of population in each quartile	
	Paranoid 15–29	Paranoid 30–64	Paranoid 15–29	Paranoid 30–64
Fourth or upper	45.2	41.6	24.9	23.0
Third	27.3	26.5	25.7	26.5
Second	19.1	19.3	26.1	25.3
First	8.4	12.6	23.3	25.2
Total	100.0	100.0	100.0	100.0

(0.11), manic-depressive psychoses (0.14), general paralysis (0.15), and
senile psychoses (0.17) show little or no correlation. The supposed tendency to mental disorders of the foreign-born populations, then, does
not appear to explain the rate patterns.

The last possibility to be discussed is that the patterns of rates reveal
that the nature of the social life and conditions in certain areas of the
city is in some way a cause of high rates of mental disorder. If there is
any truth in this hypothesis, it will be necessary to find separate explanations for each psychosis, since the distributions of rates differ both to a
large and to a small degree for each psychosis.

Although the distributions are not exactly alike, the explanations of
the concentration of general paralysis, drug addiction, and alcoholic psychoses rates according to this hypothesis are roughly similar. Different
combinations of social factors, however, are no doubt functioning in the
case of each of these psychoses. The general paralysis rates are highest
in the hobo and rooming-house areas and in the Negro areas. These are
the areas in which there is little family life, and in which the sex experience of the men is in large part with casual contacts and with prostitutes, who are relatively numerous in these districts. These conditions
make for the spread of syphilitic infection and hence for general paralysis. The dispensing and the use of drugs is very much of an underworld
activity, and this is reflected by the high rates in the zone of transition.
Lack of normal social life may underlie the dissatisfactions which cause
the use of drugs to be felt as a release, hence the slight rise in rates in the
upper-income hotel and rooming-house districts. Also, for the use of alcohol to become an appealing habit, basic dissatisfactions are often essential. High rates of alcohol consumption and of alcoholic psychoses

are in the foreign-born and rooming-house areas and may be caused by such conditions of life as monotony, insecurity, and other problems difficult to solve, from which alcohol may be a temporary relief. The significant variations of rates according to nativity and race in the different housing areas of the city indicate the greater chances for mental breakdown and personality disorganization in relation to these psychoses especially when a person is living in an area not primarily populated by members of his own group. This fact alone would appear to be the beginning for further research in these mental disorders. In the case of the alcoholic psychoses it would seem to indicate the presence of other important factors in addition to the use of alcohol.

[...]

Any factor which interferes with social contacts with other persons produces isolation. The role of an outcast has tremendous effects on the development of the personality. Lack of sufficient self-confidence and the consciousness that others do not desire one's company may act as a serious barrier to intimate social relations. The individual who feels that he is conspicuously ugly, inferior, or in disgrace may be isolated through this conception of himself.

The hypothesis that such forms of isolation are significant factors to account for the high rates of schizophrenia in certain parts of the city is strengthened by the studies which have shown that the conditions producing isolation are much more frequent in the disorganized communities.[f] Especially significant is the connection between the rates of schizophrenia, excepting the catatonic type, and indices of mobility. [...] In addition, the fact that rates for Negro, foreign-born, and native-born are all significantly higher in areas not primarily populated by their own members tends to support this isolation hypothesis. When the harmony of all these facts bearing on the isolation hypothesis is considered, the result is sufficiently impressive to make further pursuit of this lead appear to be worthwhile.

Notes

a. The seventy-five local communities, as worked out by the Local Community Research Council at the University of Chicago, were used as the basis for these rates. Some of the communities, which contained populations too small to be used as a basis for reliable rates, were combined with adjoining areas, and three of the largest communities were subdivided. This reduces the total number of communities to sixty-eight. In this manner the city was divided so that each community contains reasonably homogeneous characteristics and yet has a sufficiently large population to make possible reliable rates. [. . .]

Some of the maps for which large numbers of cases were available are based on a more detailed division of the census tracts of the city into 120 subcommunities. The use of these makes possible a somewhat finer discrimination of the differences as found in the various parts of the city. It should be noted that the rates on all the maps showing distributions in the 120 subcommunities are average rates as contrasted to total rates in the local communities. [. . .]

b. In all the following maps showing rates for the local communities the distributions are made on the basis of cases admitted to Elgin, Kankakee, and Chicago State Hospitals. The maps showing distributions in the 120 subcommunities include a minimum number of cases from Chester State Hospital, in which the criminal insane are confined. This explains the label on the maps that the distribution data are from four state hospitals.

c. A separate study of the catatonic in a foreign-born community now being conducted by Dr. H. Blumer and H. W. Dunham indicates that these persons were born in and brought up in the community. The tendency to drift into an area is more marked and has significance, for the most part, in reference to the hobo and rooming-house areas. Certainly the high schizophrenic rates in the typical foreign-born communities cannot be explained adequately by the "drifting" hypothesis.

d. It is significant to note that the maps showing the distribution of insanity and of schizophrenic rates in Providence, Rhode Island, give results which are similar to those found in the Chicago study.

e. The pattern formed by the distribution of the younger cases is not as even or consistent. Again it is necessary to point out the unreliability of the rates because of the small number of cases. The younger cases amount to 607 in number, while the older cases amount to 2,213. The correlation between the two sets of rates is .79 ± .05. In the catatonic series, presented below, the younger cases amount to 1,162 and the older cases to 789.

f. Much carefully collected evidence on this point is published in Nels Anderson, *The Hobo* (Chicago, 1923); Louis Wirth, *The Ghetto* (Chicago, 1926); Harvey W. Zorbaugh, *The Gold Coast and the Slum* (Chicago, 1927); Ruth S. Cavan, *Suicide* (Chicago, 1928); and E. Franklin Frazier, *The Negro Family in Chicago* (Chicago, 1931).

References

1. Park RE, Burgess EW. *The city.* Chicago: University of Chicago Press; 1925.

2. Park RE. Sociology. In *Research in the social sciences* (Wilson Gee, ed.). New York: Macmillan; 1929:28–29.

3. Anderson N. *The hobo*. Chicago: University of Chicago Press; 1923.

4. Zorbaugh HW. *The Gold Coast and the slum*. Chicago: University of Chicago Press; 1929.

5. Cavan RS. *Suicide*. Chicago: University of Chicago Press; 1928.

6. Wirth L. *The ghetto*. Chicago: University of Chicago Press; 1928.

7. Shaw CR, Zorbaugh FM, McKay HD, Cottrell LS. *Delinquency areas*. Chicago: University of Chicago Press; 1929.

8. Stonequist E. *The marginal man*. New York: Scribner's; 1937.

9. Frazier EF. *The Negro family in Chicago*. Chicago: University of Chicago Press; 1932.

10. Ross FA. Ecology and the statistical method. *American Journal of Sociology*. 1933;38:507–522.

11. Peters CC. Note on a misconception of statistical significance. *American Journal of Sociology*. 1933;39:231–236.

CHAPTER THREE

Selection from *Black Metropolis: A Study of Negro Life in a Northern City*

St. Clair Drake and Horace R. Cayton

Black Belt—Black Ghetto

T he deep-seated feeling that Negroes are, in the final analysis, some-
how fundamentally different from Poles, Italians, Greeks, and
other white ethnic groups finds its expression in the persistence of a
Black Belt. Midwest Metropolis seems to say: "Negroes have a right to
live in the city, to compete for certain types of jobs, to vote, to use public accommodations—but they should have a community of their own.
Perhaps they should not be segregated by law, but the city should make
sure that most of them remain within a Black Belt." As we have suggested previously, Negroes do not accept this definition of their "place,"
and while it is probably true that, if allowed free choice, the great majority would live as a compact unit for many years to come, they believe that
enforced segregation is unjust. They do not always clearly see the full
implications and consequences of residential segregation, but they are

Excerpt from St. Clair Drake and Horace R. Cayton, *Black Metropolis: A Study
of Negro Life in a Northern City* (New York: Harcourt Brace, 1945), 198–207.
Copyright © 1945 by St. Clair Drake and Horace R. Cayton. Copyright © re-
newed 1973 by St. Clair Drake and Susan Woodson. Reprinted by permission of
Houghton Mifflin Harcourt Publishing Company. All rights reserved.

generally resentful. A sampling of comments made at a time when discussion was widespread about restrictive covenants in Hyde Park will reveal the nature of this resentment. Thus, one prominent Old Settler, the daughter of a German father and a Negro mother, was vitriolic in her denunciation of residential segregation:

"I don't think we would need any housing projects on the South Side if Chicago wasn't so full of this silly old race prejudice. We ought to be able to live anywhere in the city we want to. What the government should do, or somebody with money, is to fight these restrictive covenants and let our people move where they want to. It's a dirty shame that all types of foreigners can move anywhere in the city they want to, and a colored man who has been a soldier and a citizen for his country can live only in a Black Belt. What's the use of fighting for a country that treats you that way?"

A colored "wringer man" in a laundry came to Chicago in 1921 because he had heard of "the good wages and grand opportunities." Now, having become well-adjusted, he resents residential segregation:

"Residential segregation is a big mistake. When I came here, there were white and colored living in the same neighborhood and the people seemed to understand each other. But since this neighborhood is colored only, everything is different. There are less jobs, and the neighborhood is not kept as clean as it used to be. I cannot offer any way to break down segregation. When I was married, I tried to rent houses out of the district, and the real-estate agents wouldn't rent to me. Yes, if Negroes can get houses in Hyde Park, or anywhere else, they ought to take them—for the housing condition for colored on the South Side is rotten."

Another laborer from Georgia who has been in the city nearly thirty years was also heated in his denunciation:

"Racial segregation is rotten. When white and colored both lived in this section, the rents were not so high and there seemed to be a better understanding. I have often wondered if segregation has not had a lot to do with the lack of employment, for there are certain white people that try to prove that all Negroes are bad. When they come over here, they go to the worst part of the section to prove their point."

Somewhat more moderate in his disapproval is a colored chauffeur who came to Chicago in 1912 as a Pullman porter:

"Racial segregation is something that I am not sure is a blessing. The housing proposition is serious, for the rents are very high, and the houses are not kept up as they are in white neighborhoods. On the other hand, if we were scattered among the white people there would be far less work, for by being close together we get a lot of work from the stores owned by white people that are doing business in our neighborhood. I have thought of ways to break down this segregation, but when I think that anything you do makes you a lawbreaker, you then cease to fight individuals, for then it becomes a war with the law. Remember that the police, the judges, and the strongest lawyer groups are all white and they stick together. I have seen one case of a fight between the police and the colored citizens and know that it was far from being an equal fight."

Many other Negroes, however, express a willingness to risk trouble in attacking this form of segregation. A skilled worker, a respectable church member, was very emphatic on this point:

"Hyde Park is no more than any other place in Chicago. The Negroes ought to move into Hyde Park or any other park they want to move into. I don't know of anything on earth that would keep me out of Hyde Park if I really wanted to move into it. Personally, I don't care anything about the good-will of white people if it means keeping me and my people down or in restricted neighborhoods."

A minority defends the existence of enforced residential segregation. This is done not on principle, but as a matter of expediency, or for fear of racial clashes, or because such persons feel that the time to attack segregation has not yet come. Thus, a colored waiter who blames most of the discrimination against Negroes on the Great Migration partly defends segregation:

"I myself believe segregation is good, for if the white and colored lived together there would be fights constantly. About the only business benefit we derive from a Black Belt region is from a political standpoint, for there are a lot of people working that have gotten their appointments from their power as a voting factor. I think segregation is caused by the Negro's failure to try to get out of the district. In fact, I have never tried to live out of the district. There is no reason—I just have not thought of it."

[. . .]

Most Chicago Negroes feel that the right to rent or buy a house offered to the public should be inalienable. Yet Negro businessmen and politicians will sometimes state privately that they prefer keeping the Negro population concentrated. During a campaign against restrictive covenants, one prominent Negro leader confided to an interviewer:

> "Sure, I'm against covenants. They are criminal. But I don't want Negroes moving about all over town. I just want to add little pieces to the Black Belt. I'd never get re-elected if Negroes were all scattered about. The white people wouldn't vote for me."

Most Negroes probably have a similar goal—the establishment of the *right* to move where they wish, but the preservation of some sort of large Negro community by voluntary choice. But they wish a community much larger than the eight square miles upon which Black Metropolis now stands.

[. . .]

Negro newspapers and civic leaders unanimously oppose enforced residential segregation and bitterly attack the forces that have created an overcrowded Black Belt. To them, the area is a Black Ghetto, and they insist that "new areas should be opened to break the iron ring which now restricts most Negro families to intolerable, unsanitary conditions. Restrictive-covenant agreements and the iron ring creating a Negro ghetto must be smashed."[1]

Even the Chairman of the Mayor's Committee accepted the characterization of the Black Belt as a "ghetto," and there was general agreement among the participants in the Mayor's Conference in 1944 that most of the social problems within the Black Belt were fundamentally related to the operation of restrictive covenants. (Only the spokesman for the Chicago Real Estate Board disagreed.)[a] The conference listed among the "ghetto conditions" high sickness and death rates;[b] a heavy relief load during the Depression; inadequate recreational facilities; lack of building repairs; neglect of garbage disposal and street cleaning; overcrowded schools;[c] high rates of crime and juvenile delinquency; and rough treatment by the police.

The ghetto characteristics of the Black Belt are related, in the first instance, to the poverty of its people. Here, the proportion of families on relief during the Depression was the highest for the entire city (see figure 3.1). The restricted economic base of the community was also evident in the high proportion of women doing domestic service. As a low-income area, the community was unable to maintain a high material standard of living. This poverty was aggravated by the housing problem, which caused overcrowding. Given these factors, and the lack of widespread health education among Negroes, it is not surprising that the tuberculosis death rate is five times higher than it is for whites, and that the Negro areas have the highest sickness and death rates from tuberculosis. Chicago has the highest Negro death rate from tuberculosis of any metropolitan city in the United States.[d]

The Black Ghetto also suffers from a type of social disorganization which is reflected in high illegitimacy and juvenile delinquency rates and a high incidence of insanity (see figures 3.1 and 3.2).

Restrictions upon free competition for housing, and the inability of the Black Belt to expand fast enough to accommodate the Negro population, have resulted in such a state of congestion that Negroes are living 90,000 to the square mile as compared with 20,000 to the square mile in adjacent white apartment-house areas. Since they entered the city last and are a low-income group, Negroes, in the aggregate, have inherited the worst sections of Midwest Metropolis. They have been able to "take over" some fairly decent housing in neighborhoods that were being abandoned by white residents, but these were no longer prized as residential neighborhoods. Negroes have thus become congested in undesirable residential areas.

Over half of Black Metropolis lies in that area which the city planners and real-estate interests have designated as "blighted." The "blighted areas" have come into being as a part of the process of uncontrolled city growth, for as Midwest Metropolis has grown, spontaneously and in response to economic utility, its center has become a citadel of imposing office buildings surrounded by an ever-widening belt of slums. As the city expands, this slum land becomes valuable as the site of future wholesale establishments, warehouses, transportation terminals, and light industries. No one wishes to invest in new housing upon these potentially valuable spots. Housing already there is allowed to deteriorate and is then torn down. From the standpoint of residential desirability, this entire area is "blighted."

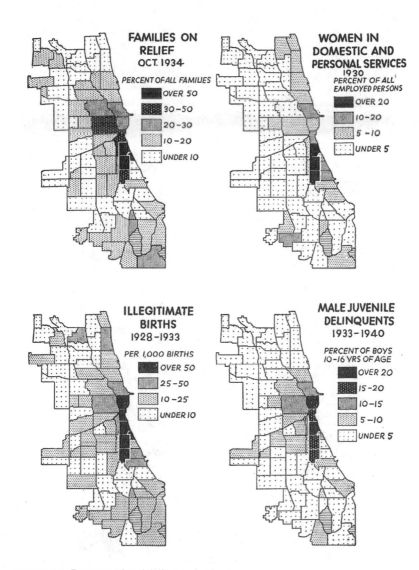

FIGURE 3.1. Poverty and social disorganization

Note: The rates for families on relief and for women employed in domestic service are from Wirth L, Furez M, eds. *Local community fact book, 1938*. Chicago: Chicago Recreation Commission; 1939. Insanity rates are from Faris REL, Dunham HW. *Mental disorders in urban areas: An ecological study of schizophrenia and other psychoses*. Chicago: University of Chicago Press; 1939. (The Black Belt community areas are those outlined in white.)

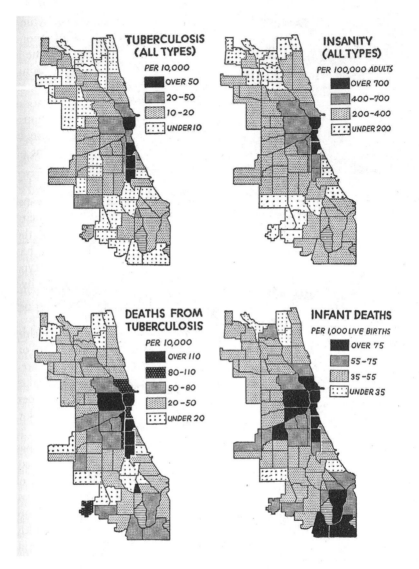

FIGURE 3.2. DISEASE AND DEATH

Note: Tuberculosis morbidity rates and infant mortality rates are from Wirth L, Furez M, eds. *Local community fact book, 1938.* Chicago: Chicago Recreation Commission; 1939. Tuberculosis mortality rates are from the records of the Municipal Tuberculosis Sanitarium. Map showing insanity rates adapted from Faris REL, Dunham HW. *Mental disorders in urban areas: An ecological study of schizophrenia and other psychoses.* Chicago: University of Chicago Press; 1939. (The Black Belt community areas are those outlined in white.)

The superficial observer believes that these areas are "blighted" because large numbers of Negroes and Jews, Italians and Mexicans, homeless men and "vice" gravitate there. But real-estate boards, city planners, and ecologists know that the Negro, the foreign-born, the transients, pimps, and prostitutes are located there because the area has already been written off as blighted. The city's outcasts of every type have no choice but to huddle together where nobody else wants to live and where rents are relatively low.

Black Metropolis has become a seemingly permanent enclave within the city's blighted area. The impecunious immigrant, once he gets on his feet, may—as we have mentioned several times—move into an area of second-settlement. Even the vice-lord or gangster, after he makes his pile, may lose himself in a respectable neighborhood. Negroes, regardless of their affluence or respectability, wear the badge of color. They are expected to stay in the Black Belt.

During the last twenty years the Negro's demand for housing has always exceeded the supply. The rental value of residential property in the Black Belt is thus abnormally high. The speculative value of the land on which the property stands is also high, and—even more than the restriction of supply—this has a tendency to drive rents up. [. . .]

Midwest Metropolis does not intend to keep on growing haphazardly. City planners and the larger real-estate interests hope some day to control its growth, and Chicago's master plan calls for the eventual reclamation of the inner city, with a garden belt of privately financed, medium-rental apartments replacing the slums. Here, it is hoped, members of the new middle class will make their homes, close to the Loop where they work, and well within the city limits. The blighted areas will thus be reclaimed. Low-cost housing nearer steel mills and industrial plants in the suburbs will be constructed (also, for the most part, with private funds) to attract the skilled and semi-skilled workers. But some question marks remain.

"What," asked an official of a Negro civic agency, "do the Chicago Real Estate Board, and the city, plan to do with the Negroes who now live in the blighted areas? Will restrictive covenants be relaxed so they, too, can move to the suburbs and near-suburbs?" This was during the Depression, when Negro labor was not in demand, and the answer of a member of the Real Estate Board was crisp: "We have no plans for them. Perhaps they can return to the South."

[. . .]

Notes

a. The real-estate interests in Midwest Metropolis insist that a general scarcity of houses is the primary problem, and that, if there were enough houses or a building program in process, middle-class white families would move away from areas close to the Black Belt and Negroes could then take over the abandoned houses. They blame New Deal restrictions and the Federal housing program for the housing shortage, charging that private capital has been made reluctant to invest. The Chicago Real Estate Board refuses, unequivocally, to sanction the abolition of restrictive covenants. Yet plenty of houses would not solve the basic question of the quality of housing available for Negro occupancy. Negroes would still be concentrated in areas of the city that have begun to deteriorate.

b. In 1925, Chicago had the lowest death rate for any American city of 1,000,000 and over, but the Negro death rate was twice that for whites. (H. L. Harris Jr., "Negro Mortality Rates in Chicago," *Social Service Review*, v. 1, no. 1, 1927.) The average standard death rate for the years 1928–1932 was 9.2 for native-whites, 10.4 for foreign-whites, and 20.0 for Negroes. (Elaine Ogden, Chicago Negro Community, WPA, 1939, p. 201.) Differences in infant mortality are reflected in the fact that 3 Negro babies die before their first birthday to every 2 white babies. Social disorganization in the Black Ghetto is reflected in deaths from homicide—six Negroes die from violent assaults for every white person who is killed.

The striking differentials in morbidity rates are those for tuberculosis (see figure 3.2) and venereal diseases. The Negro tuberculosis rate is five times the white rate, and the venereal disease rate is reported as 25 times that for whites. Both diseases are closely related to a low material standard of living and widespread ignorance of hygiene. It should be borne in mind, however, that we are dealing with rates, not absolute numbers. The actual number of Negroes who have venereal disease does not warrant the common belief that "the Negro race is eaten up with syphilis and gonorrhea." About 75 venereal disease cases were reported among every thousand Negroes in 1942, and 3 among whites.

c. Civic leaders are most bitter about the double- and triple-shift schools in the Black Belt. In 1938, thirteen of the fifteen schools running on "shifts" were in Negro neighborhoods. Pupils spent half of the day in school and were "on the streets" for the rest of the day. In 1944, the School Board alleged that this system had been abolished, but Negro leaders disputed the claim. The Board of Education consistently refused to give the authors any data on overcrowding in the schools. A building program has been projected which may relieve the situation in the future.

d. These high tuberculosis morbidity and mortality rates among Negroes may reflect the fact that Negroes as a recently urbanized group have not developed immunity to the disease. But the wide differentials also reflect the well-known fact that the care of tuberculosis demands bed rest with plenty of nutritious food.

(Rates from Dorothy J. Liveright, "Tuberculosis Mortality Among Residents of 92 Cities of 100,000 or More Population: United States, 1939–41," U. S. Public Health Reports, July 21, 1944, pp. 942–955.)

Cities of 1,000,000 and over population	Tuberculosis death rates: 1939–41	
	For Whites	For Negroes
Chicago, Illinois	45.4	250.1
New York, New York	40.4	213.0
Philadelphia, Pennsylvania	44.3	203.5
Detroit, Michigan	36.5	189.0
Los Angeles, California	49.7	137.3

Reference

1. *Chicago Defender.* July 22, 1944.

CHAPTER FOUR

Selection from *Mama Might Be Better Off Dead: The Failure of Health Care in Urban America*

Laurie Kaye Abraham

"Where Crowded Humanity Suffers and Sickens": The Banes Family and Their Neighborhood

Robert Banes sat on the edge of his hospital bed, cradling his queasy stomach. A thin cotton gown hung on him like a sack. At five feet, eleven inches, Robert weighs only 137 pounds.

Robert's kidneys stopped functioning when he was twenty-seven. He received a transplant a year later, but his body rejected the new kidney after six years. Since then he has required dialysis treatments three times a week. Dialysis clears his body of the poisonous impurities that healthy people eliminate by urinating, but the treatments cannot completely restore his health, and Robert periodically spends a couple of days in the hospital. This time, he had been admitted to the University of Illinois Hospital because he had been urinating blood for a week, a problem that did not appear terribly serious to doctors but nonetheless had to be checked.

Feeling nauseated, Robert was not paying much attention to the

Originally published as chapter 1 of Laurie Abraham, *Mama Might Be Better Off Dead: The Failure of Health Care in Urban America* (Chicago: University of Chicago Press, 1993).

game show that droned from his television. A nurse came in and stuck a thermometer in his mouth. Earlier in the day, Robert had undergone a cystoscopy, a procedure in which doctors put a miniaturized scope into his bladder to look for the source of his bleeding. He had not been told the results of the test, so he asked the nurse when his doctor would be stopping by. He also wanted to know how much longer he would have to stay in the hospital.

"You may have to go to surgery," the nurse said vaguely, flipping through his chart. A cloud passed briefly over Robert's face; the thought of surgery scared him, though he did not admit that to the nurse. Instead, he changed the subject.

"I guess I don't get dinner today," he said.

"You didn't get dinner?" she asked, surprised.

"I need some before I get sick."

"Don't do that," the nurse muttered as she walked out the door.

A minute later Robert hurried to the bathroom. "I was probably throwing up because I didn't have no food to push it down," he said, referring to the missed dinner. Robert returned to his bed and lay down, curling his knees into his stomach and pulling a blanket over his shivering body.

Four years before his kidneys failed, Robert was diagnosed with focal glomerulosclerosis, a progressive scarring of the kidneys that eventually destroys them. Focal glomerulosclerosis can be slowed, though not cured, but Robert's disease went at its own destructive pace because he did not get medical treatment until his kidneys had reached the point of no return. None of Robert's low-paying, short-term jobs had provided health insurance, and he could not wriggle into any of the narrow categories of government-sponsored insurance, which are generally reserved for very poor mothers and children, the elderly, and the permanently disabled. In other words, Robert had not been poor-parent enough, old enough, or sick enough to get care.

The game show gave way to the news and a report about a "summer virus" that was infecting children. Robert frowned. He and his wife, Jackie, have two daughters and a son: eleven-year-old Latrice, four-year-old DeMarest, and one-year-old Brianna. "Don't tell me that," he sighed. That is Robert's typical response to bad news: he prefers to avoid it.

At the moment, however, Robert would not have minded a little bad news about his own condition. Since he had been admitted to the hospital on July 5, he had not been urinating as much blood, which frustrated him and Jackie. They felt he almost had to *prove* to doctors that he was sick.

Through his open door, Robert could see his wife arrive for an early evening visit. At five feet, ten inches, Jackie is only one inch shorter than her husband, but she weighs twenty pounds more than he does. When she smiles, her pretty, heart-shaped face gets full and round, captivating her baby daughter, who pokes at her cheeks and giggles, making Jackie giggle, too.

Jackie was not smiling that day, however. When she is in public, Jackie can look impassive, even defiant, though this vanishes when her curiosity gets the better of her. She walked slowly past the nursing station looking straight ahead, moving almost regally, her muscular thighs curving beneath her slacks. Next to her husband's brittle frame, Jackie stood like an oak.

She pulled up a chair next to the hospital bed, and Robert began to relay the sketchy medical update he had heard from the nurse. Jackie listened silently; then she responded in the way she sometimes does when she feels overwhelmed.

"I'm going away for a while," Jackie said coolly. "What are you all going to do without me?"

Robert did not reply. He knew, as she did, that she wasn't going anywhere; she was just letting off steam. Today had been her day to pay the bills, which she does in person since they are usually past due, and she had ridden the bus for hours in 90-degree heat.

Jackie told her husband to call home and tell Latrice to take some drumsticks out of the freezer for dinner. Jackie's invalid grandmother, with whom the family lives in one of Chicago's poorest neighborhoods, answered the phone, so Robert gave her the instructions instead. But a few minutes later Latrice called back because she was not sure her great-grandmother had heard the message correctly. In the way other children might memorize their parents' work numbers, Latrice had memorized the phone number for the university hospital, as well as for Mount Sinai Hospital Medical Center, where her great-grandmother frequently had been hospitalized. Jackie repeated the dinner instructions and hung up the phone. "I need the bed," she said.

She began to empty the stuffed grocery bag she had carried into the hospital. It contained two new T-shirts, underwear, and socks for Rob-

ert, a day-old piece of cake from Brianna's first birthday, which he had
missed, a can of Sprite, and a bunch of grapes.

The couple watched part of another game show and talked about a
report they had heard about a family found murdered mysteriously on
the bottom of a lake. This story came from one of the tabloid news programs, whose bizarre stories the family regularly discusses. Then Jackie
called home again to check on the children, who were home with her
grandmother. The call was not reassuring: one of them had dropped
cake on the rug, the other two had stepped in it, and DeMarest report-
edly was taunting his great-grandmother.

"I need you to stay in here over the weekend so I can get things
straightened out," Jackie wearily told her husband. When one or the
other of her sick family members are hospitalized, Jackie sometimes
considers it a chance to regroup, to get things together before she has to
start taking care of everyone again.

Before Jackie left, she filled the plastic grocery bag she had emp-
tied earlier. From Robert's belated dinner, she took a wedge of leftover
chocolate cake home for DeMarest. She took packets of low-salt French
dressing, salt, and sugar that Robert had squirreled away from his meal
trays, as well as a roll of medical tape left by a nurse. Jackie carefully
folded the foil Brianna's birthday cake had been wrapped in and stashed
that in her bag, too.

Then she gave Robert $5.00 to pay for his hospital TV, which cost
$3.25 a day. Robert slowly walked Jackie to the elevator, past a dimly
lit room where the floor's patients congregated. One of the patients, a
man about Robert's age, had earlier informed Robert that he was scheduled for a second transplant the next day. He told Robert that he had
rejected his first transplanted kidney because he drank a case of beer
in one evening—the kind of story that, true or not, flies back and forth
among kidney transplant patients.

"This is my wife, Jackie," Robert said to a middle-aged woman sitting
on the edge of the day room, closest to where the couple walked. "Nice
to meet you," the woman said. Jackie smiled wanly, heading for the door.

The University of Illinois Hospital is part of what is known as the Illinois Medical Center, a 560-acre area just west of the Loop, Chicago's
downtown. The center has the highest concentration of hospital beds
in the United States, some 3,000 among its four institutions.[1] In addition to the University of Illinois, there is Cook County Hospital, one

of the best-known, last remaining, and, as the ancient edifice continues to crumble, most notorious public hospitals in the country, and Rush–Presbyterian–St. Luke's Medical Center, an institution that caters to those who, unlike Robert and Jackie, are privately insured. The Veterans Administration West Side Medical Center is also located there.

The medical and technological might of the complex contrasts dramatically with the area around it. Just past the research buildings and acres of parking lots lie some of the sickest, most medically underserved neighborhoods in the city. Medical wastelands abut abundance in American cities because health care is treated as a commodity available to those who can afford it, rather than a public good, like education. Though public schools invariably are better in prosperous suburbs than in poor city neighborhoods, every state at least provides every child with a school to attend, no matter what her family's income. The country has not even come that far with health care. Medicaid, the state and federal health insurance program intended for the poor, covers less than half of them, and much of the program is left to the states' discretion, so that a Southerner, for example, generally has to be poorer to receive Medicaid than a Northerner.

Even for those poor who manage to squeeze into Medicaid, the government's commitment to providing health care for them does not approach a commitment to equality. Just as education remains in practice separate and unequal, medical treatment for poor people with Medicaid or even Medicare (the government insurance for the elderly) is, in all but exceptional cases, conducted in a separate, second-rate environment.

The Banes family lives in the shadow of the Illinois Medical Center complex, twenty-five minutes southwest by way of the number 37 bus, which runs along Ogden Avenue. The street cuts diagonally across the city from the gentrified lakefront neighborhoods just north of the Loop to the bungalow enclaves of white ethnic suburbs that border Chicago on the southwest. Jackie and Robert live in between, on the West Side, the city's newest and poorest ghetto.

The streets were still lit by the late afternoon sun when Jackie climbed onto the bus for her trip home. Settling her bag on her lap, she fretted that doctors were going to release Robert before they figured out what was wrong with him. A person can only get so far with a "green card," she said, using the street name for the cards issued to families covered by Medicaid. "You need Palmer Courtland kind of money to get anywhere," she complained. Palmer Courtland is a self-made millionaire on "All My Children," a soap opera Jackie and Robert watch.

In addition to the hospitals and their services, programs in a clutch of other buildings near Ogden attempt to palliate what are often conditions born of poverty. There is the Illinois State Psychiatric Institute, the West Side Center for Disease Control, the Chicago Lighthouse for the Blind, and a bit further southwest, the Cook County Juvenile Court, which handles crimes by children, and those against them by their parents.

These buildings are strung along the Eisenhower Expressway, which zips from the booming Western suburbs into Chicago's downtown, whose dramatic growth in the past two decades has bypassed the West Side. Jackie rarely ventures into the Loop. From her perspective, the eight-lane highway is an escape route for the employees of the various hospitals and social service institutions, for people who do not carry poverty home with them in a plastic bag.

As Ogden turns more sharply to the west, it crosses into Jackie's neighborhood of North Lawndale, a name that carries the same ominous weight in Chicago as the South Bronx or Watts carries nationwide.[2] North Lawndale was the subject of a series in the *Chicago Tribune* in 1985 that examined the lives of the so-called underclass. Many people who work and live in North Lawndale were disturbed by what they thought was a distorted, overly negative picture of their neighborhood; the series' very name, "The American Millstone," is hated because it suggests a neighborhood that is no more than a burden to be cast off.

[. . .]

As the bus hissed and groaned up Ogden, it passed Mount Sinai Hospital, which lives the same hand-to-mouth existence as the poor blacks and Hispanics it serves. More than the University of Illinois, Mount Sinai is the Baneses' hospital. It is where Jackie's grandmother, Cora Jackson, had been repeatedly hospitalized because of complications from diabetes that eventually resulted in the amputation of her right leg. It's where Jackie's father was rushed after he suffered a stroke caused by high blood pressure. And on a happier note, it's where Jackie gave birth to Brianna a year ago.

At one time or another, the Baneses and Cora Jackson have sought (and not sought) health care in every way available to the poor. When uninsured—Robert, when his kidneys were deteriorating, and Jackie, when pregnant with Latrice—they delayed care, then went to Cook

County Hospital. Later, when Jackie went on welfare, she and the children became eligible for Medicaid.

Meanwhile, some of Mrs. Jackson's medical bills were paid by Medicare, which covers the elderly and disabled, rich and poor alike. Robert also got Medicare but only after his kidneys stopped working. People with renal failure have special status under the program: they are the only group covered on the basis of their diagnosis and regardless of age or disability. Mrs. Jackson had been sporadically eligible for Medicaid, too, which she needed because Medicare does not pay for such important things as medications. Her Medicaid coverage had been fitful because she was enrolled in what is called the "spend-down" program. She qualified for Medicaid only during the months that her medical expenses were so high they forced her income to drop below a "medically needy" level set by the state. Notably, neither Mrs. Jackson, nor anyone else in the family, had ever been covered by private insurance.

Leaving Mount Sinai, the bus cut through Douglas Park, which spreads to the north and south of Ogden. Douglas and two other West Side parks were designed in 1870 as a system of "pleasure grounds" linked together by grand boulevards. Progressive reformers came to envision them as breathing spaces to provide respite from crowded tenements and other urban ills.[3] In its heyday from 1910 until 1930, when North Lawndale was populated by first- and second-generation Jews, bands gave free concerts on weekends, couples paddled rowboats on the lagoon just to the north of Ogden Avenue, and children swam in what was one of the city's first public swimming pools—which, with its baths, was considered as important for public hygiene as it was for recreation.

Except for the players and fans at soccer and baseball games, the park these days is barely dotted with people, a young Hispanic couple walking on a path on the south side of Ogden—the Hispanic side—or several dozen black children splashing in the lagoon to the north—the African American side. Ogden is a dividing line between Hispanics and African Americans in North Lawndale, and the race line holds in the park as firmly as it does anywhere else in the neighborhood.

Though the park's glory has faded, it is the last piece of deliberately open land that Jackie passed on the Ogden bus. The rest of it consisted of a series of vacant lots, some of which run together for a block or more and which residents euphemistically call "prairies." As it was summer, some of the lots were covered with reedy grasses and weeds, frilly Queen Anne's lace, and deep brown stands of dock plant. Others were piled high with refuse—in one case, what looked like enough decaying furniture to fill an office. In another lot, a building had fallen in on itself, likely prey to the brick thieves who complete the destruction started when buildings are abandoned by landlords who can't afford their upkeep, then are stripped of sinks, stoves, and fixtures, and then finally picked apart, brick by brick. In still other lots, large fernlike weeds flourished, creating an urban jungle that suggests what a parish priest in a similar neighborhood in New Jersey called "panther beauty, beauty you don't want to mess with."[4]

As for the brick and stone two-flats, or old three-story apartment buildings still standing, it is often difficult to tell whether they are occupied or not. Rusty steel grates are locked across nearly every door, even those of the ubiquitous churches. Signs are hand painted and peeling, and since plywood is used to cover most street-level windows, even establishments that still do business have a boarded-up look.

Worse yet, dozens of storefronts have been reduced to gaping holes, outlined by shards of glass that form jagged frames for dark rooms of rubble. Only the foolhardy, or a drug addict desperate for a place to get high, would step inside.

The shrouded condition of the neighborhood unnerves Jackie. Even the local drugstore, whose windows are blocked with ugly, prehistoric stone, can seem foreboding. "You used to be able to see in the drugstore," Jackie complained. "Shoot, now you wonder if you get in somewhere, are you going to make it out safe?"

[. . .]

Currency exchanges, storefront churches, auto parts shops, liquor stores and taverns, hot dog stands, and a beauty shop or two are the only businesses left on Ogden, which used to be one of the city's major commercial streets. The largest establishment in the neighborhood, Lawndale Oldsmobile, closed more than two decades ago. Its windowless, graffitied shell has been a fixture in North Lawndale since Jackie was a child. By the time she and her grandmother moved to Chicago from Tupelo, Mississippi, in the early 1960s, the neighborhood was already in rapid decline. The Eastern European Jews who had settled the area in the early part of the century had virtually vanished by the mid-1950s, replaced by black migrants from the South. Driven by the changing nature of their businesses as well as the deteriorating neighborhood, North Lawndale's major companies fled soon after: Sears Roebuck, International Harvester, and Western Electric either departed or reduced the size of their operations. Today, the bruised and battered buildings along Ogden give sad testimony to North Lawndale's knockout blow: the ravaging riots that followed Martin Luther King Jr.'s assassination in 1968. After that, most remaining middle-class blacks fled.

In 1960, Lawndale's population peaked at 125,000; by 1980, it had plummeted to 62,000; by the end of that decade, it fell to 47,000.[5] Statistics describing the economic status of the people who remain are discouraging: almost one of every two people is on welfare; three of every five potential workers are unemployed;[6] and three of every five families are headed by women,[a] whose earning power is, of course, significantly less than that of two-parent families.

Accompanying this kind of poverty is a shocking level of illness and disability that Jackie and her neighbors merely take for granted. Her husband's kidneys failed before he was thirty; her alcoholic father had a stroke because of uncontrolled high blood pressure at forty-eight; her aunt Nancy, who helped her grandmother raise her, died from kidney failure complicated by cirrhosis when she was forty-three. Diabetes took her grandmother's leg, and blinded her great-aunt Eldora, who lives down the block.

Chicago's poor neighborhoods have always been its sickest. In 1890, a medical writer graphically described the conditions that were contributing to rampant disease among the city's immigrant industrial workers. "[Their] sole recourse usually is to the tenement where, heaped floor above floor, in a tainted atmosphere, or in low fetid hovels, amidst poverty, hunger and dirt, in foulness, want and crime, crowded humanity suffers, and sickens, and perishes; for the landlord here is also the air-lord, the lord of sunlight; lord of all the primary conditions of life and living; and these are doled out for a price, failing which the wretched tenant is turned out to seek a habitation still more miserable."[7]

The diseases that killed in the nineteenth century lent themselves to such dramatic prose. They were the great epidemics, smallpox, cholera, and typhoid fever. Such bacteria-borne infectious diseases festered because of a water supply periodically tainted by sewage and were easily spread in the crowded living quarters of poor city neighborhoods. With the coming of better sanitation methods, which included reversing the flow of the Chicago River so that the city's sewage would be sent to southern Illinois and Missouri rather than into Lake Michigan, these epidemics were largely conquered, though other age-old communicable diseases such as tuberculosis, sexually transmitted diseases, and, recently, childhood measles still disproportionately plague Chicago's poor.

One reason infectious diseases retain their foothold among the poor remains substandard housing, which is bad and getting worse in North Lawndale. A recent survey by an economic development group found that only 8% of the neighborhood's 8,937 buildings were in good to very good condition. The rest were abandoned, on the verge of collapse, or in need of repair.[6]

Dr. Arthur Jones has visited many of these decrepit buildings on house calls to patients too sick to make it into his clinic, which is located on Ogden almost directly behind Jackie's apartment. The clinic, Lawndale Christian Health Center, was founded by Dr. Jones and several other urban missionaries in 1984 and has succeeded, by most all accounts, at providing affordable and humane health care.

Dr. Jones told of one woman who was suffering a severe case of hives caused by an allergic reaction to her cat, yet repeatedly refused to get rid of the animal. "I really got kind of angry," Dr. Jones remembered, "and then she told me that if she got rid of the cat, there was nothing to protect her kids against rats." Another woman brought her two-year-old to the clinic with frostbite, so Dr. Jones dispatched his nurse practitioner to visit her home a block away from Jackie's. The nurse discovered icicles in the woman's apartment because the landlord had stopped providing heat. The stories go on, most involving landlords who cannot afford to keep up their buildings and tenants who cannot afford to leave them.

By these standards, the Baneses' apartment is in good shape. They have to contend with an occasional rat and wage a constant battle against roaches, but the landlord has kept the two-flat in decent repair; his sister lives on the first floor.

For the most part, the diseases that Jackie and her family live with are not characterized by sudden outbreaks but long, slow burns. As deadly infectious diseases have largely been eliminated or are easily cured—with the glaring exceptions of AIDS and now drug-resistant tuberculosis—chronic diseases have stepped into their wake, accounting for much of the death and disability among both rich and poor. The difference is that for affluent whites, diabetes, high blood pressure, heart disease, and the like are diseases of aging, while among poor blacks, they are more accurately called diseases of *middle*-aging.

In poor black neighborhoods on the West Side of Chicago, including North Lawndale, well over half of the population dies before the age of sixty-five, compared to a quarter of the residents of middle-class white Chicago neighborhoods.[8] Though they occur more often on the West Side, the three most common causes of premature mortality in the two areas would correspond—heart disease, diabetes, and high blood pressure—were it not for one fatal condition that increasingly is considered a major public health problem: homicide. It ranks sixth in the white neighborhoods but is the number two killer of West Siders under sixty-five.[8] Alcohol and drugs are the poisons that induce many of the West Side's deaths, whether from homicide or heart attack. Thirteen percent of fatalities in that part of the city are directly attributable to alcohol and drugs, four times the rate in white, middle-class neighborhoods.[9]

These statistics are not, of course, unique to Chicago. A study of premature mortality in Harlem showed that black men there were less likely to reach the age of sixty-five than men in Bangladesh.[10] "When sixty-seven people die in an earthquake in San Francisco, we call it a disaster and the President visits," said Dr. Harold Freeman, one of two Harlem Hospital Center physicians who conducted the study. "But here everyone is ignoring a chronic consistent disaster area, with many more people dying. And there is no question that things are getting worse."[11]

[. . .]

The starkest contrast in longevity is between white and black men, largely because of spiraling rates of homicide and AIDS among minorities. DeMarest, who was born in 1985, can be expected to live for sixty-four years and ten months, whereas an average white boy born that year will live eight years longer.[b] Jackie knows her son's chances of living a long life are not good, but she does not spend much time brooding about the dangers that await him. For now, she keeps him close to home and hopes for the best.

[. . .]

Notes

a. Personal communication with Marie Bousfield, demographer for the Chicago Department of Planning, 1991. Figure based on calculations from the 1990 U.S. Census.

b. Personal communication with Robert Armstrong, actuarial advisor, Division of Vital Statistics, National Center for Health Statistics, March 1993.

References

1. Chicago and Cook County Health Care Summit. *Chicago and Cook County health care action plan: Report of the Chicago and Cook County Health Care Summit.* Chicago: The Summit; 1990.

2. Lemann N. The origins of the underclass. *Atlantic Monthly.* June 1986:36.

3. Chicago Park District and Chicago Public Library Special Collections. *A breath of fresh air: Chicago's neighborhood parks of the Progressive Reform Era, 1900–1925.* 1989:21.

4. King W. Saving an urban wasteland. *New York Times.* August 16, 1991:B-2.

5. Chicago Department of Planning. *U.S. Census of Chicago: Race and Latino statistics for census tracts, community areas, and city wards: 1980, 1990.* Chicago: City of Chicago; 1991.

6. Chicago Tribune. *The American millstone.* Chicago: Contemporary Books; 1986.

7. Bonner T. *Medicine in Chicago, 1850–1950.* Urbana-Champaign: University of Illinois Press; 1991.

8. Chicago and Cook County Health Care Summit. Cook County Health Care Action Plan, draft appendix. 1990.

9. Chicago Department of Health. Communities Empowered to Prevent Alcohol and Drug Abuse Citywide Needs Assessment Report, working draft. 1991.

10. McCord C, Freeman HP. Excess mortality in Harlem. *New England Journal of Medicine.* 1990;322(3):173–177.

11. Rosenthal E. Health problems of inner city poor reach crisis point. *New York Times.* December 24, 1990.

CHAPTER FIVE

Selections from *Great American City: Chicago and the Enduring Neighborhood Effect*

Robert J. Sampson

Observing Chicago

Chicago is the great American city. — Norman Mailer, *Miami and the Siege of Chicago*

Enter contemporary and, yes, global Chicago.[1] Logic demands that if neighborhoods do not matter and placelessness reigns, then the city is more or less a random swirl. Anyone (or anything) could be *here* just as easily as *there*. Identities and inequalities by place should be rapidly interchangeable, the durable inequality of a community rare, and neighborhood effects on both individuals and higher-level social processes should be weak or nonexistent. The effects of spatial proximity should also be weak. And so goes much contemporary scholarship.[a]

By contrast, the guiding thesis of this book is that differentiation by neighborhood is not only everywhere to be seen, but that it is has durable properties—with cultural and social mechanisms of reproduction—and with effects that span a wide variety of social phenomena. Whether it be crime, poverty, child health, protest, leadership networks, civic

Originally published as Robert J. Sampson, *Great American City: Chicago and the Enduring Neighborhood Effect* (Chicago: University of Chicago Press, 2012), 6–20, 100–103.

engagement, home foreclosures, teen births, altruism, mobility flows, collective efficacy, or immigration, to name a few subjects investigated in this book, the city is ordered by a spatial logic ("placed") and yields differences as much today as a century ago. The effect of distance is not just geographical but simultaneously social, as described by Henry Zorbaugh in his classic treatise *The Gold Coast and the Slum*.[2] Spatially inscribed social differences, I argue, constitute a family of "neighborhood effects" that are pervasive, strong, cross-cutting, and paradoxically stable even as they are changing in manifest form.

To get an initial feel for the social and physical manifestations of my thesis and the enduring significance of place, walk with me on down the streets of this iconic American city in the first decade of the twenty-first century. I begin the tour in the heart of phantasmagoria if there ever was one—the bustling "Magnificent Mile" of Michigan Avenue, the highly touted showcase of contemporary Chicago. As we start southward from the famed Water Tower, we see mostly glitter and a collage of well-to-do people, with whites predominant among the shoppers laden with bags from the likes of Louis Vuitton, Tiffany's, Saks Fifth Avenue, Cartier, and more. Pristine stores gleam, police officers direct traffic at virtually every intersection throughout the day, and construction cranes loom in the nearby distance erecting (or in anticipation of) new condos. There is an almost complete lack of what James Q. Wilson and George Kelling famously termed "broken windows," a metaphor for neighborhood disrepair and urban neglect.[3] As I walked south on a midmorning in January of 2006, street sweepers were cleaning both sides of an already clean street as if to make the point. Whatever "disorder" exists is in fact socially organized, whether the occasional homeless asking for money in approved locations (near the river is common; in front of Van Cleef and Arpels or the Disney Store is not) or groups with a cause pressing their case with pamphlets, signs, and petitions. A favorite blip around the holidays is charity appeals mixed with the occasional hurling of abuse (or ketchup) at shoppers emerging from the furrier. I see nothing on this day but many furs. Other warmer times of the year bring out a cornucopia of causes.[b] On a warm day in late March of 2007, a homeless shelter for women presses its cause alongside an anti-Obama crusader (the latter getting many glares, in this, Obama country).

As we near the Chicago River, Donald Trump announces his vision. It is not subtle, of course, but rather a symbolic shout; in the city of skyscrapers the cranes here are busy erecting the self-described world's tallest future building, one in which "residential units on the 89th floor will break a 37-year world record held by the John Hancock Center for the world's highest homes off ground level."[4] Chicago is once again a "city on the make," as Nelson Algren put it well,[5] and so it seems perfectly fitting that Trump chose Chicago for this particular behemoth. On a cold day in March with barely a hole in the ground, international tourists were busily snapping pictures of the spectacle to be. A year later at fifteen stories and rising, and then later at almost ninety, the shutters of the tourist cameras continued to flap. In April 2009, only the height had changed, and Trump's vision was complete. Here, status is in place.

After crossing the Chicago River from the Near North Side into the Loop and passing the clash of classic architecture and Trump's monument to the future in its midst, one begins to see the outlines of the new Millennium Park in the distance, the half-billion-dollar extravaganza long championed by the second Mayor Daley and built considerably over cost with cries of corruption and cronyism.[6] Yet there is no denying the visual impact and success of Millennium Park, a Disney-like playground, all shiny and new. Even on a cold winter day there is public activity and excitement in the air. People mill about, skaters glide across the rink, and film-projected faces of average citizens stare out of the fountain's facade. Looking west from the park the skyline and bustle of the Loop stand out in a different way than the Near North—more workers and everyday business activity against the backdrop of landmark buildings and institutions.

Continuing south along Michigan Avenue past Roosevelt Road one sees more action, but with a twist. The architecture and historical pulse of the southern part of Chicago has always been different from points north. Despite its proximity to the Loop, the community of the "Near South Side" was marked by vacant rail yards, vagrants, dilapidated SRO (single-room-occupancy) hotels frequented by transients, penny arcades, and warehouses. The latter are now being redeveloped for lofts, and one old SRO building after another is being swept away for new condos and chic restaurants. Unlike the cumulative advantages being piled high atop the long-stable Gold Coast, renewal is the order of the day. Alongside and in some cases atop former railroad yards, the Near South development rose to prominence in the mid-1990s when Mayor Richard M. Daley and his wife moved there from the storied political neighborhood of Bridgeport in 1994.[c] Other developments soon took off, and today flux is readily apparent where decay once stood. Few Chicagoans just ten years ago would have imagined eating smartly at South Wabash and 21st, the former haunts of hobos and the homeless.[d] Whereas the Magnificent Mile has long anchored development and moneyed investment, the Near South Side tells a story of real change.[e]

Further down Michigan Avenue between about 35th and 47th Streets in the communities of Douglas and then Grand Boulevard, the scene is jarringly different. The transformation of the Near South has given way to what sociologists traditionally called the "slum." In a walk down Michigan Avenue in 2006 I saw what appeared to be a collapsing housing project to the left, broken glass in the street, vacant and boarded-up buildings, and virtually no people. Those I observed were walking quickly with furtive glances. On my walk in 2006 and again in early 2007, no whites were to be found, and no glimmering city parks were within sight. The cars were beat up, and there was little sign of collective gatherings or public activity, save perhaps what appeared to be a drug deal that transacted quickly. Yet even here there were stirrings of change, symbolized most dramatically by vacant lots to the west of where there once stood hulking and decaying projects built expressly to contain the city's black poor.

In fact, the South Side of Chicago once housed the most infamous slum in America. Chicago showed it knew how to build not just sky-scrapers but spectacular high-rises for the poor; the Robert Taylor Homes alone once held over twenty-five thousand residents—black, poor and isolated[7]—outdoing Cabrini Green, another national symbol of urban despair. As described by the Chicago Housing Authority itself, Robert Taylor apartments were "arrayed in a linear series of 28 16-story high-rises, which formed a kind of concrete curtain for traffic passing by on the nearby Dan Ryan Expressway."[8] The wider neighborhood of the projects—"Bronzeville," as it was named by St. Clair Drake and Horace R. Cayton in *Black Metropolis*—became infamous as one of the most dangerous and dispossessed in the country in the latter half of the twentieth century.[f] Yet in a short ten-year span the Robert Taylor Homes have been demolished (literally, blown up with dynamite) and former residents scattered throughout the metropolitan area. The tragic mistake of designed segregation became too much for even the Chicago City Council to ignore. Officially recognized as a failed policy, the last building of Robert Taylor was closed at the end of 2006.

I visited the area in March 2007 after the last building was destroyed. It was eerily quiet as I paused to contemplate and observe vast open spaces where grinding poverty once reigned amid families making the best they could out of an unforgiving environment. An especially haunting reflection came to mind, a visit in 1995 to the Robert Taylor Homes in the same exact block. Passing inoperable metal detectors and walking up urine-stenched stairs because the elevators were broken, the physical signs of degradation were overwhelming. Yet a group of us entered an apartment that was immaculate, where we met two single mothers who told a story of survival and determination to see a better day. Both of their sons had been murdered, and they had knitted a quilt with one-foot by one-foot squares honoring every other child who had also been murdered in the projects. The unfurled quilt extended nearly the length of the room. Shaken, I remember thinking at the time that surely anything would be an improvement over the prisonlike towers. On this spot one sees almost a verdant green expanse, with downtown far in the distance (figure 5.1). The "problem" is now out of sight and for many, including city leaders, out of mind.

Heading slightly east and progressing toward the lake, one sees the

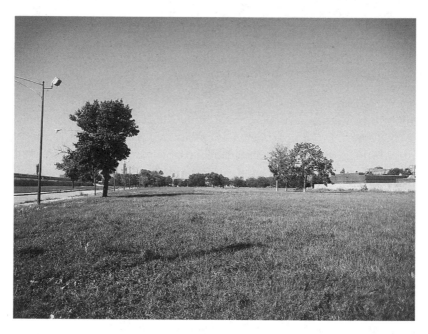

FIGURE 5.1. In the former shadows of the projects: where the Robert Taylor Homes once stood

Note: Photo by Robert J. Sampson, September 13, 2007.

emergence of a thriving black middle class amid the rubble and vacant lots adjacent to the former projects. Hard as it might be to imagine, $500,000 homes are being erected next to boarded-up buildings at the center of what was a low-rise slum just years earlier. Riders arriving by train into Chicago between the 1960s and the recent past would witness concentrated poverty up close—abandoned buildings and all the signs of decline appeared to the west of the tracks on the South Side in the small community of Oakland, which sits just north and east of Grand Boulevard. Nearby at the corner of Pershing and Langley, new homeowners are beckoned by a sign for the "Arches at Oakwood Shores"—a country club–like name—where prostitutes once roamed freely and physical destruction was rampant.[g] Vacant lots serve as reminders of the transition still in progress. At Drexel and 43rd on a day in March of 2007, a group of homeless men sit around a fire on a trash-strewn lot. At 47th and Wabash sits a huge boarded-up building, menacing in feel. Although still a work in progress, the areas in Oakland and around parts of Bronzeville represent one of the most stunning turnarounds in urban America today. How and why this happened takes on significance considering that most slums in Chicago [. . .] remain slums.

Soon after heading south from this surreal transformation to the likely "Black Gold Coast" of the future, one finds stately mansions in Kenwood and then the integrated and stable community of Hyde Park, home to passionate intellectuals and a dense organizational life. Adopted home and inspiration to President Barack Obama and other movers and shakers, almost nothing happens in Hyde Park without community input and institutional connections, visible in signs, churches, bookstores, petitions, and a wide variety of community organizations. People instantly know what you mean when you say you live in Hyde Park; the name swims in cultural meaning. [. . .]

Just west of Hyde Park, however, stark differences appear again. Across Washington Park sits a community of the same name that has seen hard times and still struggles mightily. Along the major thoroughfare of Garfield Boulevard stand burned buildings, gated liquor stores, and empty lots. At the corner of Michigan Avenue, we could not find a more apt portrayal of the second part of Zorbaugh's contrast. The inverse of Michigan Avenue north of the Loop, here we find dead spaces permeated by a sense of dread. At midday, groups of men hang out, bleary eyed and without apparent purpose. As we head further south into Woodlawn we see block after block of what most Americans would consider the classic ghetto. Black, visibly poor, and characterized by physical disrepair, west Woodlawn looks bleak to the eye. Zorbaugh might not have imagined the *Black Gold Coast and the Slum*, but today it is apparently here.

Continuing the patchwork quilt, if we head eastward to the area south of the University of Chicago, renewal announces itself once again. First one witnesses a stretch of open land where tenements once stood. Then east of the elevated tracks and former strip of decay on 63rd Street, new homes start sprouting. Around 63rd and Kimbark it looks almost like a suburb with back decks, grills, and lawns on display. On Kenwood Avenue, just south of 63rd, sit more new homes in a row. Tidy and neat, the middle class is moving in to reclaim the slums.

Heading further south to Avalon Park and Chatham we find the neighborhoods where a stable black middle class has existed for decades. Along street after street south of 79th and west of Stony Island one can see neat brick buildings, myriad neighborhood associations, and children playing happily in the streets. No new developments, no dramatic changes, and little media glare like that chronicling the disrepute of the slums. For years and like many neighborhoods across the U.S., this area has seen families raising their kids, tending to their homes, and going about quietly living the American Dream. At almost every block a sign announces a block club and shared expectations for conduct.[h]

If we head west past the Dan Ryan Expressway, we find more stability, albeit an impoverished one. Here we confront concentrated poverty stretching for hundreds of blocks. Outsiders are often surprised at how far one may drive in certain areas of Chicago's South Side and see marked signs of deterioration. Stability of change thus rules again, where neighborhoods maintain their relative positions in the overall hierarchy. Why these neighborhoods and not the ones like Oakland?

And so it goes as one continues on through the highly variegated mosaic of twenty-first-century Chicago—or Boston, New York, Los Angeles, or any other American city. Venturing down the streets of our cities, the careful observer sees what appear to be "day and night" representations of community life. There are vast disparities in the contemporary city on a number of dimensions that are anything but randomly distributed in space. Perhaps more important, the meanings that people attribute to these places and differences are salient and often highly consensual. Our walk also reveals that important as was Zorbaugh's work, the Gold Coast and the slum is not the only contrast. No matter which direction one turns in Chicago, the result will be to encounter additional social worlds—perhaps the teeming immigrant enclave of Little Village, bohemian Wicker Park, white working-class Clearing, yuppified Lincoln Park, the upper-class white community of Norwood, the incredibly diverse Uptown, or the land that time forgot, Hegewisch.

Thus while some things remain the same from Zorbaugh's day, other things have changed. The intersection of West Oak and North Cambridge in the west part of the Near North Side was considered "Death Corner" in the 1920s by Zorbaugh.[2] That maintained for decades, and the area around the infamous Cabrini Green homes was still dicey on multiple visits in the decade of the 2000s, a swelter of contradictions. Decay was present in many blocks with a large number of boarded-up buildings near Oak and Hudson. On Locust near Orleans it was common until recently to see high-rise projects with unemployed men hanging out during the day. Yet the Cabrini Green projects are in the process of being razed to be replaced by low-rise, hopefully mixed-income housing. The area sends mixed messages, and its future is one to watch, however painfully. On a brisk day in March of 2007 I witnessed a clearly emaciated and drug-addled woman begging for money a short stroll from Cabrini units near a large sign announcing new condos and a gym on North Larrabee St. with the unsubtle proclamation: "Look Better Naked." [. . .]

For now it is clear that Chicago possesses neighborhoods of nearly every ilk—from the seemingly endless bungalow belt of working-class homes to the skyscrapers of the Loop, the diversity and disparities of Chicago are played out against a vast kaleidoscope of contrasts. Indeed, the Gold Coast(s) and the slum(s)—and everything in between—represent a mosaic of contrasts that reflect the twenty-first-century city and its diversity of interrelated parts.

A Bird's-Eye View

Neighborhoods differ dramatically in their quality, feel, sights, sounds, and smells—that much is experienced in our walks. But equally remarkable is the diversity of behaviors and social actions that cluster together in space and that define the social organization of the city. At a macro level the inverse of placelessness is ecological concentration and disparity. Layering independent empirical data on top of the street observations above, I thus zoom out to take a bird's-eye view.

Consider first the apparent anomaly of the ecological concentration of disparate aspects of well-being across the neighborhoods of Chicago. Whether the measure is homicide, low birth weight, infant mortality, teen pregnancy, physical abuse, or accidental injury, there is compelling evidence pointing to geographic "hot spots" of compromised health. Figure 5.2 provides a vivid example, displaying the geographical ordering of homicide incidents and the expected health outcomes of infants over six years (2000–2005) based on the poverty rate of each of seventy-seven community areas in Chicago.[i] At first blush, what could be more different than a woman giving birth to a baby weighing less than 2,500 grams and the murder of another human being, typically by a young male? Yet homicide is highly concentrated in the same communities scoring low on infant health, with a clustering or corridor of compromised well-being on the Near South Side (e.g., the Grand Boulevard and Washington Park communities of our walk earlier), Far South Side (e.g., Riverdale, West Pullman, Roseland), and West Side (e.g., North Lawndale, West Garfield Park, and, to their south, Austin). By contrast, neighborhoods on the north and southwest sides fare much better, including some working-class communities (e.g., Portage Park), diverse communities (e.g., Lakeview), and some geographically close to high poverty and violence (e.g., Beverly, McKinley Park, and Clearing).

The reader may suspect that this spatial pattern is simply a poverty story. It is not: the infant health classification in figure 5.2 is adjusted for concentrated poverty, and alternative procedures replicate the basic pattern.[j] . . . Other commonly invoked suspects—from individual attributes and vulnerabilities on the one hand, to race/ethnic composition on the other—are insufficient to explain this stark phenomenon.[k] Equally impressive, the concentration of "death and disease," as Drake and Cayton put it over a half century earlier in *Black Metropolis*, is long-standing.[9] As shown in their original publication in 1945, whether manifested through insanity, infant mortality, delinquency, tuberculosis, or "poverty and social disorganization," the city of Chicago was highly stratified by disadvantage and ecological risk, with many high-rate communities then overlapping with those in figure 5.2. The specific communities may change, but the broader pattern of concentration is robust.

The modernist critic might give ground but view crime and disease as outliers, something out of the old "social disorganization" playbook of urban sociology.[10] So let us turn things around and look instead at the

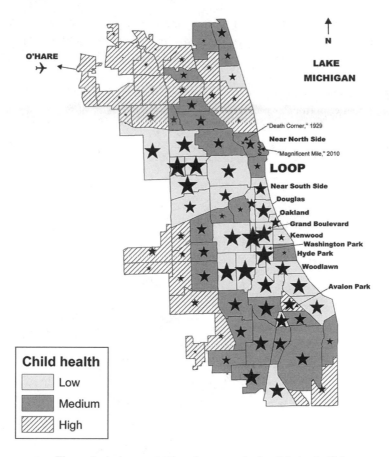

FIGURE 5.2. The ecological concentration of compromised well-being in Chicago communities: homicide predicts poor infant health, 2000–2005, poverty adjusted

Note: Stars are proportional to homicides per hundred thousand population. Adjusted child health scores are
classified into equal thirds.

American political equivalent of "apple pie"—collective civic engagement. Figure 5.3 displays the enduring association and neighborhood
concentration of collective civic events such as community festivals, fund
drives, parades, blood drives, and PTA meetings over three decades.
The data suggest that civic life is not dead but rather highly differen-
tiated and spatially ordered, with clear evidence that the clustering of
civic engagement goes well beyond chance and keeps reappearing in the
same places. Areas that generate traditional civic engagement appear

host to public protests as well, such as marches against the Vietnam or Iraq wars and protests against police brutality. Moreover, the intensity or rate of activity from 1970 to 1990 (classified into thirds) strongly predicts the initiation and location of collective civic events in 2000 that are represented as dots in figure 5.3. [. . .] This pattern of collective civic action is best explained not by race or class but the density of organizations in the community. Modern society writ large may well be an organizational one, but its manifestation has clear local imprints that are anything but random.

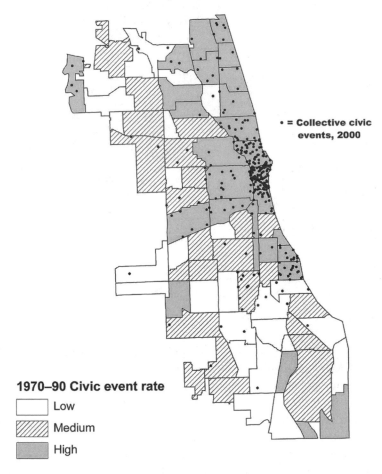

FIGURE 5.3. Spatial concentration and long-term endurance of collective civic engagement in Chicago communities, 1970–2000

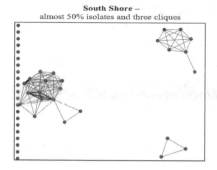
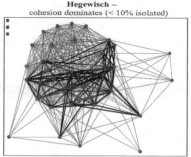

FIGURE 5.4. Community variation in network connectivity of leadership

Perhaps collective civic engagement, even impassioned protest, is not fully modern either. Maybe networks are where globalization instantiates the potential to destroy community differences.[11] As a preview of results to come, I display in figure 5.4 the pattern of "connectivity" among people to whom key leaders in two Chicago communities go in order to get things done. Each dot in the figure represents a leader, and connecting lines denote a direct or indirect tie between them. In South Shore, the ties among relevant actors are either absent, as are the "isolates" along the left (almost half of the entire set), or they collapse into one of three distinct "cliques" that are disconnected from each other. By contrast, in Hegewisch ties are very dense, with only three isolates and over 90% of leaders deeply embedded in an overlapping structure of ties. Chicago is composed of marked variations in structural configurations such as these, with consequences for key dimensions of city life, especially including political power and the allocation of resources (e.g., funds for economic development, parks, and cultural affairs).

As a further and distinctly contemporary example, figure 5.5 maps the distribution of income-adjusted Internet use in 2002 alongside the concentration of "bohemians" (artists and related workers, designers, actors, producers and directors, dancers and choreographers, musicians, singers, writers and authors, and photographers) in Chicago in 2000. The economist Richard Florida posits bohemians as a leading indicator of the "creative class," that group of intellectuals, writers, artists, and scientists who seek to live alongside other creative people.[12,13] According to Florida, the creative class is the driving engine for economic growth—one that is transforming work, leisure, and community. Whatever one makes of this causal claim about growth, figure 5.5 clearly reveals that they cluster together—cyberspace use and the creative class reflect residential sorting into distinct spatial communities. Like the other social phenomena considered so far, this concentration is highly nonrandom, and the story is not reducible to economics. One might worry about differential access to the Internet, for example, the so-called digital divide. But figure 5.5 shows the frequency of Internet use that is expected based on the community's income level and median rent. When we remove these economic correlates in further analysis, a persistent connection remains.[1] A form of cultural sorting appears to be present. Even the dis-

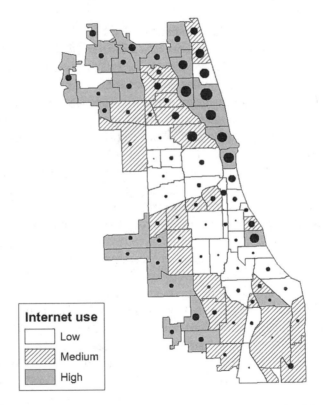

FIGURE 5.5. Local cosmopolitans: income-adjusted Internet use and "Bohemia"

Note: Communities classified in equal thirds according to Internet usage reported in 2001–2002 community survey, 0–9% (light), 9–17% (medium), and 17–50% (dark) using Internet more than five hours per week. Internet use rate adjusted for median income and median rent of the community in 2000. Circles proportional to "Bohemians" per hundred thousand, defined as artists, designers, actors, producers and directors, dancers and choreographers, musicians, singers, writers and authors, and photographers.

tribution of Starbucks in Chicago is similarly clustered and tracks closely the density of bohemians, perhaps much to their chagrin.[m,14]

A final example takes us out of the Windy City. Even though my earlier observations of neighborhood disparity and social distance by place reflect several dimensions, and despite the bird's-eye maps of the city thus far, the stubborn reader might still object that this is just a Chicago story. Or perhaps a peculiar "state" effect of American policy rather than a neighborhood effect.[15] So let us peek ahead and compare Chicago to an exemplar of modern efficiency, cultural sophistication, state planning, and cutting edge technology—Stockholm, Sweden. It is hard to imagine two cities more different than Chicago and Stockholm, not to mention the countries within which they are situated. Stockholm certainly doesn't have concentrated poverty the likes of Chicago, and more people are murdered in Chicago in a single year than over the last fifty years in Stockholm. But surprising similarities emerge despite the radical differences in state policies.

As an initial demonstration, I assess whether concentrated poverty is similarly related to violence, each defined the same way, in both cities. Figure 5.6 shows a similar decreasingly positive association of violence with disadvantage in both cities. To be sure, there are many more disadvantaged neighborhoods in Chicago, where the association with violence begins to tail off. There are also more concentrated *affluent* neighborhoods in Chicago as well (note the areas to the left of the graph). In this sense, figure 5.6 reflects "inequality compression" in Stockholm, characterized by restricted variation in disadvantage and lower violence. Indeed, Chicago "sits atop" Stockholm at virtually every level of disadvantage, and its extended range of concentrated disadvantage is pronounced. Yet as disadvantage rises, violence does as well in both cities in a nonlinear way, a distinct pattern unlikely to arise by chance.[16] Detailed research by Swedish criminologists further shows the concentration of homicides (albeit fewer in number, of course) in a disproportionately small number of neighborhoods, just like Chicago.[17]

These distinct ecological patterns provide a tantalizing hint that larger principles of societal organization, such as equality of housing and racial stratification, are etched in place and that they may explain city differences in violence. It remains to be seen how well this framework stands up to further tests, but it appears that there is something fundamental about place stratification and violence that cuts across international boundaries

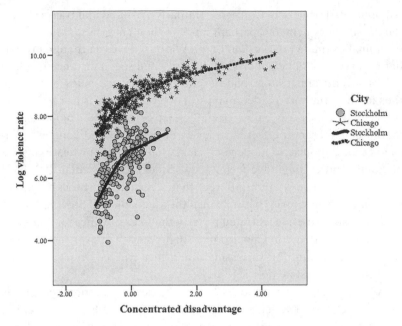

FIGURE 5.6. Similar prediction of violence rates by concentrated disadvantage in highly divergent contexts: Chicago and Stockholm neighborhoods

and yet is locally manifested in its distributional form. The larger point is that Chicago is not just a lens through which to view contemporary American cities; instead it can provide a platform for investigating cross-national or comparative questions as well. [. . .]

[. . .]

Things Go Together

As Clifford Shaw and Henry D. McKay argued in the Chicago of the 1920s and 1930s, Drake and Cayton in the mid-twentieth century, and William Julius Wilson and Douglas Massey near century's end, many social problems typically considered "outcomes" cluster together.[9,18–20] This pattern continues. Violence, a leading indicator of neighborhood viability, remains concentrated in early twenty-first-century Chicago and cities as different as Stockholm. [. . .] Incidents of low birth weight map onto the location of violence (figure 5.2), and when I extend the data through

2005 this same relationship remains (correlation of 0.77, $p < 0.01$). Other indicators of well-being tell the same story. For example, the infant mortality rate is correlated 0.76 with the teenage birth rate, which is in turn highly correlated with the homicide rate at 0.89 (both $p < 0.01$). There is a deep and divided structure in the concentration of well-being across multiple dimensions of the contemporary city.

What are often considered *sources* of compromised well-being—such as unemployment, segregation, poverty, and family disruption—are equally clustered in space. The basics of these patterns are common to many cities and extend across multiple ecological units of analysis ranging from census tracts to metropolitan areas and even states.[21,22] I illustrate and update this phenomenon here by considering empirical patterns for a core set of socioeconomic indicators in both Chicago and the U.S. I argue that disadvantage is not encompassed in a single characteristic but rather is a synergistic composite of social factors that mark the qualitative aspects of growing up in severely disadvantaged neighborhoods. My colleagues and I investigated this idea by examining six characteristics of census tracts nationwide, taken from the 1990 and 2000 censuses, to create a measure of concentrated disadvantage: *welfare receipt, poverty, unemployment, female-headed households, racial composition* (percentage black), and *density of children*. These indicators all loaded on a single principal component we called "concentrated disadvantage" in both decades and both Chicago and the rest of the U.S. (altogether some sixty-five thousand census tracts).[23] The main difference of note between the U.S. and Chicago neighborhoods is that the exposure of children under eighteen years of age to concentrated economic disadvantage and racial segregation is more pronounced in Chicago. The data thus confirm that neighborhoods that are both black *and* poor, and that are characterized by high unemployment and female-headed families, are ecologically distinct, a characteristic that is not simply the same thing as low economic status. In this pattern Chicago is not alone.

[...]

Concentrated Incarceration: A New "Pathology"?

There is a new kind of social distortion that has come to characterize the national scene that might surprise even Moynihan, were he alive today.

From the 1920s to the early 1970s, the incarceration rate in the United States averaged 110 inmates per one hundred thousand persons. This rate of incarceration varied so little both here and abroad that many scholars believed that the nation and the world were experiencing a stable equilibrium of punishment. But beginning in the mid-1970s, the incarceration rate in the United States accelerated dramatically, reaching the unprecedented rate of 197 inmates per one hundred thousand persons in 1990 and the previously unimaginable rate of 504 inmates per one hundred thousand persons in 2008.[24] Incarceration in the United States is now so prevalent that it has become a normal stage in the life course for many disadvantaged young men, with some segments of the population more likely to end up in prison than attend college. Scholars have broadly described this national phenomenon as *mass incarceration*.[25]

Yet, in fact, mass incarceration has a local concentration, what Charles Loeffler and I have called "Punishment's Place."[26] Obscured by a focus on national trends are profound variations in incarceration rates by communities within cities, especially by their racial composition. Like the geographically concentrated nature of criminal offending by individuals, a small proportion of communities bear the disproportionate brunt of U.S. crime policy's experiment with mass incarceration. In Chicago, we can see this by calculating the rate of incarceration for each census tract in Chicago and comparing it to the level of concentrated disadvantage and percentage black.[n] The correlation of incarceration rates in 1990–95 with concentrated disadvantage and percentage black at the neighborhood level in 1990 is 0.82 and 0.75, respectively. The corresponding correlations for 2000 disadvantage and percentage black predicting incarceration in 2000–2005 are 0.80 and 0.74. The persistence over time at the census-tract level is, by implication, very strong (0.86, all coefficients $p < 0.01$). Because of this ecological concentration, large swaths of the city, especially in the southwest and northwest, are relatively untouched by the imprisonment boom no matter which period we examine, with almost no one sent to prison in some areas. By contrast, there is a dense and spatially contiguous cluster of areas in the near west and south central areas of Chicago that have rates of incarceration many times higher. This pattern of concentration results in a racialized configuration of the city—the correlation between concentrated disadvantage and the incarceration rate in white areas is no different than zero, but in black, Latino, and mixed areas the correlation is over 0.6 ($p < 0.01$).

Once again, then, "things go together," but the strength of the connection, especially among social dislocations like poverty, crime, infant mortality, low birth weight, incarceration, and unemployment, is decidedly stronger in communities of color.

Notes

a. The "Los Angeles School" of urban sociology might be thought to be the leading proponent of this view, but I refer broadly to current thinking across the social sciences, including sociology, political science, epidemiology, and perhaps especially economics. [. . .]

b. During a street observation on another walk in 2006 (March 10), I witnessed a protest march replete with drummers, chanting, and dissemination of a statement from the Dalai Lama. Leading the march were monks who sought to draw attention to Tibetan dissidents on the occasion of the forty-seventh anniversary of the Tibetan National Uprising Day. [. . .]

c. Bridgeport, an iconic working-class white neighborhood that produced generations of political heavyweights, sits south and west of the Dan Ryan, within earshot of the Chicago White Sox's Comiskey Park. The Daleys' move away from Bridgeport to a nearly half-million-dollar townhouse in Central Station Townhouse (in 1994 dollars) was the subject of much consternation among locals and widely reported in the local media. It was not the price so much as the identity of location—the beers and brats of Richard M. Daley's father in Bridgeport were given a symbolic punch. Daley #2 has been reported as intending to move up even more, quite literally, to a high-rise perch across from Millennium Park, smack in the heart of the Loop. Rising over a former Dunkin' Donuts near the corner of Wabash and Randolph, the Heritage at Millennium Park commands stunning views of the park and Lake Michigan to the east.

d. Nels Anderson's *On Hobos and Homelessness* is widely considered the major "Chicago School" take on the homeless. [. . .] He studied the West Madison Street Area, but the Near South was another favorite haunt of hobos in the early years. At the current intersection stands a Latin American and Caribbean fusion restaurant, where I dined twice in 2007 with many well-heeled and fashionable people out on the town.

e. [. . .] It is not clear the term [*gentrification*] fits the Near South. Gentrification is commonly thought to mean areas where the lower-income residents are pushed out. Many areas here had no permanent residents. The South Loop has seen a net loss of thousands of SRO units since 1990.

f. Whether [because of] crime, school dropout, mortality, or disease, the Wentworth district long stood out. [. . .]

g. Field observations, 2007.

h. Typical is the 8000 South Avalon block club, welcoming visitors but "no ball playing, car washing, speeding, loud music, loitering or littering." Nearly every block club declares the same.

i. I define child health as the standardized combination of infant mortality and low-birth-weight babies—these two indicators are very highly correlated ($0.81, p < 0.01$). As expected based on prior research, poverty is significantly correlated ($0.78, p < 0.01$) with poor infant health. [. . .]

j. Another way to demonstrate the spatial link is to estimate the association of homicide with infant mortality and low birth weight while directly controlling for poverty. When I do so, the partial correlation is 0.60 ($p < 0.01$). Poverty thus does not explain away the clustering.

k. Population size cannot explain the patterning of events either as that is also adjusted. Interestingly, even *within* the highest-crime-rate community of Chicago, crime is highly concentrated by time and place, almost as if the wider citywide patterns of ecological concentration are refracted onto the microlocal level of a single block. [. . .]

l. The partial correlation of rates of Internet use and bohemians across communities, controlling for median rent and median income, is 0.55 ($p < 0.01$). [. . .]

m. As of the mid-2000s there were only a handful of Starbucks south of Roosevelt Road in Chicago; most cluster on the North Side. A Starbucks in Wicker Park was visibly defaced with graffiti on a visit in 2007. Clashes of culture were readily apparent. Exiting Myopic Books, where one can buy any number of dog-eared radical treatises, a perfectly opulent woman from American Apparel stared down at me from a billboard.

n. We measure the imprisonment rate by the number of unique Chicago-residing felony defendants sentenced to the Illinois Department of Corrections from the Circuit Court of Cook County divided by the number of Chicago inhabitants ages eighteen to sixty-four in the 2000 census. We use adults "at risk" in the denominator in order to rule out confounding variations in the prevalence of children age eighteen that are not eligible for prison. Similarly, we exclude those at the older end because, while society is aging, very few prisoners are over sixty-five. [. . .]

References

1. Abu-Lughod J. *New York, Chicago, Los Angeles: America's global cities.* Minneapolis: University of Minnesota Press; 1999.

2. Zorbaugh H. *The Gold Coast and the slum: A sociological study of Chicago's Near North Side.* Chicago: University of Chicago Press, 1929.

3. Wilson JQ, Kelling G. Broken windows: The police and neighborhood safety. *Atlantic.* 1982;127:29–38.

4. Emporis Buildings. 2007. http://www.emporis.com/en/wm/bu/?id=102119.

5. Algren N. *Chicago: City on the make*. Chicago: University of Chicago Press; 1951.

6. Gilfoyle T. *Millennium Park: Creating a Chicago landmark*. Chicago: University of Chicago Press; 2006.

7. Venkatesh SA. *American project: The rise and fall of a modern ghetto*. Cambridge, MA: Harvard University Press; 2000.

8. Chicago Housing Authority. 2007. http://www.thecha.org/housingdev/robert_taylor.html.

9. Drake SC, Cayton HR. *Black metropolis: A study of Negro life in a northern city*. Chicago: University of Chicago Press; 1945 [1993].

10. Kornhauser RR. *Social sources of delinquency: An appraisal of analytic models*. Chicago: University of Chicago Press; 1978.

11. McCarthy H, Miller P, Skidmore P, eds. *Network logic: Who governs in an interconnected world?* London: Demos; 2004.

12. Florida R. *The rise of the creative class: And how it's transforming work, leisure, community and everyday life*. New York: Basic; 2002.

13. Graif C. From diversity to the rise of creative hotspots of artists and non-profit art organizations. Cambridge, MA: Harvard University, Department of Sociology; 2010.

14. Sampson RJ. After-school Chicago: Space and the city. *Urban Geography*. 2008;29:127–137.

15. Wacquant L. *Urban outcasts: A comparative sociology of advanced marginality*. Cambridge: Polity; 2008.

16. Sampson RJ, Wikström PO. The social order of violence in Chicago and Stockholm neighborhoods: A comparative inquiry. In *Order, conflict, and violence* (Kalyvas SN, Shapiro I, Masoud T, eds.). New York: Cambridge University Press; 2008.

17. Wikström PO. *Urban crime, criminals, and victims*. New York: Springer; 1991.

18. Shaw CR, McKay HD. *Juvenile delinquency and urban areas*. Chicago: University of Chicago Press; 1942 [1969].

19. Wilson WJ. *The truly disadvantaged: The inner city, the underclass, and public policy*. Chicago: University of Chicago Press; 1987.

20. Massey DS. American apartheid: Segregation and the making of the underclass. *American Journal of Sociology*. 1990;96(2):329–357.

21. Sampson RJ, Morenoff JD, Gannon-Rowley T. Assessing "neighborhood effects": Social processes and new directions in research. *Annual Review of Sociology*. 2002;28:443–478.

22. Land KC, McCall PL, Cohen LE. Structural covariates of homicide rates: Are there any invariances across time and space? *American Journal of Sociology*. 1990;95(4):922–963.

23. Sampson RJ, Sharkey P, Raudenbush SW. Durable effects of concen-

trated disadvantage on verbal ability among African-American children. *Proceedings of the National Academy of Sciences.* 2008;105:845–852.

24. Bureau of Justice Statistics. Prisoners in 2008. 2010. https://www.bjs.gov/content/pub/pdf/p08.pdf.

25. Western B. *Punishment and inequality in America.* New York: Sage; 2006.

26. Sampson RJ, Loeffler C. Punishment's place: The local concentration of mass incarceration. *Daedalus.* 2010;139:20–31.

PART II

The Health Gap

This second part includes empirical studies describing health inequities in Chicago. These studies emphasize the importance of place and, in particular, the importance of race/racism as a social determinant of health. They focus on a wide range of conditions, including cancer, birth weight, AIDS, breast cancer, and hypertension, but our emphasis is not on the conditions themselves but, rather, on how these health outcomes reflect social inequalities.

Consider a *Chicago Sun-Times* story reporting "Racial, Economic Chasm in Chicago's Health Seen in Study" (see figure 3). It summarized research from the Sinai Urban Health Institute (SUHI), one of the leading research groups in Chicago, that showed that Puerto Rican children had the highest prevalence of asthma in the city. This finding generated an important discussion, and the community asked questions with no simple answers. Why did this health gap exist? What was causing the health gap? And how could it be eliminated?

This part of the *Reader* offers a sampling of the complexity involved in measuring health gaps. How do we account for the importance of place? How do we go beyond thinking of poor health as an individual-level *risk*, something to be addressed through behavioral change? How do we incorporate time into our analyses, recognizing the dynamic nature of health inequities (acknowledging that changes in policy and developments in technology can lead to unforeseen/unintended *increases* in health inequities)? And, perhaps most importantly, how do we conceptualize *race* in health research?

This part begins with the work of Clyde Phillips and Loretta Lacey, who published a descriptive epidemiologic study detailing cancer profiles in "high-risk" communities—predominantly African American neighbor-

Puerto Rican, black child asthma soaring

Racial, economic chasm in Chicago's health seen in study

BY JIM RITTER
Health Reporter

A new study has found that 34 percent of Puerto Rican children in Chicago have asthma, the highest rate on record.

Twenty-five percent of Chicago's African American kids also have asthma, the study found. The highest rate previously documented, 25 percent, is in New York's Harlem neighborhood.

The Chicago study also found a huge racial divide in other health areas. An adult in mostly Hispanic South Lawndale is about nine times more likely to be uninsured than an adult in mostly white Norwood Park. Blacks are more than three times as likely to be diagnosed with diabetes as whites. And 37 percent of blacks are smokers, compared to the national rate of 23 percent.

Previous studies have documented similar disparities. But lead researcher Steven Whitman said he was shocked at how wide the racial divide is in Chicago. The study recommended reforms to ensure that "health and even life and death are not driven by the color of one's skin or how much money one has."

Researchers from Sinai Urban Health Institute conducted in-depth surveys of 1,699 adults and 811 children in South Lawndale, Norwood Park, Humboldt Park (mostly black and Hispanic), West Town (Hispanic and white), North Lawndale (black) and Roseland (black).

BY THE NUMBERS

Percentage of children under 12 who have asthma*:

Norwood Park (15%)

Humboldt Park (28%)

West Town (28%)
N. Lawndale (23%)
S. Lawndale (12%)

Roseland (23%)

U.S. average: 12 percent*
* Includes children diagnosed by a doctor and children suspected of having asthma based on answers to screening questions.
** Includes only cases diagnosed by doctor

PERCENT, BY RACE
Puerto Rican: 34%
African American: 25%
Mexican: 14%
White: 14%
SOURCE: Improving Community Health Survey
–SUN-TIMES

For each child age 12 and younger, researchers asked whether he or she has been diagnosed with asthma or has asthma symptoms.

The 54-page study was funded by a $750,000 grant from the

Robert Wood Johnson Foundation.

No one knows for certain why asthma rates in inner-city neighborhoods in Chicago and other cities are increasing. Several factors probably combine to trigger asthma in kids predisposed to the disease or to make symptoms worse in those who already have the condition, said Dr. Jay Shannon, an asthma specialist at Cook County's Stroger Hospital and a board member of the American Lung Association of Metropolitan Chicago.

Shannon said these inner-city asthma triggers include:
♦ Cockroach droppings and body parts.
♦ High mold counts in poorly maintained housing.
♦ Secondhand smoke. The Sinai study found that between 48 percent and 59 percent of the asthma kids in North Lawndale, Roseland and Humboldt Park live with smokers.
♦ Air pollution from industries, coal-burning power plants and other sources.
♦ Inadequate health care.
♦ Stress, depression and anxiety.

The study recommended "intensive education efforts" to control childhood asthma. It noted that a Mount Sinai Hospital study found that even a brief session with an asthma educator reduces trips to the emergency room. Monthly sessions and a case manager reduce trips further.

Mount Sinai's education program has helped keep 4-year-old Wilfredo Couret Jr.'s asthma under control. Wilfredo, who is half Puerto Rican and half Mexican, once was so prone to asthma attacks that his mother put him in a high chair to prevent him from running around.

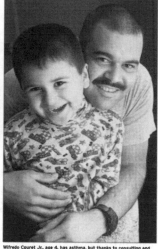

Wifredo Couret Jr., age 4, has asthma, but thanks to consulting and medication, his wheezing has stopped. –RICHARD A. CHAPMAN/SUN-TIMES

An asthma educator showed the family how to avoid asthma triggers by, for example, removing rugs, drapes and stuffed animals and dusting every two days. Wilfredo also takes a daily asthma-control drug. He hasn't had an attack in five months, and can play tag with his sister without wheezing.

The report also found racial and income disparities in diabetes, smoking, adult asthma, depres-

sion, obesity, HIV/AIDS and overall mental and physical health.

The Chicago Public Health Department is trying to reduce such disparities, a spokesman said. Most department clinics are in minority neighborhoods. And in North and South Lawndale, the Health Promotion Project is attempting to prevent and control diabetes and heart disease by improving the general health of the community.

FIGURE 3. "Racial, economic chasm"
Source: Chicago Sun-Times. January 8, 2004.

hoods. Their assessment was clear: "The excess black cancer mortality rates are directly linked to the multiple problems of the socioeconomically disadvantaged, who are unable to purchase or gain access to state-of-art medical services."

What drives the association between a social determinant such as race (which we understand as a social construct, not a biological category) and a health outcome is not so clear. For instance, Richard David and James Collins conducted seminal work in understanding that race is a multidimensional social construct. They examined racial differences in birth weight of infants based on the mother's race and place of birth, contrasting US-born white and black women as well as African-born mothers living in Illinois. Among women at low risk, the birth-weight patterns for infants of African-born black women were more closely related to US-born white women and that the rate in US-born black women was twofold higher than African-born black women and threefold higher than US-born white women. The work of David and Collins directly challenged genetic explanations for health inequities and gave support for social and psychophysiological theories. For example, David and Collins noted: "A woman's exposure as a young child to the effects of poverty or racial discrimination could adversely affect birth weight in the next generation."

Later in this part of the *Reader*, we include studies that explore community-level data as well as black-white health gaps. Ami Shah and her colleagues at SUHI document the geographic and racial/ethnic health disparities that can be hidden in aggregate-level data. The SUHI survey— one of the most important household surveys carried out in Chicago— was developed and administered by door-to-door engagement in six of the seventy-seven Chicago communities (Norwood Park, Humboldt Park, West Town, North Lawndale, South Lawndale, and Roseland). It enabled intercommunity comparisons along with comparisons to findings for the entire city of Chicago for health conditions, health behaviors, and health care access.

Small area analysis of disparities in common health conditions was then further developed in the work of Edward Naureckas and Sandra Thomas, who highlight the need to consider health care utilization data. Naureckas and Thomas found that inequalities in asthma-related mortality and hospitalization utilization rates by race did not diminish in the years following the release of the National Asthma Education and Prevention Program guidelines. This work demonstrated how health gaps persist despite the availability of effective medications and evidence-based treatment guidelines.

Also in this part of the *Reader*, we see the work of Steven Whitman et al., which highlights the interplay between place, time, and technological advances. As mammography for early detection became more common in the 1990s, Whitman et al. measured breast cancer mortality rate ratios in Chicago against those in New York City and the United States as a whole. Their analysis revealed that the black-white gap was not statistically significant in Chicago or New York City or the United States in 1980 but that it increased and became significant by 2005 in all regions, but especially Chicago. Like the work of David and Collins on birth weight, the Whitman et al. study challenged genetic or biological explanations for black-white differences in health outcomes and poignantly explained: "Racial disparities in breast cancer mortality cannot be viewed outside the context of racism in the US." Other research from

SUHI has gone on to explore black-white rate ratios in the fifty most populous cities in the United States, focusing on mortality from heart disease,[1] breast cancer,[2] prostate cancer,[3] and lung cancer.[4]

Similarly, Girma Woldemichael et al. examined the correlations between race/ethnicity, age, and gender on survival among persons who died from AIDS-related causes and the modifying impact of the recommendation in December 1995 that highly active antiretroviral therapy (HAART) should be the standard of care. Using Chicago Department of Public Health data from 1993 to 2001, they found that the gap in survival between non-Hispanic blacks and whites increased from 1.18 in the pre-HAART era to 1.50 in the post-HAART era. In this case, the introduction of an effective therapy led to the widening of health disparities in outcomes, which was posited to be due to higher rates of access to care for socially advantaged groups (mirroring the results of Whitman et al.).

While most of the work in this part of the *Reader* is quantitative, we know that this style of research by itself is not the only way to understand health gaps. In their work on breast cancer mortality in Chicago, Karen Kaiser et al. reported the results of four focus groups with black women about their views of breast cancer. The work highlighted the gap between the community's understanding of breast cancer and what we know about the epidemiology of cancer mortality. For instance, the study found that a majority of black women believed that all women have the same chance of dying from breast cancer (as one women explained, "Cancer is an equal opportunity, evil attacker") and that individual lack of awareness or follow-through on screening was the cause of higher breast cancer mortality in blacks. The structural and social determinants of health—while consistently documented in the scientific literature—are not always front and center in public thinking about disease.

As a whole, these selections give a glimpse of the large literature that has developed in Chicago to describe health gaps. These selections emphasize Chicago's experience with studies that value local data (community-level data) as well as studies that acknowledge the importance of race/racism as a social determinant of health.

References

1. Benjamins MR, Hirschtick JL, Hunt BR, Hughes MM, Hunter B. Racial disparities in heart disease mortality in the 50 largest U.S. cities. *Journal of Racial and Ethnic Health Disparities*. 2017;4(5):967–975.

2. Hunt B, Hurlbert MS. Black:white disparities in breast cancer mortality in the 50 largest cities in the United States, 2005–2014. *Cancer Epidemiology*. 2016;45:169–173.

3. Benjamins MR, Hunt BR, Raleigh SM, Hirschtick JL, Hughes MM. Racial disparities in prostate cancer mortality in the 50 largest US cities. *Cancer Epidemiology*. 2016;44:125–131.

4. Hunt B, Balachandran B. Black:white disparities in lung cancer mortality in the 50 largest cities in the United States. *Cancer Epidemiology*. 2015; 39(6):908–916.

CHAPTER SIX

Cancer Profiles from Several High-Risk Chicago Communities

Clyde W. Phillips and Loretta F. Prat Lacey

C hicago is similar to other major American urban centers in its cultural, demographic, socioeconomic, and ethnic diversity; therefore, it serves as an excellent model for studying typical life patterns, including health, of various populations.

The authors share the concern of many worldwide investigators who realize that cancer incidence and eradication can be improved if better screening, early detection, and follow-up methods can be developed. This is particularly true for the segments of the world population that are at high risk for cancer. It is noteworthy that the persons who comprise the majority of the high-risk category are usually from the lower level of the socioeconomic scale and are generally minorities—blacks, Hispanics, and other disadvantaged racial and ethnic groups.

This study details some of the results of an ongoing epidemiologic survey of three high-density population tracts in Chicago, primarily black, where cancer incidence, morbidity, and mortality statistics are highest for the city at large.

[...]

Originally published in *Journal of the National Medical Association* 79, no. 7 (1987): 701–4. Copyright Elsevier 1987.

Study of Cancer Deaths

In 1980, the Chicago Department of Health, upon recommendation of its Cancer Advisory Committee, initiated a study of cancer deaths in the city. Cancer had already been determined as the second leading cause of death for a number of years, a pattern no different from the national vital statistics. The members of the Cancer Advisory Committee realized that if a major impact against cancer was to be accomplished, then the communities with the highest cancer mortality rates would have to be brought under careful surveillance and their residents directed to health facilities where state-of-the-art screening, detection, and therapy could be provided.

Cancer profiles for the communities with the highest cancer mortality rates were developed. Three communities, each predominantly black, were determined to be most in need of interventions.[1]

Demography

Since the 1980 census, Chicago's population has remained at a total of approximately 3 million people. However, certain shifts in the racial and ethnic population have been noted during the current decade. In 1980, blacks represented 39.8% of the total population, whites and others (Asians and Pacific Islanders) represented 46.1%, and Hispanics comprised 14.1% of people. In 1985, the percentage of blacks had increased to 41.3% of the population, while whites and others had decreased to 42.5%, and Hispanics had increased to 16.2% (figure 6.1). Therefore, it is apparent that Chicago's racial composition is changing in a manner similar to other major urban centers in our nation, with a decrease in the white population and an increase in minorities, particularly blacks and Hispanics. This shift is directly related to the apparent increasing incidence of diseases such as cancer among the minority populations, who also are at the lowest level of the socioeconomic scale and cannot afford proper health care.

Cancer Profiles

The three communities with the highest cancer mortality rates among blacks are all on the south side of Chicago, and two are contiguous. In

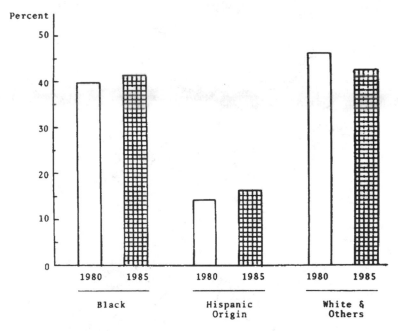

FIGURE 6.1. Racial and ethnic composition of Chicago in 1980 and 1985

1982, the cancer mortality rate for the city of Chicago was 194.8 per 100,000 population. This figure had remained within this range for the five-year period previous to the study. The community with the highest cancer mortality rate among blacks was Woodlawn, 316.5 per 100,000 population. Greater Grand Crossing, a community contiguous to Woodlawn, was next with a black cancer mortality rate of 302.3 per 100,000 population. The third community was Kenwood, with a black cancer mortality rate of 299.6 per 100,000 population (figure 6.2). Total deaths from cancer for all races in 1982 was 5,853, and blacks represented 2,014 of this figure.

Epidemiology

Health care is a commodity that is purchased at great cost from entrepreneurs by the privileged. William Darity, Dean of the School of Public Health at the University of Massachusetts, has conducted detailed studies that demonstrate the marked disparity in health status between the privileged and those who are either at or below the poverty level.[2]

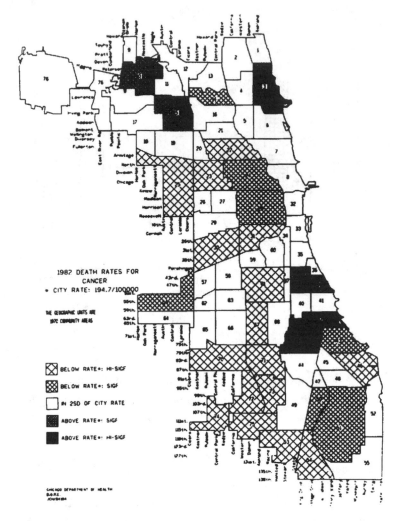

FIGURE 6.2. Map of Chicago communities showing death rates from cancer in 1982

As blacks constitute the largest segment of the nation's poor, it is obvious that their health status would be at the lowest level. This was highlighted 20 years ago when the first nationwide conference on "The Health Status of the Negro" was conducted at Howard University College of Medicine, March 13–14, 1967. At this historic meeting, Dr. Paul B. Comely, Professor and Head of the Department of Preventive Medicine and Public Health at Howard, directed attention to the "widening gap between Negro and white morbidity and mortality."

The participants at this conference determined that "the unfavorable morbidity and mortality experiences of the Negro population were not due to any genetic differences, but rather to housing, unemployment, non-availability and/or inaccessibility of health service facilities, discrimination and segregation and inadequate family structure."[3]

Knowledge, Attitudes, and Practices

Documentation of blacks' knowledge, attitudes, and practices about cancer is meager; however, in 1980, the American Cancer Society (ACS) commissioned EVAXX, Inc., a black-owned evaluation organization, to study black Americans' attitudes toward cancer and cancer tests. These findings were then compared with a similar ACS-sponsored study conducted earlier among a sample of the general population.

The findings confirmed the impressions of many black health professionals, and others, that black Americans underestimate the prevalence of cancer and have a false belief that they will not become a cancer patient. This is in direct contrast to whites, who believe the opposite. Further, blacks are pessimistic, in general, about the possibility of a cure for cancer, and tend to view its diagnosis as a death sentence. Blacks are less aware than whites about cancer's warning signs, and procrastinate more about visiting a physician, even when ominous symptoms are present. Socioeconomic status is an important factor in this mix, and the lower income black knows less and does less about cancer than those with higher income.[4] These false beliefs and similar myths among black Americans probably make a major contribution to the differential deficit ratio for cancer between blacks and whites. These beliefs, in addition to the inaccessibility of adequate health care for the economically deprived, compound the problem.[5]

Intervention efforts to reach groups at increased risk require use of comprehensive and innovative strategies that dictate close cooperation between health care providers and those groups being served. These interventions include health education techniques to improve awareness levels; support strategies that encourage acceptance and compliance to recommended health regimens; and methods to assist in the adaptation of lifestyle modifications that will thereby reduce cancer risks.

Conclusions

Chicago is a typical major American urban center with a diverse ethnic, cultural, and socioeconomic population. Blacks represent a large percentage of Chicago's total population, and comprise a disproportionately high segment of the low socioeconomic group. Persons in low socioeconomic groups have the highest incidence, morbidity and mortality rates from all diseases, including cancer, because of limited access to state-of-the-art medical services.

An epidemiologic study of cancer deaths in Chicago, conducted by the Department of Health, determined that the three communities with the highest cancer death rates in the city were each predominantly black.

Blacks are generally less aware of cancer's major threat to good health, and tend to be fatalistic about the ultimate outcome of a cancer patient.

If the goal of the National Cancer Institute (to reduce cancer mortality 50% by the year 2000) is to be realized, then the marked differentials in cancer incidence, morbidity, survival, and mortality rates between blacks and whites must be attacked by significantly improved cancer prevention and control interventions in the black community.

References

1. Chicago Department of Health. *Cancer profiles for municipal neighborhood health centers.* Chicago: Bureau of Operations Research and Epidemiology; 1982.

2. Darity WA. Socio-economic factors influencing the health status of black Americans. *International Quarterly of Community Health Education.* 1986; 7(2):91–108.

3. Cornely PB. The health status of the Negro today and in the future. *American Journal of Public Health.* 1968;58(4):647–654.

4. Black Americans' attitudes toward cancer and cancer tests: Highlights of a study. *CA: A Cancer Journal for Clinicians.* 1981;31(4):212–218.

5. Baquet C, Ringen K. Cancer control in blacks: Epidemiology and NCI program plans. *Progress in Clinical and Biological Research.* 1986;216:215–227.

CHAPTER SEVEN

Differing Birth Weight among Infants of U.S.-Born Blacks, African-Born Blacks, and U.S.-Born Whites

Richard J. David and James W. Collins Jr.

During the past 40 years, epidemiologic research has elucidated many important associations between the sociodemographic characteristics of mothers and the birth weight of infants.[1–4] For example, the extremes of childbearing age,[1] cigarette smoking,[2] inadequate prenatal care,[3] urban poverty,[4] and black race[5] are well-documented risk factors for low birth weight. Other obstetrical risk factors account for part of the racial disparity in birth weights, but differences persist.[6–9]

Although the incidence of low birth weight decreases in both blacks and whites as the number of risk factors declines, the improvement is faster among whites, resulting in a wider birth-weight gap between blacks and whites among infants of low-risk women.[1,4] This has led some investigators to believe that genetic factors associated with race influence birth weight.[10–15] In the 1967 National Collaborative Perinatal Project, only 1% of the total variance in birth weight among 18,000 infants was accounted for by socioeconomic variables, leading the authors to conclude that "race behaves as a real biological variable in its effect on birth weight. This effect of race [is] presumably genetic."[10] The assumption that black women differ genetically from white women in their ability to bear normal or large infants persists in more recent studies of fetal

Originally published in the *New England Journal of Medicine* 337, no. 17 (1997): 1209–14. Copyright © 1997, Massachusetts Medical Society.

growth,[13,16] one of which, for example, refers to "genetic factors affecting growth, such as neonatal sex and race."[16]

Few data have been published on the birth weights of infants born to African-born women in the United States. Most African Americans trace their origins to western Africa, where the slave trade flourished in the 17th and 18th centuries.[17,18] It is estimated that U.S. blacks derive about three-quarters of their genetic heritage from West African ancestors and the remainder from Europeans.[18–21] To the extent that population differences in allele frequency underlie the observed differences in birth weight between blacks and whites in the United States, one would expect women of "pure" West African origin to bear smaller infants than comparable African Americans, considering the European genetic admixture in the latter. However, to our knowledge, no population of West African women delivering infants in the United States has been studied. We therefore undertook an analysis of racial differences in birth weight based on U.S.-born and African-born women giving birth in Illinois.

Methods

Study Population

We obtained data on the birth weights of singleton black and white infants born in Illinois and the birthplaces of their mothers, using birth-certificate tapes for 1980 through 1995 from the Illinois Department of Public Health. All the white infants studied had U.S.-born mothers and were not of Latino origin. The mothers of the black infants fell into two groups: women born in sub-Saharan Africa and those born in the United States. We selected random samples of the white and black U.S.-born women in order to have groups convenient for analysis; these groups included 2.5% of white births and 7.5% of black births.

Black women born in the Western Hemisphere but not in the United States (i.e., born in Canada, the Caribbean, or South America) were excluded from the study. Such designations of maternal origin were available for the period 1980 through 1988. During that period, birth records were coded with three separate fields: the mother's race, the mother's place of birth, and the mother's origin or descent. Women whose race was coded as "black," whose place of birth was coded as "not in Western Hemisphere," and whose origin or descent was coded as "Africa, excluding northern Africa" were considered to have immigrated from sub-Saharan Africa. According to the 1990 Census, 66% of African-born blacks living in Illinois for whom a sub-Saharan country of birth was recorded came from either Nigeria or Ghana.[22] From 1989 on, the variable indicating origin or descent was replaced by a variable specifically pertaining to Hispanic origin, but a new, detailed set of birthplace codes allowed us to identify births on the basis of the mother's country of birth. We therefore selected births from 1989 through 1995 in which the mother's birthplace was 1 of 17 present-day countries corresponding to the area from which African slaves originated in the 17th and 18th centuries.[18,20]

Analysis of Birth Weights

As a first step toward exploring the possible contribution of genetic factors to the racial disparity in outcomes of pregnancy, we compared the curves for the distribution of birth weight, the mean birth weights, and the rates of low birth weight (defined as the number of births of infants weighing less than 2500 g per 100 live births) of infants born to U.S.-born blacks, African-born blacks, and U.S.-born whites. In addition, we computed rates of moderately low (1500 to 2500 g) and very low (< 1500 g) birth weight. Next, we determined the distribution of sociodemographic risk factors (the mother's age, education, and marital status, the trimester of first prenatal care, and the father's education) and reproductive risk factors (the overall number of pregnancies and whether there was a history of fetal loss or infant death) in the three groups of women. For the risk factors and outcomes, we calculated relative risks and 95% confidence intervals, using the infants of U.S.-born white women as the reference group.[23]

[...]

Results

The mean birth weight of the white infants was 3446 g, as compared with 3333 g for the infants of the African-born black women and 3089 g for the infants of the U.S.-born black women (table 7.1). The proportion of very-low-birth-weight infants was similar for African-born blacks and U.S.-born blacks. Even though the infants born to African-born blacks

TABLE 7.1 **Birth-weight data in Illinois, 1980–1995, according to the mother's race and place of birth**

Variable	Subgroup of mothers			Relative risk (95% CI) in black mothers[†]	
	U.S.-born whites	African-born blacks	U.S.-born blacks	African born	U.S. born
Raw data					
No. of births	44,046	3,135	43,322		
Mean birth weight (g)	3,446	3,333	3,089		
Low birth weight (% of infants)	4.3	7.1	13.2	1.6 (1.4–1.9)	3.1 (2.9–3.2)
Moderately low	3.6	4.8	10.6	1.3 (1.1–1.6)	3.0 (2.8–3.1)
Very low	0.7	2.3	2.6	3.2 (2.5–4.1)	3.5 (3.1–4.0)
Matched cases[‡]					
No. of births	2,950	2,950	2,950		
Mean birth weight (g)	3,475	3,341	3,195		
Low birth weight (% of infants)	3.6	6.9	8.5	1.9 (1.5–2.4)	2.4 (1.9–2.9)
Moderately low	3.1	4.7	6.1	1.5 (1.2–2.0)	2.0 (1.5–2.5)
Very low	0.5	2.2	2.4	4.1 (2.4–7.0)	4.5 (2.6–7.7)

Note: Data on birth weight were missing for 19 infants (0.02 percent of the total). Low birth weight was defined as a weight of less than 2500 g, moderately low birth weight as a weight of 1500–2499 g, and very low birth weight as a weight of less than 1500 g.

†Relative risks shown are for the risk of low birth weight in the infants of women in the group shown as compared with the infants of U.S.-born white women. CI denotes confidence interval.

‡In this analysis, each African-born black woman was matched with one U.S.-born white woman and one U.S.-born black woman for age, marital status, education and spouse's education, prenatal care, parity, and the presence or absence of previous fetal loss.

had a slightly lower mean birth weight than the white infants, the overall distribution of birth weights was similar in the two groups and was different from that among the infants of U.S.-born blacks (figure 7.1).

Table 7.2 shows the distribution of selected risk factors in the three groups of women. The African-born black women delivered the highest proportion of infants who were their mothers' fourth or subsequent children and had the highest proportion of previous fetal and infant deaths. The U.S.-born black women were the youngest, the least likely to be married, the least well educated, and the most likely to have received prenatal care late or not at all. The white women surpassed both groups of black women with regard to only one risk factor—primigravidity.

When the infants of African-born black women were compared with those of U.S.-born women matched for the mother's age, marital status, education, prenatal care, parity, and prior fetal loss and the father's edu-

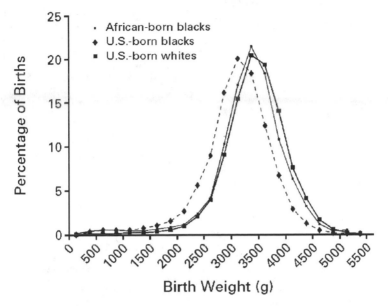

FIGURE 7.1. Distribution of birth weights among infants of U.S.-born white and black women and African-born black women in Illinois, 1980–1995

Note: The calculation of frequencies was based on all singleton births in Illinois. The study population included the infants of 3,135 black women born in sub-Saharan Africa, 43,322 black women born in the United States (a sample that included 7.5% of the total number of black women giving birth in Illinois), and 44,046 U.S.-born white women (2.5% of the total number of white women giving birth in Illinois).

cation, the differences between the groups narrowed somewhat, but their relation did not change (table 7.1). With white infants as the reference group, the relative risks for low and moderately low birth weight were both significantly higher among infants of U.S.-born blacks than among infants of African-born blacks. However, the relative risk of very low birth weight was similar in the two groups of infants born to blacks.

To gain more insight into the relative importance of the risk factors in the three groups, we used multiple-regression analysis to study the changes in birth weight predicted by each factor. The models we constructed (table 7.3) all showed a positive effect of being married (an increase of 60 to 124 g in predicted birth weight), having had one or two previous pregnancies (an increase of 29 to 50 g), and having no previous fetal loss (an increase of 19 to 55 g). Of the risk factors, only marital status had a statistically significant effect among the infants of African-born blacks.

TABLE 7.2 **Distribution of selected risk factors in the study population according to the mother's race and place of birth**

Variable	Subgroup of mothers (rate per 100)			Relative risk (95% CI) in black mothers[†]	
	U.S.-born whites	African-born blacks	U.S.-born blacks	African born	U.S. born
Maternal age < 20 yr.	8.8	1.5	28	0.2 (0.1–0.2)	3.1 (3.0–3.2)
Education < 12 yr.					
Mother	13	8	36	0.6 (0.5–0.7)	2.9 (2.8–3.0)
Father	11	6	34	0.5 (0.4–0.6)	2.9 (2.9–3.0)
Mother unmarried	14	24	76	1.7 (1.6–1.8)	5.3 (5.2–5.4)
Late prenatal care or none	15	26	36	1.7 (1.6–1.8)	2.3 (2.3–2.4)
Gravidity					
1	34	22	29	0.6 (0.6–0.7)	0.9 (0.8–0.9)
> 3	15	31	26	2.0 (1.9–2.1)	1.7 (1.6–1.7)
Prior death					
Fetus[‡]	24	39	28	1.6 (1.5–1.7)	1.1 (1.1–1.2)
Infant	1.7	3.0	2.9	1.8 (1.5–2.2)	1.7 (1.6–1.9)

Note: Data on the number of previous pregnancies were obtained for 44,053 U.S.-born white women, 3,135 African-born black women, and 43,334 U.S.-born black women. For the other variables shown, there were missing data, as follows: maternal age, 0.01 percent; maternal education, 0.26 percent; paternal education, 16.4 percent; marital status, 0.05 percent; start of prenatal care, 1.38 percent; previous fetal death, 0.07 percent; and previous death of an infant, 0.36 percent.

†Relative risks shown are for the risk of low birth weight in the infants of women in the group shown as compared with the infants of U.S.-born white women. CI denotes confidence interval.

‡This category includes spontaneous and induced abortions, miscarriages, and stillbirths, regardless of the period of gestation.

TABLE 7.3 **Regression models showing the predicted effects of low-risk sociodemographic and reproductive variables in the mother on the birth weight of infants in each subgroup defined according to the mother's race and place of birth**

Variable	Subgroup of mothers (grams)		
	U.S.-born whites (N = 44,046)	African-born blacks (N = 3,135)	U.S.-born blacks (N = 43,322)
Birth weight with no protective factors present	3,144[†]	3,130[†]	2,942[†]
Maternal age > 19 yr.	0	+146[†]	−25[†]
Maternal education > 11 yr.	+128[†]	−26	+82[†]
Mother married	+118[†]	+60[‡]	+124[†]
Prenatal care in 1st 3 mo.	+60[†]	−4	+47[†]
Gravida 2 or 3	+50[†]	+41	+29[†]
No prior fetal loss	+19[§]	+36	+55[†]

Note: The values in the table show the increase or decrease in the predicted birth weight in each group, as estimated by arithmetically combining the predicted birth weight with no protective factors present with the sum of the protective factors, each multiplied by 1 if the factor was present or by 0 if it was absent. P values indicate the stability of these point estimates; the greater the standard error of the coefficient, the less the statistical significance.

†$P < .001$; ‡$P < .05$; §$P < .01$

On the basis of the multivariable models in table 7.3, the birth weight of the infants of African-born blacks was 14 g less than that of the infants of U.S.-born whites after we controlled for risk factors. In another model, we looked at only the U.S.-born white women and the African-born black women, with race included as a dichotomous variable. In that analysis, the infants of the U.S.-born whites weighed 98 g more than the infants of the African-born blacks after adjustment for age, education, marital status, gravidity, prenatal care, and a history of fetal loss. In a similar model that included only women born in the United States, the white infants weighed 248 g more than the black infants after adjustment for the same six variables.

Table 7.4 shows the mean birth weights and rates of low birth weight among infants born to the women at lowest risk—those 20 to 39 years of age who began their prenatal care in the first trimester, had at least 12 years of education, and were married to men who also had at least 12 years of education. Sixty-six percent of the white women fit this pro-

TABLE 7.4 **Mean birth weights and rates of low birth weight among infants with mothers at low risk, according to the mother's race and place of birth**

	Subgroup of mothers			Relative risk (95% CI) in black mothers*	
Low-risk variables studied	U.S.-born whites	African-born blacks	U.S.-born blacks	African born	U.S. born
Sociodemographic variables only[†]					
No. of births	29,012	1,577	6,181		
Mean birth weight (g)	3,497	3,344	3,243		
Low birth weight (rate per 100)	3.3	7.0	9.0	2.2 (1.8–2.6)	2.8 (2.5–3.1)
Very low birth weight (rate per 100)	0.6	2.4	1.8	4.3 (3.4–6.2)	3.3 (2.6–4.2)
Reproductive variables added[‡]					
No. of births	12,361	608	2,670		
Mean birth weight (g)	3,551	3,454	3,299		
Low birth weight (rate per 100)	2.4	3.6	7.5	1.5 (1.0–2.4)	3.0 (2.5–3.5)
Very low birth weight (rate per 100)	0.4	0.5	1.3	1.3 (0.4–4.2)	3.3 (2.2–5.2)

*Relative risks shown are for the risk of low birth weight in the infants of women in the group shown as compared with the infants of U.S.-born white women. CI denotes confidence interval.

†This analysis was limited to women 20–39 years of age who began their prenatal care in the first trimester of pregnancy, had at least 12 years of education, and were married to men who also had at least 12 years of education.

‡This analysis was limited as described in the preceding note but also excluded primigravidas and mothers with a history of fetal or infant loss.

file, as compared with 50% of the African-born black women and 14% of the U.S.-born black women. The mean birth weight and rates of low birth weight of the infants born to African-born blacks were interme-diate between the values in U.S.-born whites and those in U.S.-born blacks. However, when reproductive risk factors were included in the se-lection of low-risk women, the differences between the infants of U.S.-born whites and the infants of African-born blacks in mean birth weight and rates of both low and very low birth weight were narrowed, whereas the differences between the infants of U.S.-born whites and U.S.-born blacks were unchanged. The greatest change was in very low birth weight; the exclusion of women with a history of fetal loss resulted in nearly identical rates among infants of African-born blacks and those of U.S.-born whites, eliminating the significant excess of infants with very low birth weight born to African-born blacks.

Discussion

The distribution of birth weights among infants of African-born black women approximated that among infants of U.S.-born white women. The rate of low-birth-weight births for African-born black women was between the rate for U.S.-born white women and that for U.S.-born black women. Adjusting for maternal risk factors in three ways shifted the magnitude of the differences in birth weight but did not alter the basic pattern. Among infants of African-born black women and those of U.S.-born black women, very low birth weight occurred at a similar frequency. Nevertheless, these data provide some evidence against the theory that there is a genetic basis for the disparity between white and black women born in the United States in the mean birth weights of their infants.

According to most studies, racial differences in birth weight per-sist independently of numerous social and economic risk factors.[8,9] This has led some investigators to suggest that the differences have a genetic basis.[11–14] Our findings challenge the genetic concept of race as it relates to birth weight. The African-born women in our study were new im-migrants from the same region from which the ancestors of most U.S. blacks came, but without the estimated 20 to 30% admixture of Euro-pean genetic material that has occurred since the mid-17th century.[18–21] If genetics played a prominent part in determining black–white dif-ferences in birth weight, the infants of the African-born black women should have had lower birth weights than those of the U.S.-born black women. We found the opposite: regardless of socioeconomic status, the infants of black women born in Africa weighed more than the infants of comparable black women born in the United States.

[...]

As data inconsistent with the genetic hypothesis of racial differences accumulate, social and psycho-physiologic hypotheses are advanced.[5,24–28] A woman's exposure as a young child to the effects of poverty or racial discrimination could adversely affect birth weight in the next generation.[29,30] The high educational level of African-born black women in Illinois indicates that rigorous selection occurs among African immigrants and suggests an overrepresentation of women born into affluent families, an elite subgroup in any developing nation.

[...]

References

1. Kleinman JC, Kessel SS. Racial differences in low birth weight: Trends and risk factors. *New England Journal of Medicine.* 1987;317(12):749–753.

2. Fox SH, Koepsell TD, Daling JR. Birth weight and smoking during pregnancy—effect modification by maternal age. *American Journal of Epidemiology.* 1994;139(10):1008–1015.

3. Murray JL, Bernfield M. The differential effect of prenatal care on the incidence of low birth weight among blacks and whites in a prepaid health care plan. *New England Journal of Medicine.* 1988;319(21):1385–1391.

4. Collins JW Jr., David RJ. The differential effect of traditional risk factors on infant birthweight among blacks and whites in Chicago. *American Journal of Public Health.* 1990;80(6):679–681.

5. David RJ, Collins JW Jr. Bad outcomes in black babies: Race or racism? *Ethnicity and Disease.* 1991;1(3):236–244.

6. Lieberman E, Ryan KJ, Monson RR, Schoenbaum SC. Risk factors accounting for racial differences in the rate of premature birth. *New England Journal of Medicine.* 1987;317(12):743–748.

7. Rawlings JS, Rawlings VB, Read JA. Prevalence of low birth weight and preterm delivery in relation to the interval between pregnancies among white and black women. *New England Journal of Medicine.* 1995;332(2):69–74.

8. Klebanoff MA, Shiono PH, Berendes HW, Rhoads GG. Facts and artifacts about anemia and preterm delivery. *Journal of the American Medical Association.* 1989;262(4):511–515.

9. Sheehan TJ, Gregorio DI. Low birth weight in relation to the interval between pregnancies. *New England Journal of Medicine.* 1995;333(6):386–387.

10. Naylor AF, Myrianthopoulos NC. The relation of ethnic and selected socio-economic factors to human birth-weight. *Annals of Human Genetics.* 1967;31(1):71–83.

11. Little RE, Sing CF. Genetic and environmental influences on human birth weight. *American Journal of Human Genetics.* 1987;40(6):512–526.

12. Magnus P. Further evidence for a significant effect of fetal genes on variation in birth weight. *Clinical Genetics.* 1984;26(4):289–296.

13. Hulsey TC, Levkoff AH, Alexander GR. Birth weights of infants of black and white mothers without pregnancy complications. *American Journal of Obstetrics and Gynecology.* 1991;164(5 pt. 1):1299–1302.

14. Goldenberg RL, Cliver SP, Cutter GR, et al. Black-white differences in newborn anthropometric measurements. *Obstetrics and Gynecology.* 1991;78 (5 pt. 1):782–788.

15. Wildschut HI, Lumey LH, Lunt PW. Is preterm delivery genetically determined? *Paediatric and Perinatal Epidemiology.* 1991;5(4):363–372.

16. Amini SB, Catalano PM, Hirsch V, Mann LI. An analysis of birth weight by gestational age using a computerized perinatal data base, 1975–1992. *Obstetrics and Gynecology.* 1994;83(3):342–352.

17. Oliver R, Fage JD. *A short history of Africa.* 6th ed. New York: Facts on File; 1988.

18. Reed TE. Caucasian genes in American Negroes. *Science.* 1969;165(3895): 762–768.

19. Chakraborty R, Kamboh MI, Ferrell RE. "Unique" alleles in admixed populations: A strategy for determining "hereditary" population differences of disease frequencies. *Ethnicity and Disease.* 1991;1(3):245–256.

20. Adams J, Ward RH. Admixture studies and the detection of selection. *Science.* 1973;180(4091):1137–1143.

21. Glass B, Li CC. The dynamics of racial intermixture: An analysis based on the American Negro. *American Journal of Human Genetics.* 1953;5(1):1–20.

22. Bureau of the Census. *1990 Census of Population: Social and economic characteristics: Illinois, section 1 of 2.* CP-2-15. Washington, DC: US Government Printing Office; 1993.

23. Schlesselman JJ. *Case control studies: Design, conduct, analysis.* New York: Oxford University Press; 1982.

24. Cooper R. A note on the biologic concept of race and its application in epidemiologic research. *American Heart Journal.* 1984;108(3 pt. 2):715–722.

25. Witzig R. The medicalization of race: Scientific legitimization of a flawed social construct. *Annals of Internal Medicine.* 1996;125(8):675–679.

26. Rowley DL, Hogue CJ, Blackmore CA, et al. Preterm delivery among African-American women: A research strategy. *American Journal of Preventive Medicine.* 1993;9(6 suppl.):1–6.

27. Krieger N, Rowley DL, Herman AA, Avery B, Phillips MT. Racism, sexism, and social class: Implications for studies of health, disease, and well-being. *American Journal of Preventive Medicine.* 1993;9(6 suppl.):82–122.

28. Geronimus AT. The weathering hypothesis and the health of African-American women and infants: Evidence and speculations. *Ethnicity and Disease.* 1992;2(3):207–221.

29. Valanis BM, Rush D. A partial explanation of superior birth weights among foreign-born women. *Social Biology.* 1979;26(3):198–210.

30. Emanuel I, Filakti H, Alberman E, Evans SJ. Intergenerational studies of human birthweight from the 1958 birth cohort: 1, Evidence for a multigenerational effect. *British Journal of Obstetrics and Gynaecology.* 1992;99(1):67–74.

CHAPTER EIGHT

Variations in the Health Conditions of Six Chicago Community Areas

A Case for Local-Level Data

Ami M. Shah, Steven Whitman, and Abigail Silva

Until recently, local-level public health data have not been routinely collected and thus are not readily available. Existing data that can be geocoded to the county, city, or community level are derived from traditional surveillance systems (e.g., vital records and communicable disease registries), and provide information on small-area trends and variances in mortality,[1-3] measures related to birth outcomes,[4] and infectious diseases.[5] However, they offer little local information on the determinants of morbidity and mortality.[6,7] Such information is derived from health surveys, often conducted at the national (e.g., National Health Interview Survey [NHIS]) and state (e.g., Behavioral Risk Factor Surveillance System [BRFSS]) levels. Although these data are essential in terms of national public health policies and health monitoring, they are typically not available at the local level.

Social epidemiologists and public health practitioners have responded to this growing need for local health data.[8-10] For instance, Northridge et al., gathering data at the local level, found that the smoking prevalence rate in Harlem (42%) was notably different from the rate in New York State as a whole (25%) and the rate among non-Hispanic Blacks resid-

Originally published in the *American Journal of Public Health* 96, no. 8 (August 2006): 1485–91, by the American Public Health Association.

ing in the state (25%).[11] Others have conducted health surveys designed to gather these important data at the county (e.g., Los Angeles County Health Survey[12] and Seattle–King County Survey),[13] city,[14] and community or neighborhood[15,16] levels. Even the Centers for Disease Control and Prevention, which conducts state-based health surveys (i.e., BRFSS surveys), has recognized the importance of local-level data, designing the Selected Metropolitan/Micropolitan Area Risk Trends Project to mathematically estimate health-related prevalence proportions in smaller geographic areas.[17,18]

As urban settings become increasingly diverse and certain populations are disproportionately affected by disease,[19,20] variations in the health status of these smaller geographic areas may be substantial,[2] and such variations must be considered if true advances in disease prevention and control are to be achieved.[8–10,21–23] To explore such differences, we conducted a household survey in 6 diverse communities of Chicago to examine health profile differences.

Methods

Community Areas

Chicago is divided into 77 officially designated community areas that are often used as a basis for describing the city's health conditions, delivering health care services, and implementing community-based interventions.[24] Figure 8.1 shows the 6 community areas selected for this survey, and table 8.1 presents some of their demographic and socioeconomic characteristics.

We selected these community areas for various social and political reasons, but our primary interest was their role in shaping local policies and developing community interventions. We selected North Lawndale and South Lawndale because we are affiliated with the Sinai Health System, which serves these communities (figure 8.1). The population of North Lawndale is almost entirely Black, and the median household income is $18,000; South Lawndale is predominantly Mexican, with a median household income of $32,000.

The contiguous communities of West Town and Humboldt Park, located west of downtown Chicago, are interesting in an epidemiological sense in that they are both facing transitions related to urban development. In addition, they are home to energetic and dedicated community-

TABLE 8.1 **Demographic characteristics of 6 Chicago community areas compared with Chicago overall and the United States: Improving Community Health Survey, 2002–2003**

	Humboldt Park	North Lawndale	Norwood Park	Roseland	South Lawndale	West Town	Chicago	United States
Total population	65,836	41,768	37,669	52,723	91,071	87,435	2,896,016	281,421,906
Race/ethnicity (%)								
Non-Hispanic Black	47	94	1	98	13	9	36	12
Non-Hispanic White	3	1	88	1	4	39	31	69
Hispanic	48	5	6	1	83	47	26	13
Mexican	24	3	3	0	76	25	18	7
Puerto Rican	18	0	0	0	1	16	4	1
Median household income ($)	28,728	18,342	53,402	38,237	32,320	38,915	38,625	41,994
High school diploma (%)[a]	50	60	83	77	37	70	72	80
Unemployment rate (%)[b]	18	26	3	17	12	7	10	6
Individual poverty rate (%)[c]	31	45	4	18	27	21	20	12

Note: Data for Chicago and the United States were derived from the 2000 census.

[a]Among those 25 years or older.

[b]Percentage of resident civilians older than 16 years who did not have a job and were actively seeking work.

[c]Percentage of residents with annual incomes below the federally defined poverty level in 1999.

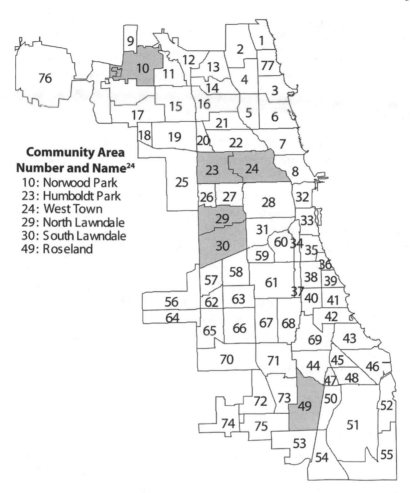

FIGURE 8.1. Six of Chicago's 77 community areas

based organizations that were eager to use the data gathered here to implement changes. The population of West Town is one-half White, one-quarter Mexican, and one-quarter Puerto Rican, whereas that of Humboldt Park is one-half Black, one-quarter Mexican, and one-quarter Puerto Rican. Finally, we selected Roseland, a predominantly Black community on the south side, and Norwood Park, a predominantly White community on the north side, because they represented 2 geographically and racially disparate communities.

According to 2000 US census data, median household incomes in the

6 study communities ranged from \$18,000 to \$53,000, compared with \$39,000 for Chicago and \$42,000 for the United States as a whole. Overall, the communities were reflective of different geographic areas but were not selected to be representative of the city of Chicago.

Sample

The sample was composed of adults living in households situated in each of the 6 community areas. We employed a 3-stage probability sampling design to ensure community representation.[25] First, we selected 15 census blocks from each community area using probability proportional to size sampling,[26] meaning that the blocks in each community area were selected in a manner proportionate to the number of individuals 18 years or older who lived on these blocks according to the 2000 US census. Second, we randomly selected households from each block. Third, a screener enumerated all household members and identified a random adult respondent using the Troldahl-Carter-Bryant methodology.[27] Eligibility was limited to selected individuals between the ages of 18 and 75 years who resided in one of the targeted community areas, were physically and mentally able to answer the interview questions in English or Spanish, and provided consent to participate.

[. . .]

Data Collection

The survey was administered face to face in respondents' homes from September 2002 through April 2003. Interviewers were hired and trained by the Survey Research Laboratory, which has been involved in conducting a number of such household surveys. Interviewers were either members of or culturally familiar with the communities surveyed. Interviewers underwent 21 hours of formal training, and roughly one-third were native Spanish speakers or bilingual.

Community leaders from the survey design committee sent an advance letter to households selected for the survey. Interviewers made at least 12 attempts to screen and interview the randomly selected adult from each household at different times of the day and different days of the week. Most (85%) of the interviews, which were approximately 1 hour in duration, were conducted during evening and weekend hours.

Interviewees received a health information packet (in Spanish or English) along with $40 for their time.

The survey was administered via computer-assisted personal interviewing techniques to reduce the potential for errors related to data entry or skip patterns. Ten percent of each interviewer's work was validated at random for quality assurance purposes. The goal of conducting at least 300 face-to-face interviews in each community area was met in 5 of the 6 communities. Only 190 interviews were completed in Norwood Park, the predominantly White community area with the highest median household income.

Response Rate

Interviews were attempted at 4,888 households. Of the original list of addresses derived from census data, only 89.5% were occupied. We were able to make contact in the case of 76.3% of these households, and 76.5% of households successfully contacted cooperated with the screening. A total of 1953 eligible individuals were contacted, of whom 1699 (87%) agreed to participate and completed the survey.

The overall response rate, based on a conservative calculation procedure outlined by the American Association for Public Opinion Research,[28] was 43.2%. In this procedure, all originally sampled buildings and households were included in the denominator.[29] That is, unoccupied housing, households that no longer existed, and households where interviewers were not able to locate residents were included, in addition to individuals who refused to participate.

[…]

Statistical Analysis

The 2000 US population was used as the standard in directly age-adjusting health condition prevalence proportions to be consistent with comparison data. The sampling weights used in our analysis accounted for differential probabilities of selection and post-stratification so that the sample would resemble the distribution of each community area's population according to the 2000 census. For each measure, we assessed differences in community area pairwise prevalence rates using z tests for proportions. We examined 15 comparisons for each measure (e.g., South

Lawndale vs. North Lawndale, South Lawndale vs. Norwood Park) in terms of their statistical significance.

In addition, we compared prevalence rates for each community area measure with rates for Chicago as a whole and evaluated statistical significance at the .05 α level. Although we conducted a number of significance tests, we did not adjust the overall significance level (e.g., via a Bonferroni inequality calculation) because we viewed this analysis as exploratory and did not examine any formal hypotheses regarding community differences. We analyzed the data using Stata, version 8.0, to account for sampling design effects.[30]

Results

Table 8.2 presents the data for the 13 health conditions, health behaviors, and health care access measures assessed in our analyses. Most of the differences in these measures between the community areas themselves and between the community areas and Chicago as a whole were statistically significant. For example, the percentage of people reporting that they had been diagnosed with high blood pressure ranged from 17% in South Lawndale to 41% in North Lawndale, and 13 of the 15 pairwise comparisons made between the different community areas were statistically significant. Furthermore, high blood pressure prevalence rates in 5 of the 6 community areas were statistically different from the overall Chicago rate of 23%.

In a similar manner, and consistent with data on insurance coverage, Norwood Park residents were more likely than residents of other communities to obtain needed dental care and prescription medicines. Only 9% of these individuals, compared with 34% in West Town and 33% in Humboldt Park, had not obtained needed dental care in the previous 12 months because they could not afford it. Of the 15 pairwise comparisons made for this measure, 5 were statistically significant. Similarly, 4% of Norwood Park residents, compared with 24% of North Lawndale and 23% of Humboldt Park residents, had not obtained needed prescription medicines in the previous 12 months because they could not afford them. In this case, 9 of 15 pairwise comparisons were significant. Chicago data were not available for either of these variables.

Of the total of 195 tests (15 pairwise comparisons for each of the 13 measures) examining differences between measures, 108 were statistically

TABLE 8.2 **Prevalence of selected health conditions, health behaviors, and measures of health care access among adults in 6 Chicago community areas, 2002–2003**

	No. of significant pairwise comparisons[a]	Prevalence (95% CI)						
		Humboldt Park	North Lawndale	Norwood Park	Roseland	South Lawndale	West Town	Chicago
Health condition								
High blood pressure	13	35b (32.6, 37.2)	41b (37.8, 44.6)	26 (23.6, 28.6)	39b (36.2, 40.7)	17b (12.7, 20.5)	28b (24.7, 31.2)	23 (20.6, 25.2)
Arthritis	9	23 (20.0, 25.8)	25b (22.6, 26.8)	18 (16.1, 19.8)	25b (22.4, 26.8)	10b (7.8, 11.2)	27b (24.0, 29.6)	20 (17.9, 21.7)
Asthma	11	17b (14.8, 19.3)	18b (15.7, 19.9)	12 (10.4, 14.3)	13 (10.8, 15.1)	1b (0.6, 1.2)	21b (17.9, 23.4)	11 (10.2, 12.4)
Depression	12	21 (18.8, 22.6)	15 (13.2, 17.1)	9 (7.2, 9.8)	13 (11.1, 13.9)	21 (18.1, 23.3)	23 (19.9, 26.6)	…
Diabetes	11	16b (13.3, 18.5)	10b (8.1, 12.4)	4b (3.5, 5.2)	12b (10.0, 13.1)	6 (3.8, 7.3)	14b (11.4, 16.0)	7 (6.6, 8.4)
Obese (body mass index ≥ 30 kg/m²)	9	36b (33.3, 39.5)	41b (37.6, 44.9)	20 (18.3, 22.6)	38b (35.5, 40.3)	37b (31.3, 42.8)	31b (27.4, 34.8)	22 (20.0, 23.2)
Health behaviors								
Engages in 30 min of moderate activity 5 times per week	7	34 (28.9, 38.8)	30 (26.0, 33.6)	30 (22.3, 37.4)	27 (22.6, 31.0)	15b (7.7, 21.6)	36 (30.1, 41.4)	30 (25.4, 35.7)
Current smoker	8	35b (26.8, 43.4)	39b (33.7, 44.8)	18b (15.7, 21.2)	33b (24.9, 41.6)	20 (15.0, 25.3)	32b (25.4, 38.1)	24 (21.6, 28.9)
Health care access								
Currently insured (adults 18–64 yr.)	11	61b (53.6, 69.1)	61b (52.0, 69.1)	93b (88.7, 97.5)	70 (62.6, 76.9)	46b (30.2, 61.0)	73 (68.4, 77.9)	73 (69.6, 77.4)
Did not obtain needed dental care in past year	5	33 (29.5, 36.5)	28 (21.8, 34.8)	9 (6.4, 12.0)	30 (21.8, 39.2)	25 (13.1, 36.5)	34 (26.4, 41.4)	…
Did not obtain needed prescription medications in past year	9	23 (18.7, 27.1)	24 (18.2, 29.9)	4 (2.2, 6.2)	15 (9.2, 20.9)	12 (7.1, 16.5)	18 (11.9, 23.8)	…
Mammogram in past year (women ≥ 40 yr.)	3	56 (35.2, 76.1)	65 (52.9, 76.6)	65 (52.6, 77.9)	61 (52.2, 69.7)	38b (28.2, 47.5)	47b (31.4, 63.5)	67 (46.6, 74.0)
Colonoscopy/sigmoidoscopy in past year (adults ≥ 50 yr.)	0	16 (7.2, 25.1)	13 (4.8, 20.8)	18 (9.1, 27.2)	25 (12.6, 36.6)	14 (0.0, 27.8)	16 (5.2, 27.4)	…

Note: CI = confidence interval. Pairwise comparisons were made between community areas themselves and between community areas and Chicago as a whole. Health conditions prevalence data were age adjusted to the 2000 census standard population.

[a] Out of a possible 15 between-community comparisons.

[b] Significantly different ($P < .05$) from overall Chicago rate.

significant (10 would have [been] expected by chance alone from the unadjusted significance levels used). Finally, of the 54 tests (9 measures with
available Chicago data for each of the 6 community areas) involving comparisons with Chicago data, 35 were significant (3 would have been expected by chance).

Discussion

The overarching question addressed in this analysis was whether there
were substantial variations in the health measures assessed between the
community areas themselves and between the community areas and
Chicago as a whole. Our data indicate that considerable variations existed in both instances. However, it should be noted that our analyses
were exploratory and that the sample size was not selected to detect a
particular effect size. As such, it is possible that any differences we have
described here as statistically significant may not be meaningful or important, but it is also possible that meaningful or important differences
did not reach the level of statistical significance. The variations identified demonstrate that existing national and even state surveys may not
reflect the health conditions of local (often diverse) communities and
suggest that available Chicago data may be inadequate in terms of representing the health of the city's 77 community areas.

Previous analyses of vital statistics and communicable disease registry data have revealed considerable variations in health among these
Chicago communities as well.[3] Our survey data supplement such information and further identify substantial differences in the current status and determinants of health among these populations. For instance,
North Lawndale and South Lawndale are adjacent to one another, yet
they have very different health profiles. To consider just 1 measure, 39%
of the former community's residents are smokers, compared with only
20% of those of the latter community. If data are examined in an aggregated fashion, contextual differences in the demographic and health profiles of specific communities will not be identified, leading to difficulties
in identifying and mounting effective community-based public health
and public policy programs.

Another example of the importance of community-level data can be
found in comparisons of North Lawndale and Roseland. Although both

are composed virtually entirely of African American residents, Roseland has a much higher median household income level ($38,000), one that is similar to Chicago and national levels. North Lawndale's median household income ($18,000), in contrast, makes it one of the poorest of Chicago's 77 community areas. Despite this substantial economic difference, Roseland's residents exhibited statistically significant advantages on only 4 of the 13 health measures assessed in this study (asthma, depression, insurance, and access to prescription medicines). These similarities, as opposed to the much larger differences that one might expect on the basis of the 2 communities' median household incomes, raise important questions about the relation between race and class.[31-35] Again, such a provocative finding can be obtained only through disaggregation of data at the community level.

Although it is one of the largest cities in the United States and its population is diverse, Chicago—labeled in a seminal study as "hypersegregated"[36] (i.e., segregated on many dimensions simultaneously)—has proven to be an ideal setting for small area studies. A strength of this study is that some of the community areas assessed were homogeneous, lending valuable information to assessments of racial and ethnic health disparities. In fact, recent reports[37,38] based on health status indicators drawn solely from vital records and communicable disease registries have demonstrated substantial and even increasing Black-White disparities at the city level in Chicago. Our study adds to a more general picture of the city's health conditions in that we examined disparities at the community area level and analyzed health measures not available in existing databases. The kinds of disaggregated data used in our investigation are necessary to fully appreciate and ultimately remedy disparities in communities such as those assessed here.

Although it is not surprising that individuals of lower socioeconomic status fare worse than those in better financial situations in terms of health measures, the extent of such inequities has rarely been documented. Researchers can use the present local-level data to continue to investigate how people's place of residence may affect their health,[39,40] how socioeconomic factors correlate with health risk factors,[41] and how self-reported survey data combined with analyses of existing birth and death certificates can provide in-depth profiles of community health conditions.[2,3,5,42,43]

[...]

References

1. *Shaping a health statistics vision for the 21st century.* Washington, DC: US Department of Health and Human Services; 2002.

2. Fang J, Bosworth W, Madhavan S, Cohen H, Alderman MH. Differential mortality in New York City (1988–1992): 2, Excess mortality in the south Bronx. *Bulletin of the New York Academy of Medicine.* 1995;72(2):483–499.

3. Whitman S, Silva A, Shah A, Ansell D. Diversity and disparity: GIS and small-area analysis in six Chicago neighborhoods. *Journal of Medical Systems.* 2004;28(4):397–411.

4. Krieger N, Chen JT, Waterman PD, Soobader MJ, Subramanian SV, Carson R. Choosing area based socioeconomic measures to monitor social inequalities in low birth weight and childhood lead poisoning: The Public Health Disparities Geocoding Project (US). *Journal of Epidemiology and Community Health.* 2003;57(3):186–199.

5. Krieger N, Waterman PD, Chen JT, Soobader MJ, Subramanian SV. Monitoring socioeconomic inequalities in sexually transmitted infections, tuberculosis, and violence: Geocoding and choice of area-based socioeconomic measures—the Public Health Disparities Geocoding Project (US). *Public Health Reports.* 2003;118(3):240–260.

6. McGinnis JM, Foege WH. Actual causes of death in the United States. *Journal of the American Medical Association.* 1993;270(18):2207–2212.

7. Mokdad AH, Marks JS, Stroup DF, Gerberding JL. Actual causes of death in the United States, 2000. *Journal of the American Medical Association.* 2004;291(10):1238–1245.

8. Frieden TR. Asleep at the switch: Local public health and chronic disease. *American Journal of Public Health.* 2004;94(12):2059–2061.

9. Simon PA, Wold CM, Cousineau MR, Fielding JE. Meeting the data needs of a local health department: The Los Angeles County Health Survey. *American Journal of Public Health.* 2001;91(12):1950–1952.

10. Fielding JE, Frieden TR. Local knowledge to enable local action. *American Journal of Preventive Medicine.* 2004;27(2):183–184.

11. Northridge ME, Morabia A, Ganz ML, et al. Contribution of smoking to excess mortality in Harlem. *American Journal of Epidemiology.* 1998;147(3): 250–258.

12. *The health of Angelenos: A comprehensive report of the health of residents of Los Angeles County.* Los Angeles: Los Angeles County Department of Health Services; 2000.

13. Public Health—Seattle and King County Epidemiology, Planning and Evaluation Unit. *Communities Count 2000: Social and health indicators across King County.* http://www.communitiescount.org/uploads/pdf/archives/FullReport .final.pdf.

14. New York City Department of Health and Mental Hygiene. New York City Health and Nutrition Examination Survey (NYC HANES). http://nychanes.org.

15. Karpati A, Kerker B, Mostashari F, et al. *Health disparities in New York City*. New York City Department of Health and Human Hygiene; 2004. https://www.commonwealthfund.org/sites/default/files/documents/___media_files_publications_other_2004_jul_health_disparities_in_new_york_city_karpati_disparities_pdf.pdf.

16. New York City Department of Health and Human Hygiene. New York City Community Health Survey 2002. 2002. https://www1.nyc.gov/site/doh/data/data-sets/community-health-survey.page.

17. Centers for Disease Control and Prevention. *SMART: Selected metropolitan and micropolitan area risk trends*. https://www.cdc.gov/brfss/smart/Smart_data.htm.

18. Centers for Disease Control and Prevention. *2002 IL BRFSS SMART (selected metropolitan/micropolitan area risk trends for Illinois)*. 2002. https://www.cdc.gov/brfss/smart/Smart_data.htm.

19. Fullilove RE, Fullilove MT, Northridge ME, et al. Risk factors for excess mortality in Harlem: Findings from the Harlem Household Survey. *American Journal of Preventive Medicine*. 1999;16(3 suppl.):22–28.

20. Northridge ME, Meyer IH, Dunn L. Overlooked and underserved in Harlem: A population-based survey of adults with asthma. *Environmental Health Perspectives*. 2002;110(suppl. 2.):217–220.

21. American Public Health Association. *Healthy communities 2000: Model standards: Guidelines for community attainment of the year 2000 national health objectives*. Washington, DC; 1991.

22. Brownson RC, Bright FS. Chronic disease control in public health practice: Looking back and moving forward. *Public Health Reports*. 2004;119(3):230–238.

23. Howell EM, Pettit KL, Ormond BA, Kingsley GT. Using the National Neighborhood Indicators Partnership to improve public health. *Journal of Public Health Management and Practice*. 2003;9(3):235–242.

24. Chicago Fact Book Consortium. *Local community fact book: Chicago metropolitan area, 1990*. Chicago: Academy Chicago; 1995.

25. Kish L. *Survey sampling*. New York: Wiley; 1965.

26. Sudman S. *Applied sampling*. New York: Academic; 1976.

27. Troldahl V, Carter RE. Random selection of respondents within households in phone surveys. *Journal of Marketing Research*. 1964;1(2):71–76.

28. American Association for Public Opinion Research. *Standard definitions: Final dispositions of case codes and outcome rates for surveys*. Ann Arbor, MI: American Association for Public Opinion Research; 2000.

29. Johnson TP, Owens L. Survey response rate reporting in the professional literature. In *Proceedings of the 2003 American Statistical Association Conference*. Alexandria, VA: American Statistical Association; 2004:127–133.

30. *Stata statistical software, version 8.0* [computer program]. College Station, TX: Stata Corp.; 2003.

31. Krieger N, Rowley DL, Herman AA, Avery B, Phillips MT. Racism, sexism, and social class: Implications for studies of health, disease, and well-being. *American Journal of Preventive Medicine.* 1993;9(6 suppl.):82–122.

32. Navarro V. Race or class versus race and class: Mortality differentials in the United States. *Lancet.* 1990;336(8725):1238–1240.

33. Kaufman JS, Cooper RS. Seeking causal explanations in social epidemiology. *American Journal of Epidemiology.* 1999;150(2):113–120.

34. Muntaner C. Invited commentary: Social mechanisms, race, and social epidemiology. *American Journal of Epidemiology.* 1999;150(2):121–126; discussion 127–128.

35. Ren XS, Amick BC, Williams DR. Racial/ethnic disparities in health: The interplay between discrimination and socioeconomic status. *Ethnicity and Disease.* 1999;9(2):151–165.

36. Massey DS, Denton NA. *American apartheid: Segregation and the making of the underclass.* Cambridge, MA: Harvard University Press; 1993.

37. Silva A, Whitman S, Margellos H, Ansell D. Evaluating Chicago's success in reaching the Healthy People 2000 goal of reducing health disparities. *Public Health Reports.* 2001;116(5):484–494.

38. Margellos H, Silva A, Whitman S. Comparison of health status indicators in Chicago: Are black-white disparities worsening? *American Journal of Public Health.* 2004;94(1):116–121.

39. Acevedo-Garcia D, Lochner KA. Residential segregation and health. In *Neighborhoods and health* (Kawachi I, Berkman LF, eds.). New York: Oxford University Press; 2003:265–287.

40. Diez Roux AV. The examination of neighborhood effects on health: Conceptual and methodological issues related to the presence of multiple levels of organization. In *Neighborhoods and health* (Kawachi I, Berkman L, eds.). New York: Oxford University Press; 2003:45–64.

41. Barbeau EM, Krieger N, Soobader MJ. Working class matters: Socioeconomic disadvantage, race/ethnicity, gender, and smoking in NHIS 2000. *American Journal of Public Health.* 2004;94(2):269–278.

42. O'Campo P. Invited commentary: Advancing theory and methods for multilevel models of residential neighborhoods and health. *American Journal of Epidemiology.* 2003;157(1):9–13.

43. Kawachi I, Berkman LF. *Neighborhoods and health.* New York: Oxford University Press; 2003.

CHAPTER NINE

Demographic Characteristics and Survival with AIDS

Health Disparities in Chicago, 1993–2001

Girma Woldemichael, Demian Christiansen, Sandra Thomas, and Nanette Benbow

Several factors have led to increases in survival among persons with AIDS, including the use of immunologic criteria to define AIDS, earlier identification of and treatment for opportunistic diseases, and widespread use of highly active antiretroviral therapy (HAART).[1-4] Although the expansion in the case definition and improvements in diagnosing and treating diseases resulted in modest improvements in survival times before the advent of HAART, controlled trials, clinic-based studies, and surveillance data found dramatic improvements in survival after December 1995, when HAART was recommended as the standard of care for persons with AIDS.[3,5-14] The effect of the new treatment on AIDS mortality become apparent almost immediately. National HIV/AIDS-related mortality declined 28% from 1995 to 1996, an additional 45% from 1996 to 1997, and 28% from 1997 to 1998.[15]

Large urban centers have had the highest AIDS incidence rates since the disease was first described in 1981, and the city of Chicago is no exception. From 1981 through 2006, more than 23,000 AIDS cases were reported.[16,17] Nearly 56% of those persons had died by 2006.[18] After 1980,

Originally published in the *American Journal of Public Health* 99, supp. 1 (2009): S118–23, by the American Public Health Association.

Chicago became unique among large US cities because its population was comprised of roughly equal numbers of non-Hispanic blacks, non-Hispanic whites, and Hispanics. In 1993, non-Hispanic blacks and whites each comprised approximately 38% of the population; 19% of city residents were Hispanic (predominately Mexican and Puerto Rican). Although non-Hispanic white adults in Chicago were more likely than were whites across the nation to lack a high school diploma, they had a higher per capita income than did non-Hispanic whites nationally. Non-Hispanic blacks and Hispanics had per capita incomes similar to their counterparts nationally and substantially lower than that of non-Hispanic whites.

By the end of 2001, Chicago's non-Hispanic white population had declined by 17% and its non-Hispanic black population by 6%. The Hispanic population grew by 33%, with a declining proportion having a Puerto Rican background and increasing numbers originating from Central and South America. Although Chicago's non-Hispanic white population decreased in size, its relative wealth increased, with a per capita income 40% higher than that of non-Hispanic whites nationally. The per capita incomes of non-Hispanic blacks and Hispanics continued to mirror those of their counterparts nationally, and the income gap between these groups and Chicago's non-Hispanic white population increased.

Minorities, particularly non-Hispanic blacks, are disproportionately affected by AIDS. For example, one-third of the citizens of Chicago and nearly two-thirds of its AIDS patients are non-Hispanic blacks.

Because of the disproportionate effect of HIV/AIDS on some of Chicago's demographic groups and because we were aware of no previous studies that analyzed cause-specific AIDS mortality in relation to survival time, we conducted a survival analysis among persons diagnosed with AIDS between January 1993 and December 2001. Individuals were followed through 2003 to identify factors that predicted increased survival and to examine disparities in survival, particularly by demographic characteristics.

Disparities in AIDS survival may be influenced by many factors. Disparities in screening and early diagnosis can be caused by differences in recognition of risk; the importance of health relative to other concerns, such as economic subsistence and violence; negative consequences, such as social stigma, associated with receiving an HIV or AIDS diagnosis; and access to providers of screening services. For persons diagnosed with AIDS, survival may be influenced by differences in access to care providers; the quality of care provided, including the cultural competence of care providers and medical appropriateness of treatment; and the patient's ability to successfully adhere to treatment regimens. Health literacy has been shown to be an important mediator of disparities in adherence to AIDS medical treatment.[19] Differences in health literacy between ethnic groups can be influenced by local structural factors. For example, urban public schools (including the Chicago public schools) have long been known for providing significantly lower-quality education in predominately minority than in white neighborhoods.[20]

Methods

Data Sources and Study Population

The HIV/AIDS Reporting System database, developed by the Centers for Disease Control and Prevention and maintained by the Chicago Department of Public Health's Office of HIV/AIDS Surveillance, was the source of data on survival with AIDS. The state of Illinois requires that all cases of AIDS be reported within 7 days of diagnosis, regardless of whether the individual has been reported previously by another provider.[21] Adults and adolescents (i.e., those 13 years and older) who were diagnosed with AIDS between January 1993 and December 2001 and reported to the Chicago Department of Public Health through June 2006 were eligible for inclusion.

We restricted our analyses to persons who identified themselves as non-Hispanic white, non-Hispanic black, or Hispanic. These 3 groups represented 94% of the general population of Chicago and 99% of AIDS cases diagnosed between 1993 and 2001.[18,22] In addition, we limited the study population to individuals who acquired AIDS through 3 major exposure categories: male-to-male sexual contact, injection drug use, or heterosexual contact.

[...]

Results

Demographic and risk characteristics for individuals diagnosed with AIDS in the pre-HAART era (1993–1995) and HAART era (1996–2001) are shown in table 9.1. Overall, 11022 adults and adolescents were diagnosed with AIDS between January 1, 1993, and December 31, 2001.

TABLE 9.1 **Demographic and risk characteristics of persons diagnosed with AIDS before and after the introduction of highly active antiretroviral therapy: Chicago, 1993–2001**

Characteristic	Pre-HAART era, 1993–1995 (no. [%])	HAART era, 1996–2001 (no. [%])	Total (no. [%])
Gender			
Male	4,353 (83.5)	4,514 (77.8)	8,867 (80.5)
Female	863 (16.6)	1,292 (22.3)	2,155 (19.6)
Race/ethnicity			
Non-Hispanic black	2,966 (56.9)	3,858 (66.5)	6,824 (61.9)
Non-Hispanic white	1,527 (29.3)	1,102 (19)	2,629 (23.9)
Hispanic	723 (13.9)	846 (14.6)	1,569 (14.2)
Mode of transmission			
Male-to-male sexual contact	2,524 (51.1)	2,250 (42.8)	4,774 (46.8)
Injection drug use	2,040 (41.3)	2,218 (42.2)	4,258 (41.8)
Heterosexual contact	376 (7.6)	790 (15)	1,166 (11.4)
Age at diagnosis (yr.)			
13–29	735 (14.3)	736 (12.8)	1,471 (13.5)
30–49	3,849 (74.5)	4,248 (73.6)	8,097 (74.1)
≥ 50	573 (11.1)	788 (13.7)	1,361 (12.5)
Opportunistic diseases			
Pneumocystis carinii pneumonia	489 (9.4)	469 (8.1)	958 (8.7)
Kaposi's sarcoma	88 (1.7)	67 (1.2)	155 (1.4)
Other[a]	2,865 (54.9)	2,496 (43.8)	5,361 (48.6)
No disease specified	1,774 (34)	2,774 (47.8)	4,548 (41.3)
Vital status			
Alive	1,681 (32.2)	3,628 (62.5)	5,309 (48.2)
Deceased	3,535 (67.8)	2,178 (37.5)	5,731 (51.2)
Deaths from AIDS	2,159 (41.4)	1,157 (19.9)	3,316 (30.1)
Deaths from other causes	1,376 (26.4)	1,021 (17.6)	2,397 (21.8)
Total	5,216 (47.3)	5,806 (52.7)	11,022 (100)

Note: HAART = highly active antiretroviral therapy.

[a]All diseases except *Pneumocystis carinii* pneumonia and Kaposi's sarcoma.

Of these, 5731 (51%) had died by December 31, 2003. Approximately 30% of deaths were attributable to causes related to AIDS. Most of the AIDS patients studied were male (81%) and non-Hispanic black (62%). Nearly three-quarters of the study population were aged 30 to 49 years at the time they were diagnosed with AIDS. Approximately 47% of cases were attributed to male-to-male sexual contact and 42% to injection drug use.

Cumulative adjusted 1-, 3-, and 5-year AIDS survival probabilities are shown in table 9.2. Overall, 5-year survival improved from 49% in the pre-HAART era to 76% in the HAART era. Figure 9.1 shows adjusted AIDS survival curves in the pre-HAART and HAART eras. All

TABLE 9.2 **Adjusted probability estimates of 1-, 3-, and 5-year survival among persons diagnosed with AIDS before and after the introduction of highly active antiretroviral therapy: Chicago, 1993–2001**

Characteristics	Pre-HAART era, 1993–1995			HAART era, 1996–2001		
	1 year	3 years	5 years	1 year	3 years	5 years
Gender						
Male	0.81	0.58	0.51	0.86	0.77	0.72
Female	0.78	0.55	0.49	0.88	0.82	0.77
Race/ethnicity						
Non-Hispanic black	0.78	0.54	0.46	0.87	0.79	0.73
Non-Hispanic white	0.79	0.56	0.52	0.90	0.86	0.83
Hispanic	0.80	0.59	0.55	0.88	0.83	0.79
Mode of transmission						
Male-to-male sexual contact	0.77	0.53	0.48	0.90	0.85	0.81
Injection drug use	0.79	0.57	0.49	0.86	0.77	0.70
Heterosexual contact	0.85	0.59	0.53	0.90	0.83	0.78
Age of diagnosis (yr.)						
13–29	0.85	0.60	0.53	0.92	0.87	0.81
30–49	0.78	0.56	0.49	0.89	0.82	0.77
≥ 50	0.68	0.45	0.41	0.76	0.66	0.63
Total	0.78	0.55	0.49	0.88	0.81	0.76

Note: HAART = highly active antiretroviral therapy.

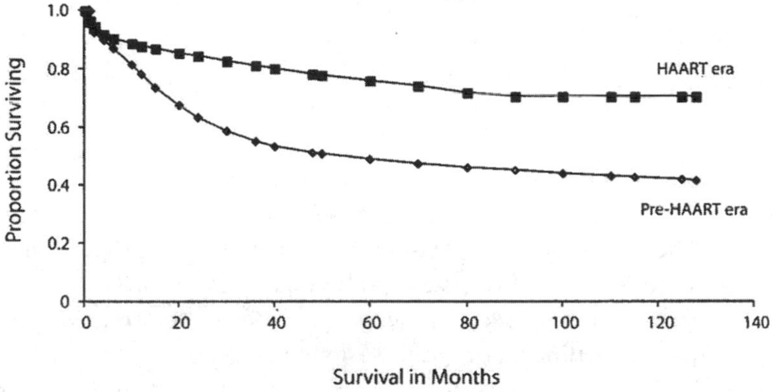

FIGURE 9.1. Adjusted survival curves of AIDS patients in Chicago before (1993–1995) and after (1996–2001) the introduction of highly active antiretroviral therapy (HAART)

groups experienced increases in AIDS survival across these 2 periods, but not all at the same rate.

Table 9.3 shows adjusted hazard ratios for AIDS death and 95% confidence intervals by era for variables included in our final model, includ-

TABLE 9.3 **Adjusted hazard ratios for survival for persons diagnosed with AIDS before and after the introduction of highly active antiretroviral therapy: Chicago, 1993–2001**

	Pre-HAART era, 1993–1995		HAART era, 1996–2001	
Characteristic	HR (95% CI)	P	HR (95% CI)	P
Gender				
Male (ref.)	1.00		1.00	
Female	0.90 (0.79, 1.03)	.12	1.20 (1.03, 1.40)	.02
Race/ethnicity				
Non-Hispanic black	1.18 (1.06, 1.31)	<.01	1.51 (1.26, 1.80)	<.01
Non-Hispanic white (ref.)	1.00		1.00	
Hispanic	0.94 (0.81, 1.09)	>.05	1.22 (0.97, 1.53)	.10
Mode of transmission				
Male-to-male sexual contact (ref.)	1.00		1.00	
Injection drug use	0.94 (0.85, 1.04)	.22	1.30 (1.14, 1.49)	<.01
Heterosexual contact	0.89 (0.74, 1.08)	.25	0.94 (0.76, 1.16)	.54
Age of diagnosis (yr.)				
13–29 (ref.)	1.00		1.00	
30–49	1.19 (1.05, 1.35)	.01	1.23 (1.02, 1.49)	.03
≥ 50	1.63 (1.38, 1.93)	<.01	2.28 (1.82, 1.49)	<.01
Opportunistic diseases				
Pneumocystis carinii pneumonia (ref.)	1.00		1.00	
Kaposi's sarcoma	1.11 (0.79, 1.55)	.55	0.99 (0.53, 1.85)	.97
Other	1.15 (0.99, 1.33)	.07	1.50 (1.22, 1.86)	.01
None	0.50 (0.43, 0.59)	<.01	0.55 (0.44, 0.69)	<.01

Note: HAART = highly active antiretroviral therapy; HR = hazard ratio; CI = confidence interval. Cox regression model used to adjust for gender, race/ethnicity, mode of transmission, age at diagnosis, and opportunistic diseases.

ing gender, race/ethnicity, age, mode of transmission, and type of opportunistic disease. In almost every instance, the hazard ratio increased from the pre-HAART to the HAART era, implying disproportionate rates of improvement in AIDS survival times across eras.

After we adjusted for race/ethnicity, age, mode of transmission, and type of first opportunistic disease, we found that in the pre-HAART era, women were 10% less likely than were men to die from AIDS. However, in the HAART era, females were 20% more likely than were men to die from AIDS.

Similarly, in the pre-HAART era, the hazard of AIDS death was 18% greater for non-Hispanic blacks and 6% lower for Hispanics than for non-Hispanic whites. In the HAART era, however, the hazard of death for both non-Hispanic blacks and Hispanics increased in comparison with the hazard for non-Hispanic whites: non-Hispanic blacks were

51% more likely to die and Hispanics were 22% more likely to die than were non-Hispanic whites.

In both the pre-HAART and HAART eras, the hazard of death from AIDS increased with age at AIDS diagnosis. There was little difference in the hazard of death among persons aged 30 to 49 years and those aged 13 to 29 years by era, but the risk of AIDS death among persons aged 50 years and older compared with those aged 13 to 29 years increased considerably by era (table 9.3). Persons 50 years and older were 63% more likely to die in the pre-HAART era and were 128% more likely to die in the HAART era than were those aged 13 to 29 years. There was no statistically significant difference in AIDS survival between heterosexuals or injection drug users and men who had sex with men in the pre-HAART era. In the HAART era, however, drug users were 30% more likely to die from AIDS than were men who had sex with men, after adjustment for gender, race/ethnicity, and age at AIDS diagnosis.

Discussion

Our study showed increased survival times with AIDS in the HAART era compared with the pre-HAART era, a result that is consistent with the results of several similar analyses.[5,23,24] Each group studied had improved 1-, 3-, and 5-year survival rates from the pre-HAART era to the HAART era. These improvements were likely a result of increased provider recognition of and treatments for opportunistic diseases, particularly *Pneumocystis carinii* pneumonia and *Mycobacterium avium* complex. Also, AIDS diagnoses made earlier in the course of the disease, resulting from inclusion of immunologic criteria in the AIDS case definition, likely increased survival.[1]

[...]

Although our data indicated significant improvement in survival among all groups studied, the rate at which survival improved was not uniform. Furthermore, it was these differences in the rate of improvement that accounted for higher hazard rates in the HAART era. For example, the hazard of death among non-Hispanic blacks compared with non-Hispanic whites increased from 18% in the pre-HAART era to 51% in the HAART era. However, the disparity stemmed not from decreases in survival among non-Hispanic blacks but from disproportionate gains in survival among non-Hispanic whites, a disparity we also observed for other demographic characteristics. This pattern echoed patterns in survival observed in the early 1990s. A nationally representative study of persons with HIV showed that women and non-Hispanic blacks received a lower quality of care than did other HIV-infected persons.[25]

Non-Hispanic blacks were found to have poorer survival than whites because they had more-advanced disease when they sought care and treatment; they also had less exposure to *Pneumocystis carinii* pneumonia prophylaxis.[26] Of 9 studies published between 1985 and 1991, 4 found a decrease in survival for non-Hispanic blacks compared with non-Hispanic whites,[25-31] 4 found no difference in survival,[29,32-34] and 1 found an increase in survival.[29,35] In several of these studies, after control for socioeconomic differences, there was no difference found in survival by race/ethnicity.[36]

A survival analysis of HIV to AIDS progression from 1994 to 2005 showed that non-Hispanic blacks and Hispanics were 45% more likely to progress to AIDS within 12 months than were non-Hispanic whites. This suggests that non-Hispanic blacks may have been unaware of their HIV status longer, or entered primary care later, than non-Hispanic whites.[37] If non-Hispanic whites were more likely to seek health care earlier in the course of their disease, there might have been more time to manage treatment effectively. It is not clear, however, to what degree, if any, delayed progression from HIV to AIDS among non-Hispanic whites contributed to increases in survival. HIV reporting in Illinois began in 1999, which provided only 2 years of overlap with our data.

[...]

Conclusions

We found significantly increased survival with AIDS in the HAART era compared with the pre-HAART era. All groups we studied had improved survival rates, although not all groups benefited to the same extent. Differential rates in improvement, rather than increased morbidity and mortality, explain the disparities in the hazard ratios by race/ethnicity across eras. These findings have significant implications for prevention and care organizations: rather than focusing on the reasons for disparities, examining protective factors in non-Hispanic whites and emulating them in other populations may prove more effective. In Chicago, for example, a useful strategy may be to assess protective factors in both blacks and whites and tailor interventions that will extend these protections to the Hispanic population.

Enhancing existing efforts to prevent HIV-infected individuals from infecting susceptible individuals and developing new interventions to increase early recognition of disease and to remove barriers to accessing care will help Chicago's disadvantaged population to achieve even greater increases in survival. In addition, effective community-level interventions to reduce health disparities require public engagement and support, but the frequency and appropriateness of media coverage of disparities are inadequate, despite a growing body of academic literature.[38] This is another issue that should be addressed in intervention development and planning.

References

1. Centers for Disease Control and Prevention. 1993 revised classification system for HIV infection and expanded surveillance definition for AIDS among adolescents and adults. *MMWR Recommendations and Reports.* 1992; 41(RR-17):1–19.

2. Centers for Disease Control and Prevention. USPHS/IDSA guidelines for the prevention of opportunistic infections in persons infected with human immunodeficiency virus: A summary. *MMWR Recommendations and Reports.* 1995;44(RR-8):1–34.

3. Centers for Disease Control and Prevention. Guidelines for the use of antiretroviral agents in IIIV infected adults and adolescents. *MMWR Recommendations and Reports.* 1998;47(RR-5):43–82.

4. Porter K, Babiker A, Bhaskaran K, et al. Determinants of survival following HIV-1 seroconversion after the introduction of HAART. *Lancet.* 2003; 362(9392):1267–1274.

5. Lee LM, Karon JM, Selik R, Neal JJ, Fleming PL. Survival after AIDS diagnosis in adolescents and adults during the treatment era, United States, 1984–1997. *Journal of the American Medical Association.* 2001;285(10):1308–1315.

6. Pallela FJ, Delaney KM, Moorman AC, et al. Declining morbidity and mortality among patients with advanced human immunodeficiency virus infection. *New England Journal of Medicine.* 1998;338:853–860.

7. Pezzotti P, Napoli PA, Acciai S, et al. Increasing survival time after AIDS in Italy: The role of new combination antiretroviral therapies: Tuscany AIDS Study Group. *AIDS.* 1999;13(2):249–255.

8. McNaghten AD, Hanson DL, Jones JL, Dworkin MS, Ward JW. Effects of antiretroviral therapy and opportunistic illness primary chemoprophylaxis on

survival after AIDS diagnosis: Adult/Adolescent Spectrum of Disease Group. *AIDS*. 1999;13(13):1687–1695.

9. Vittinghoff E, Scheer S, O'Malley P, Colfax G, Holmberg SD, Buchbinder SP. Combination antiretroviral therapy and recent declines in AIDS incidence and mortality. *Journal of Infectious Diseases*. 1999;179(3):717–720.

10. Detels R, Munoz A, McFarlane G, et al. for the Multicenter AIDS Cohort Study Investigators. Effectiveness of potent antiretroviral therapy on time to AIDS and death in men with known HIV infection duration. *Journal of the American Medical Association*. 1998;280(17):1497–1503.

11. Harper DM, Thomas SD. *Leading causes of death in Chicago, 1989–1999*. Chicago: Department of Public Health Epidemiology Program; 2002.

12. Minino AM, Arias E, Kochanek KD, Murphy SL, Smith BL. Deaths: Final data for 2000. *National Vital Statistics Reports*. 2002;50(15):1–119.

13. Hoyert DL, Arias E, Smith BL, Murphy SL, Kochanek KD. Deaths: Final data for 1999. *National Vital Statistics Reports*. 2001;49(8):1–113.

14. Murphy SL. Deaths: Final data for 1998. *National Vital Statistics Reports*. 2000;48(11):1–105.

15. Centers for Disease Control and Prevention. Slidesets. N.d. https://www.cdc.gov/mmwr/preview/mmwrhtml/mm5021a2.htm.

16. Centers for Disease Control and Prevention. Pneumocystis pneumonia—Los Angeles. *Morbidity and Mortality Weekly Report*. 1981;30:250–252.

17. Steinberg S, Fleming P. The geographic distribution of AIDS in the United States: Is there a rural epidemic? *Journal of Rural Health*. 2000;16(1):11–19.

18. STD/HIV/AIDS Chicago—Winter 2006. Chicago: Office of HIV/AIDS Surveillance; 2007.

19. Osborn CY, Paasche-Orlow MK, Davis TC, Wolf MS. Health literacy: An overlooked factor in understanding HIV health disparities. *American Journal of Preventive Medicine*. 2007;33(5):374–378.

20. Darling-Hammond L. Unequal opportunity: Race and education. 1998. https://www.brookings.edu/articles/unequal-opportunity-race-and-education.

21. Ill Admin Code tit 77 x693 (2001) http://www.ilga.gov/commission/jcar/admincode/077/077006930000200R.html.

22. US Bureau of the Census. 2000 Census: Internet release A, 2001. https://factfinder.census.gov/faces/nav/jsf/pages/index.xhtml.

23. Karon JM, Rosenberg PS, McQuillan G, Khare M, Gwinn M, Petersen LR. Prevalence of HIV infection in the United States, 1984 to 1992. *Journal of the American Medical Association*. 1996;276(2):126–131.

24. Lemp GF, Payne SF, Neal D, Temelso T, Rutherford GW. Survival trends for patients with AIDS. *Journal of the American Medical Association*. 1990;263(3):402–406.

25. Easterbrook PJ, Keruly JC, Creagh-Kirk T, Richman DD, Chaisson RE, Moore RD. Racial and ethnic differences in outcome in zidovudine-treated pa-

tients with advanced HIV disease: Zidovudine Epidemiology Study Group. *Journal of the American Medical Association.* 1991;266(19):2713–2718.

26. Walensky RP, Paltiel AD, Losina E, et al. The survival benefits of AIDS treatment in the United States. *Journal of Infectious Diseases.* 2006;194(1):11–19.

27. Chang HG, Morse DL, Noonan C. Survival and mortality patterns of an acquired immunodeficiency syndrome (AIDS) cohort in New York State. *American Journal of Epidemiology.* 1992;138(5):341–349.

28. King WD, Wong MD, Shapiro MF, Landon BE, Cunningham WE. Does racial concordance between HIV-positive patients and their physicians affect the time to receipt of protease inhibitors? *Journal of General Internal Medicine.* 2004;19(11):1146–1153.

29. Curtis JR, Patrick DL. Race and survival time with AIDS: A synthesis of the literature. *American Journal of Public Health.* 1993;83(10):1425–1428.

30. Moore RD, Hidalgo J, Sugland BW, Chaisson RE. Zidovudine and the natural history of the acquired immunodeficiency syndrome. *New England Journal of Medicine.* 1991;324(20):1412–1416.

31. Harris JE. Improved short-term survival of AIDS patients initially diagnosed with Pneumocystis carinii pneumonia, 1984 through 1987. *Journal of the American Medical Association.* 1990;263(3):397–401.

32. Creagh-Kirk T, Doi P, Andrews E, et al. Survival experience among patients with AIDS receiving zidovudine: Follow-up of patients in a compassionate plea program. *Journal of the American Medical Association.* 1988;260(20): 3009–3015.

33. Lagakos S, Fischl MA, Stein DS, Lim L, Volberding P. Effects of zidovudine therapy in minority and other subpopulations with early HIV infection. *Journal of the American Medical Association.* 1991;266(19):2709–2712.

34. Justice AC, Feinstein AR, Wells CK. A new prognostic staging system for the acquired immunodeficiency syndrome. *New England Journal of Medicine.* 1989;320(21):1388–1393.

35. Friedland GH, Saltzman B, Vileno J, Freeman K, Schrager LK, Klein RS. Survival differences in patients with AIDS. *Journal of Acquired Immune Deficiency Syndromes.* 1991;4(2):144–153.

36. Chaisson RE, Keruly JC, Moore RD. Race, sex, drug use, and progression of human immunodeficiency virus disease. *New England Journal of Medicine.* 1995;333(12):751–756.

37. Christiansen D, Benbow N. Race/ethnicity and time from HIV diagnosis to AIDS, Chicago, 1999–2005. Annual Conference of State and Territorial Epidemiologists; June 2007; Atlantic City, NJ.

38. Amzel A, Ghosh C. National newspaper coverage of minority health disparities. *Journal of the National Medical Association.* 2007;99(10):1120–1125.

CHAPTER TEN

The Racial Disparity in Breast Cancer Mortality

Steven Whitman, David Ansell, Jennifer Orsi, and Teena Francois

Introduction

It is frequently noted that black women die from breast cancer at a higher rate than white women.[1-3] In addition, some analyses suggest that there are racial differences in biological characteristics of breast tumors.[4,5] These two matters are often then conflated to suggest that differential biology may be a risk factor for the racial disparity in breast cancer mortality.[6-8] We believe that such a syllogism is faulty and is proven wrong by an examination of the data underlying this disparity. The purpose of this article is to present data relevant to this issue from the United States, New York and Chicago regarding the racial disparity in breast cancer mortality and to suggest systems-based hypotheses that might be examined in order to delineate the factors responsible for this disparity.

Methods

Deaths where the cause was malignant neoplasm of the breast (ICD-9 = 174, ICD-10 = C50) were included in this analysis. There was an ICD version change in 1999; however, we did not apply a comparability ratio

Originally published in the *Journal of Community Health* 36 (2011): 588–96.
© Springer Science+Business Media, LLC 2010. Reprinted with permission.

to 1998 breast cancer deaths because there was no statistically significant difference in the number of cases captured between versions 9 and
10 based on coding changes (the comparability ratio for malignant neoplasm of breast = 1.01, 95% CI: 1.00–1.01).[9]

United States Data

All US numerators were abstracted from death files maintained by the
National Center for Health Statistics. Population-based denominators
for 1980, 1990, and 2000 were derived from Census data. Population-
based denominators for non-Hispanic white in 2005 were gathered from
the American Community Survey. Population-based denominators
for the non-Hispanic black population in 2005 were not readily available, so we estimated this population using the same methodology employed to estimate the 2005 non-Hispanic black population in Chicago.
Population-based denominators for years other than 1980, 1990, 2000,
and 2005 were estimated using exponential interpolation. For 1980 denominator data and 1980–1989 we utilized data on black and white persons (which included Hispanics) because Hispanic origin data were not
available for the US overall during that time period.

New York City Data

New York City numerator data for the years 1980–1989 and 2005 were
obtained through a special request to the New York Department of Mental Health and Hygiene. Numerator data for the years 1990–2004 were
abstracted from death files maintained by the National Center for Health
Statistics. Population-based denominators for 1980, 1990, 2000, and 2005
were obtained via the same avenues as for Chicago (below). Population-
based denominators for the non-Hispanic black population in 2005 were
not readily available, and thus we used the same estimating techniques as
for the non-Hispanic black population in Chicago to estimate this population. Population-based denominators for years other than 1980, 1990,
2000, and 2005 were estimated using exponential interpolation.

Chicago Data

All Chicago numerators were abstracted from the vital records (birth
and death) files maintained by the Illinois Department of Public Health

and provided to us by the Chicago Department of Public Health. Denominators for population-based rates in Chicago in 1980, 1990, and
2000 were gathered from the Census. Denominators for non-Hispanic
white (NHW) in 2005 were gathered from the American Community
Survey.[10] Denominators for the non-Hispanic black (NHB) population
in 2005 were not readily available, so we estimated the population using
an age-specific ratio calculated by dividing the number of non-Hispanic
blacks by total blacks in the 2000 Census and multiplying the proportion
by the number of all blacks in 2005 from the American Community Survey for each age group. Denominators for years other than 1980, 1990,
2000, and 2005 were estimated using exponential interpolation.

Analysis of Trends

To measure disparity we calculated the rate ratio between the NHB and
NHW rates. The rate ratio is greater than 1.00 if the NHB rate is higher
than the NHW rate and less than 1.00 if the NHW rate is higher than the
NHB rate.

Statistical Analyses

To determine if a disparity widened or narrowed significantly between
1980 and 2005 we calculated a two-sided z-score using a bootstrap tech-
nique developed by Keppel and colleagues[11] and examined the corresponding P-value for the z-score. A P-value of < 0.05 was considered
significant for all analyses. The significance of trends was tested using
joinpoint analysis.[12] Each joinpoint represents a significant change in the
trend, denoted as a straight line on a log scale. The overall significance
was set at $P = 0.05$. No more than three joinpoints were allowed.

Results

Figure 10.1a presents results for the United States. As table 10.1 indicates, the graph for white women contains 4 segments, the last 3 of which
indicate significant declines (the first corresponds to a significant increase). For black women there is a significant upward slope for 1980–
1993 and a significant downward slope after that. The black breast cancer mortality rate was 31.8 in 1980, and the NHB rate was 35.6 in 2005,

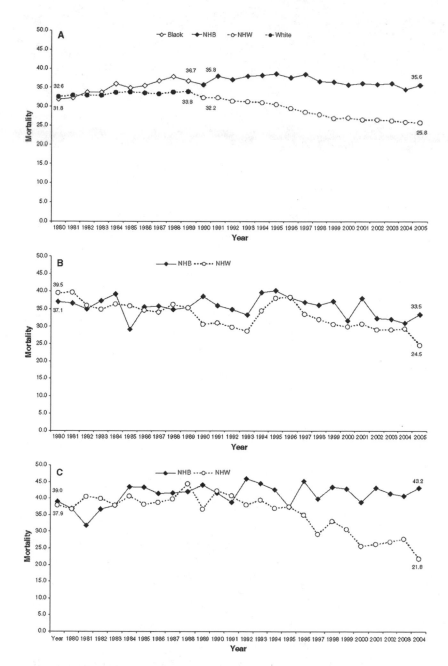

FIGURE 10.1. Age-adjusted female breast cancer mortality rates. *A*, United States, by race, 1980–2005. *B*, New York City, by race, 1980–2005. *C*, Chicago, by race, 1980–2005.

Note: Open diamonds represent black data that includes Hispanics, and closed circles represent white data that includes Hispanics (1980–1989). Closed diamonds represent non-Hispanic blacks, and open circles represent non-Hispanic whites (1990–2005).

TABLE 10.1 Joinpoint analysis of trends in breast cancer mortality rates for the United States, New York City, and Chicago, 1980–2005

Race/place	Segment 1			Segment 2			Segment 3			Segment 4		
	Years	APC	95% CI	Years	APC	95% CI	Years	APC	95% CI	Years	APC	95% CI
US white	1980–88	0.4	(0.0, 0.7)*	1988–95	−1.5	(−2.0, −1.0)*	1995–99	−2.9	(−4.3, −1.4)*	1999–2005	−0.8	(−1.3, −0.3)*
US black	1980–93	1.3	(0.9, 1.7)*	1993–2005	−0.8	(−1.2, −0.5)*						
NYC white	1980–92	−2.2	(−2.9, −1.4)*	1992–95	6.6	(−8.3, 24.0)	1995–2003	−3.3	(−4.5, −2.1)*			
NYC black	1980–2005	−0.3	(−0.7, 0.01)									
Chicago white	1980–92	0.7	(−0.2, 1.7)	1992–2005	−4.1	(−5.1, −3.1)*						
Chicago black	1980–82	−9.2	(−24.4, 9.0)	1982–85	9.4	(−8.4, 30.6)	1985–2005	−0.1	(−0.05, 0.3)			

*Statistically significant annual percentage change, $P < .05$.

a statistically significant increase ($P < 0.001$). The white rate was 32.6 in 1980, and the NHW rate was 25.8 in 2005, a statistically significant decrease ($P < 0.001$). Since 1982 the black/NHB rates have been higher than the white/NHW rates.

Figure 10.1b contains NHW and NHB rates for NYC. There are 3 segments for NHW women, two of which show significant declines. There was a statistically significant decrease in the NHW rates between 1980 (39.5) and 2005 (24.5) ($P < 0.001$). There was only 1 segment for NHB women, and it showed no significant change over the 25 years (table 10.1). The rate changed from 37.1 in 1980 to 33.5 in 2005, but the difference was not statistically significant ($P > 0.05$).

Figure 10.1c presents the breast cancer mortality rates for Chicago from 1980 to 2005. In 1980 the rates for NHB and NHW women were essentially equal at about 38. The rates remained more or less constant until the early 1990s, when the NHW rate began to decline. By 2005 the NHW rate was 21.8, a decline of 42% ($P < 0.001$), while the NHB rate had increased (a non-significant amount) to 43.2.

The associated joinpoint analysis (table 10.1) locates three trend lines for NHB mortality, none of them with a significant slope, indicating that there has been no change in the breast cancer mortality rates for black women in Chicago over the past 25 years. Table 10.1 also indicates a constant trend for NHW women in Chicago from 1980 to 1992 and a significant downward trend after that associated with an annual change of −4.1% ($P < 0.05$).

Table 10.2 presents selected data points from these three graphs. All three begin in 1980 with the NHB and NHW breast cancer mortality rates being approximately equal, and each ends in 2005 with the NHB rate being much higher than the NHW rate. Over time, the NHB:NHW relative risk (RR) in the US increased from 0.98 to 1.38; in NYC from 0.94 to 1.36; and in Chicago from 1.03 to 1.98. Each of the 2005 RRs within each location is significantly different than the 1980 RR ($P < 0.001$). For the US as a whole the NHB:NHW RRs have remained rather constant in recent years (2000 and 2005) but are significantly different than 1.00 ($P < 0.001$). Changes in New York City NHB:NHW RRs have varied over time with only the RRs for 1990 and 2005 being significantly different from 1.00 ($P < 0.001$). In Chicago, the NHB:NHW RRs have increased steadily over time, with the RRs for 2000 and 2005 being significantly different than 1.00 ($P < 0.001$).

TABLE 10.2 **Breast cancer mortality rates for the United States, New York City, and Chicago, non-Hispanic black (NHB) and non-Hispanic white (NHW) women, selected years**

Year	Location	NHB	NHW	Rate ratio (RR) (95% CI)	Change in RR**
1980*	US	31.8	32.6	0.98 (0.94–1.01)	—
1990	US	35.8	32.2	1.11 (1.08–1.15)	
2000	US	35.7	27.0	1.32 (1.28–1.36)	
2005	US	35.6	25.8	1.38 (1.34–1.42)	(<.001)
1980	NYC	37.1	39.5	0.94 (0.82–1.08)	—
1990	NYC	38.5	30.6	1.26 (1.10–1.44)	
2000	NYC	31.6	29.8	1.06 (0.93–1.21)	
2005	NYC	33.5	24.5	1.36 (1.19–1.56)	(<.001)
1980	Chicago	39.0	37.9	1.03 (0.85–1.25)	—
1990	Chicago	44.0	36.7	1.20 (1.00–1.44)	
2000	Chicago	42.9	30.6	1.40 (1.15–1.70)	
2005	Chicago	43.2	21.8	1.98 (1.58–2.49)	(<.001)

*Data for 1980 for the United States are for black and white women regardless of Hispanic ethnicity.
**Values in parentheses indicate whether RR in 2005 is significantly different from the one in 1980.

Discussion

The image portrayed by the three graphs could not be explained by biological differences. In all three locations the black and white rates were similar in the 1980s and then started to diverge, just as the benefits from early detection via mammography[13] and treatment[14] were manifesting themselves. In all cases this divergence took place because the white rate started improving and the black rate did not. For the US and Chicago the black rate is higher than it was 25 years ago. In NYC it is lower but only by a small, non-significant amount. Although there may be differences between the races in tumor biology, these explanations would be inadequate to explain why the mortality disparity has been growing rapidly in Chicago but remaining rather constant in NYC and the US. Biology also cannot explain the variability in the disparities in the three areas.

A recent article addressing this issue has reached the same conclusion based on a specific database from Louisiana.[15] Another recent article has found that for many cancers, including breast cancer, disparities in survival actually increase as "amenability to medical interventions" increases.[16] That is, as we become more able to improve cancer outcomes, racial disparities widen because more privileged groups are able to gain access to these interventions. This is precisely what has happened with breast cancer mortality in the three geographies analyzed above.

Since differential biology can't explain these racial disparities, what might? We have been able to identify three hypotheses.[2]

Differential Access to Mammography

Most surveys of self-reported mammography utilization have shown that black and white women have equal screening rates at about the national goals.[17,18] However, several studies of medical records and chart reviews demonstrate that self-report of mammography utilization is substantially inaccurate because many women over-report utilization.[19,20] A recent comprehensive meta-analysis indicates that poor women, and thus black women, over-report more than other (white) women, rendering the equality of self-reported mammography use a misleading measure and leaving a substantial racial gap.[21] If mammography is an effective screening tool, then differential access favoring white women would contribute to the disparity in breast cancer mortality. For example, we know that breast cancers detected by screening are smaller, less likely to be estrogen receptor negative, and less likely to be undifferentiated than unscreened cancers.[22]

Differential Quality of Mammography

There are a number of different measures of mammography quality,[23,24] but we focus on just one here as an example of how such thinking might proceed. The literature suggests that for every 1,000 screening mammograms we should expect to find about 6 breast cancers. This rate of 0.006 is an average that is based on millions of mammogram exams worldwide.[25–27] The detection rate will be lower for women who are screened regularly (as low as 2 breast cancers per 1,000) and higher for women who are rarely screened (10 per 1,000).[15] For example, the National Breast and Cervical Cancer Early Detection Program, which provides mammograms to poor women who tend not to receive regular screening, found a breast cancer detection rate of 0.0094 based upon the experiences of about 1.2 million women between 1991 and 2002.[28] Breast cancer screening programs that find cancer detection rates well below 0.006 may suffer from quality problems.

A well-publicized example may be suggestive of our hypothesis. In

October of 2002 the *New York Times* ran a very long front page story about a woman who obtained a mammogram at a city clinic, was told she was fine and 8 months later was diagnosed with breast cancer. The clinic that missed the cancer was investigated and found to be detecting breast cancers at a rate of only 1 per 1,000 screening mammograms. As a result, the State Department of Health offered free mammograms to women who had been seen recently by the clinic. Over 4,500 women returned and were re-screened, and 25 cancers that had been missed were detected.[29,30]

Substantial information suggests that there is variation in the quality of the mammography process.[31] If this quality tended to be inferior at institutions that serve poorer women, then this would contribute to the racial disparity in breast cancer mortality. Despite the logic to this argument we have been able to locate only one paper that investigated this hypothesis, and it found negative results.[32] We thus discuss this topic in somewhat greater detail.

Some reports have found that radiologists who spend more time (variously defined) reading mammograms tend to find more tumors and to find them smaller.[19] However, this relationship between volume and quality is not uniformly agreed upon.[33,34] It has also been found that breast imaging specialists find more cancers than general radiologists. For example, Sickles and his colleagues reported that specialists found breast cancers at a rate almost twice as high as general radiologists when reading screening mammograms (6.0/1,000 compared with 3.4—our calculations).[27] Breast imagers tend to do better when seeking to resolve diagnostic mammograms as well.[27,31] Again, if such imagers tended to work at institutions that served wealthier women, then this too would serve to increase disparities in mammography interpretation, cancer detection and ultimately mortality.

But the reading is just one part of the mammography process. Another is recalling women who have had abnormal mammograms that require follow-up. In our experience it is not uncommon for the lost to follow-up rate at community institutions for this group to be as high as 33%.[35] Reports in the literature have found similar results with varying definitions, resulting in 28% without diagnostic resolution within 6 months[36] and 16% for which a final diagnosis was not recorded.[25] Such loss to follow-up and/or an incomplete diagnostic process would also decrease the cancer detection rates found by screening mammography.

Furthermore, it has been documented that black women experience longer delays between an initial abnormal finding on a mammogram and obtaining a diagnosis.[37] There are other issues as well. For example, a recent study found that black women were twice as likely not to be notified about an abnormal result or to not correctly be able to interpret the information they received.[38]

Differential Access to Quality Treatment

Multiple studies have demonstrated that black people receive inferior medical care for almost every medical condition.[39–41] Breast cancer is no exception.[37,42,43] The disparities in breast cancer treatment occur for various reasons such as delays in treatment, inadequate access to adjuvant therapy, non-receipt of designated care, co-morbidities, financial barriers, etc.[44–47] Certainly such disparate treatment would contribute to the racial disparity in breast cancer mortality.

The Biological Explanation

Taken together, these three hypotheses might be enough to explain the racial disparity in breast cancer mortality without invoking genetic etiologies. This is certainly the view of the Metropolitan Chicago Breast Cancer Task Force which has been organizing from this point of view.[48] It is nonetheless instructive to review the biological explanation. The fabric of this argument has two main threads that are sometimes presented simultaneously.

Racial Differences in Tumor Biology

Studies have revealed racial differences in diagnosed tumor size, stage, lymph node involvement, grade, estrogen receptor status, etc.[7,49,50] However, in some cases these differences might be generated by the later detection of tumors in black women and thus be a function of the detection process and not the race of the women. A recent prominent study lends support to this view.

Smith-Bindman and her colleagues examined data on over 1,000,000 women. Unadjusted data revealed statically significant black:white differences in tumor size, stage, grade, and lymph node involvement. However, these observed differences "were attenuated or eliminated after the cohort was stratified by screening history."[51] Specifically, after mammography history was taken into account racial differences in tumor size, stage and lymph node involvement disappeared. Only tumor grade remained significant, though the differences varied in inexplicable ways (some significant, some not significant) across mammography history.[51]

The Independent Predictor Explanation

Even if there were innate racial differences in breast cancer biology it would still be necessary to tie these to disparities in breast cancer mortality to complete the syllogism. This is the task that generally falls to various versions of regression analysis. In such analyses researchers gather data for breast cancer mortality, race and other variables (confounders), notably some measure of socioeconomic status. Initially racial differences in breast cancer mortality are observed. If after "adjustment" or "correction" for these other confounders race remains statistically significant, then these researchers conclude that race is an independent (i.e., innate) risk factor for breast cancer mortality. Consider a recent example, simply one among many.

Woodward and her colleagues compared two independent cohorts (consisting of NHB and NHW women, among others) attending the same university hospital. The two cohorts were defined based upon their treatment needs. After adjustment for many biological variables black race remained an independent predictor of lower overall survival in both cohorts. The authors note that "such differences in tumor biology, as well as previously described socioeconomic factors, likely contribute to the lower rate of survival in the AA breast cancer population." They then reflect on the following: "It is clear that, as with any cohort grouped by self-reported race, those who self-report their race as AA or black represent a genetically and culturally diverse group. *Therefore, explaining how AA race is associated with biologically more aggressive breast cancer will likely be difficult*"[6] (our italics). Similar analyses are employed by other authors.[8]

Two major factors suggest that the analytical structure used in these studies is faulty. First, it is not clear that there exists a biological black or African American race/grouping. Such a construct is heatedly debated in the medical literature,[52,53] while the social science literature has virtually unanimously agreed that this race is a social (not biological) construct.[54,55] If such a genetic group does not exist, then of course genetics could not be responsible for the mortality disparity.

Second, the mathematical assumptions underlying this type of "independence after regression analysis" and the "problem of residual confounding" are troublesome to say the least, involving issues such as difficulties with categorization, measurement, aggregation and non-commensurate indicators, in addition to contributors to racial differences not even touched on by measures of socioeconomic status (e.g., racism).[56] We have not been able to locate even one paper that has used this "independence after regression" model that has even noted these issues, let alone tried to explain how they might affect their findings as they cited biology as a risk factor for the mortality disparity.

The causes of the black:white disparity in breast cancer mortality is a complex matter that deserves serious analysis. We would like to make it clear that we are not suggesting that there are no racial biological differences in tumor characteristics. Biological risk factors other than tumor histology which could affect the observed mortality disparity might involve issues like obesity and estrogen status. Another possible factor involved in the racial disparity in breast cancer mortality is the use of hormone replacement therapy (HRT). It is established that white women use HRT more. In fact, since the Women's Health Initiative's report the use of HRT has declined a great deal, and following this so has the incidence of breast cancer among white (but not black) women.[57] This will decrease the breast cancer mortality rate among white women and thus increase the racial disparity.

However, we cannot see how these could generate the racial disparities in mortality that are the subject of this report, most of which have appeared recently and which vary substantially by the three analyzed geographies. Some authors discuss the possibility of a gene-environment interaction.[58] This may be a possibility, but here too we cannot envision how such an interaction would produce the nature of the racial disparities delineated in this paper. Rather, we hypothesize that these disparities are a function of racial disparities in screening and treatment. Such hypotheses are, of course, subject to empirical analysis. Until empirical verification these hypotheses remain just that.

Conclusion

Racial disparities in breast cancer mortality cannot be viewed outside the context of racism in the US. Misdirected focus on biological causes places the burden of this disparity on the innate genetic characteristics of the woman and not on external modifiable factors such as access and quality. As Sankar and her colleagues have written, "Overemphasis on genetics as a major explanatory factor in health disparities could lead researchers to miss factors that contribute to disparities more substantially and may also reinforce racial stereotypes, which may contribute to disparities in the first place."[59]

In a more general sense Cooper and his colleagues have noted that: "Minority groups, particularly blacks in the United States, are assumed to be genetically predisposed to virtually all common chronic diseases. The correlation between the use of unsupported genetic inferences and the social standing of a group is glaring evidence of bias and demonstrates how race is used both to categorize and to rank order subpopulations."[60]

It is easy for us to look back now and see the folly—and racism—of the claim that differential racial biology was responsible for the elevated prevalence of syphilis among black people in Alabama—so much so that it had to be studied as a unique entity.[61] We fear that current research claims about race, biology and breast cancer mortality similarly perpetuate racial stereotypes about disease and have the potential to harm black people still once again. This is why we must get this correct. As Brawley and Freeman have pointed out: "Deep ethical and moral questions [are raised] concerning how the research community, the American health care system, and society as a whole will move toward providing remedies for this unacceptable reality [of disparities in health]."[62] It is our hope that the analyses presented in the current report will help move this pursuit ahead.

References

1. Howlader N, Ries LA, Stinchcomb DG, Edwards BK. The impact of underreported Veterans Affairs data on national cancer statistics: Analysis using population-based SEER registries. *Journal of the National Cancer Institute.* 2009;101(7):533–536.

2. Hirschman J, Whitman S, Ansell D. The black:white disparity in breast cancer mortality: The example of Chicago. *Cancer Causes and Control.* 2007; 18(3):323–333.

3. Brawley OW. Disaggregating the effects of race and poverty on breast cancer outcomes. *Journal of the National Cancer Institute.* 2002;94(7):471–473.

4. Olopade OI, Fackenthal JD, Dunston G, Tainsky MA, Collins F, Whitfield-Broome C. Breast cancer genetics in African Americans. *Cancer.* 2003;97(1 suppl.):236–245.

5. Cunningham JE, Butler WM. Racial disparities in female breast cancer in South Carolina: Clinical evidence for a biological basis. *Breast Cancer Research and Treatment.* 2004;88(2):161–176.

6. Woodward WA, Huang EH, McNeese MD, et al. African-American race is associated with a poorer overall survival rate for breast cancer patients treated with mastectomy and doxorubicin-based chemotherapy. *Cancer.* 2006;107(11): 2662–2668.

7. Carey LA, Perou CM, Livasy CA, et al. Race, breast cancer subtypes, and survival in the Carolina Breast Cancer Study. *Journal of the American Medical Association.* 2006;295(21):2492–2502.

8. Albain KS, Unger JM, Crowley JJ, Coltman CA, Hershman DL. Racial disparities in cancer survival among randomized clinical trials patients of the Southwest Oncology Group. *Journal of the National Cancer Institute.* 2009; 101(14):984–992.

9. Anderson RN, Minino AM, Hoyert DL, Rosenberg HM. Comparability of cause of death between ICD-9 and ICD-10: Preliminary estimates. *National Vital Statistics Reports.* 2001;49(2):1–32.

10. US Bureau of the Census. 2000 Census: Internet release A, 2001. https://factfinder.census.gov/faces/nav/jsf/pages/index.xhtml.

11. Keppel KG, Pearcy JN, Klein RJ. Measuring progress in healthy people 2010. *Healthy People 2010 Statistical Notes.* 2004;25:1–16.

12. Kim HJ, Fay MP, Feuer EJ, Midthune DN. Permutation tests for join-point regression with applications to cancer rates. *Statistics in Medicine.* 2000; 19(3):335–351.

13. Jones BA, Patterson EA, Calvocoressi L. Mammography screening in African American women: Evaluating the research. *Cancer.* 2003;97(8):2047–2048.

14. Berry DA, Cronin KA, Plevritis SK, et al. Effect of screening and adjuvant therapy on mortality from breast cancer. *New England Journal of Medicine.* 2005;353(17):1784–1792.

15. Chu QD, Smith MH, Williams M, et al. Race/ethnicity has no effect on outcome for breast cancer patients treated at an academic center with a public hospital. *Cancer Epidemiology Biomarkers and Prevention.* 2009;18(8):2157–2161.

16. Tehranifar P, Neugut AI, Phelan JC, et al. Medical advances and racial/ethnic disparities in cancer survival. *Cancer Epidemiology Biomarkers and Prevention.* 2009;18(10):2701–2708.

17. Centers for Disease Control and Prevention. Breast cancer screening and socioeconomic status—35 metropolitan areas, 2000 and 2002. *Morbidity and Mortality Weekly Report.* 2005;54(39):981–985.

18. Whitman S, Shah AM, Silva A, Ansell D. Mammography screening in six diverse communities in Chicago—a population study. *Cancer Detection and Prevention.* 2007;31(2):166–172.

19. Smith-Bindman R, Chu P, Miglioretti DL, et al. Physician predictors of mammographic accuracy. *Journal of the National Cancer Institute.* 2005;97(5): 358–367.

20. Kagay CR, Quale C, Smith-Bindman R. Screening mammography in the American elderly. *American Journal of Preventive Medicine.* 2006;31(2):142–149.

21. Rauscher GH, Johnson TP, Cho YI, Walk JA. Accuracy of self-reported cancer-screening histories: A meta-analysis. *Cancer Epidemiology Biomarkers and Prevention.* 2008;17(4):748–757.

22. Olivotto IA, Gomi A, Bancej C, et al. Influence of delay to diagnosis on prognostic indicators of screen-detected breast carcinoma. *Cancer.* 2002;94(8): 2143–2150.

23. American College of Radiology (ACR). *Breast imaging reporting and data system (BI-RADS).* 4th ed. Reston, VA: American College of Radiology; 2003.

24. Rosenberg RD, Yankaskas BC, Abraham LA, et al. Performance benchmarks for screening mammography. *Radiology.* 2006;241(1):55–66.

25. May DS, Lee NC, Richardson LC, Giustozzi AG, Bobo JK. Mammography and breast cancer detection by race and Hispanic ethnicity: Results from a national program (United States). *Cancer Causes and Control.* 2000;11(8): 697–705.

26. Wang H, Karesen R, Hervik A, Thoresen SO. Mammography screening in Norway: Results from the first screening round in four counties and cost-effectiveness of a modeled nationwide screening. *Cancer Causes and Control.* 2001;12(1):39–45.

27. Sickles EA, Wolverton DE, Dee KE. Performance parameters for screening and diagnostic mammography: Specialist and general radiologists. *Radiology.* 2002;224(3):861–869.

28. Ryerson AB, Bernard VB, Major AC. *National breast and cervical cancer early detection program: 1991–2002 national report.* Atlanta: Centers for Disease Control and Prevention, National Center for Chronic Disease Prevention and Health Promotion, Division of Cancer Prevention and Control; 2005.

29. Moss M, Steinhauer J. Mammogram clinic's flaws highlight gaps in US rules. *New York Times.* October 24, 2002:A1.

30. Centers for Disease Control and Prevention. Breast cancer—screening data for assessing quality of services—New York, 2000–2003. *Morbidity and Mortality Weekly Report.* 2004;53(21):455–457.

31. Miglioretti DL, Smith-Bindman R, Abraham L, et al. Radiologist characteristics associated with interpretive performance of diagnostic mammography. *Journal of the National Cancer Institute.* 2007;99(24):1854–1863.

32. Jones BA, Culler CS, Kasl SV, Calvocoressi L. Is variation in quality of mammographic services race linked? *Journal of Health Care for the Poor and Underserved.* 2001;12(1):113–126.

33. Institute of Medicine and National Research Council. *Improving breast imaging quality standards.* Washington, DC: National Academies Press; 2005.

34. Barlow WE, Chi C, Carney PA, et al. Accuracy of screening mammography interpretation by characteristics of radiologists. *Journal of the National Cancer Institute.* 2004;96(24):1840–1850.

35. Hirschman J, Whitman S, Ansell D, Grabler P, Allgood K. *Breast cancer in Chicago: Eliminating disparities and improving mammography quality.* Chicago: Sinai Urban Health Institute; 2006.

36. Kerner JF, Yedidia M, Padgett D, et al. Realizing the promise of breast cancer screening: Clinical follow-up after abnormal screening among black women. *Preventive Medicine.* 2003;37(2):92–101.

37. Elmore JG, Nakano CY, Linden HM, Reisch LM, Ayanian JZ, Larson EB. Racial inequities in the timing of breast cancer detection, diagnosis, and initiation of treatment. *Medical Care.* 2005;43(2):141–148.

38. Jones BA, Reams K, Calvocoressi L, Dailey A, Kasl SV, Liston NM. Adequacy of communicating results from screening mammograms to African American and white women. *American Journal of Public Health.* 2007;97(3):531–538.

39. Smedley BD, Stih AY, Nelson AR, eds. *Unequal treatment: Confronting racial and ethnic disparities in health care.* Washington, DC: National Academies Press; 2003.

40. Epstein AM, Ayanian JZ, Keogh JH, et al. Racial disparities in access to renal transplantation—clinically appropriate or due to underuse or overuse? *New England Journal of Medicine.* 2000;343(21):1537–1544, 1532 preceding 1537.

41. Trivedi AN, Zaslavsky AM, Schneider EC, Ayanian JZ. Relationship between quality of care and racial disparities in Medicare health plans. *Journal of the American Medical Association.* 2006;296(16):1998–2004.

42. Gross GR, Smith BD, Wolf E, Andersen M. Racial disparities in cancer therapy—did the gap narrow between 1992 and 2002? *Cancer.* 2008;112(4):900–908.

43. Li CI, Malone KE, Daling JR. Differences in breast cancer stage, treatment, and survival by race and ethnicity. *Archives of Internal Medicine.* 2003;163(1):49–56.

44. Gorin SS, Heck JE, Cheng B, Smith SJ. Delays in breast cancer diagnosis and treatment by racial/ethnic group. *Archives of Internal Medicine.* 2006;166(20):2244–2252.

45. Schleinitz MD, DePalo D, Blume J, Stein M. Can differences in breast cancer utilities explain disparities in breast cancer care? *Journal of General Internal Medicine.* 2006;21(12):1253–1260.

46. Breen N, Wesley MN, Merrill RM, Johnson K. The relationship of socioeconomic status and access to minimum expected therapy among female breast cancer patients in the National Cancer Institute Black-White Cancer Survival Study. *Ethnicity and Disease.* 1999;9(1):111–125.

47. Institute of Medicine. *Committee on Quality of Health Care in America: Crossing the quality chasm: A new health system for the 21st century.* Washington, DC: National Academy Press; 2006.

48. Ansell D, Grabler P, Whitman S, et al. A community effort to reduce the black/white breast cancer mortality disparity in Chicago. *Cancer Causes and Control.* 2009;20(9):1681–1688.

49. Chlebowski RT, Chen Z, Anderson GL, et al. Ethnicity and breast cancer: Factors influencing differences in incidence and outcome. *Journal of the National Cancer Institute.* 2005;97(6):439–448.

50. Curtis E, Quale C, Haggstrom D, Smith-Bindman R. Racial and ethnic differences in breast cancer survival: How much is explained by screening, tumor severity, biology, treatment, comorbidities, and demographics? *Cancer.* 2008;112(1):171–180.

51. Smith-Bindman R, Miglioretti DL, Lurie N, et al. Does utilization of screening mammography explain racial and ethnic differences in breast cancer? *Annals of Internal Medicine.* 2006;144(8):541–553.

52. Freeman HP. The meaning of race in science—considerations for cancer research: Concerns of special populations in the National Cancer Program. *Cancer.* 1998;82(1):219–225.

53. Hunt LM, Megyesi MS. The ambiguous meanings of the racial/ethnic categories routinely used in human genetics research. *Social Science and Medicine.* 2008;66(2):349–361.

54. Duster T. *Backdoor to eugenics.* 2nd ed. New York: Routledge; 2003.

55. Allen TW. *The invention of the white race.* New York: Verso; 1997.

56. Kaufman JS, Cooper RS, McGee DL. Socioeconomic status and health in blacks and whites: The problem of residual confounding and the resiliency of race. *Epidemiology.* 1997;8(6):621–628.

57. Krieger N, Chen JT, Waterman PD. Decline in US breast cancer rates after the Women's Health Initiative: Socioeconomic and racial/ethnic differentials. *American Journal of Public Health.* 2010;100(suppl. 1):S132–S139.

58. McClintock MK, Conzen SD, Gehlert S, Masi C, Olopade F. Mammary cancer and social interactions: Identifying multiple environments that regulate gene expression throughout the life span. *Journals of Gerontology Series B, Psychological Sciences and Social Sciences.* 2005;60(special no. 1):32–41.

59. Sankar P, Cho MK, Condit CM, et al. Genetic research and health disparities. *Journal of the American Medical Association.* 2004;291(24):2985–2989.

60. Cooper RS, Kaufman JS, Ward R. Race and genomics. *New England Journal of Medicine.* 2003;348(12):1166–1170.

61. Jones JL. *Bad blood.* New York: Free Press; 1993.

62. Brawley OW, Freeman HP. Race and outcomes: Is this the end of the beginning for minority health research? *Journal of the National Cancer Institute.* 1999;91(22):1908–1909.

Black Women's Awareness of Breast Cancer Disparity and Perceptions of the Causes of Disparity

Karen Kaiser, Kenzie A. Cameron, Gina Curry,
and Melinda Stolley

Introduction

Black women face the greatest breast cancer mortality burden of any racial or ethnic group in the United States.[1] The black-white breast cancer disparity is particularly pronounced in Chicago: in 2007, black women in Chicago were 62% more likely to die of breast cancer than their white counterparts.[2] A city-wide task force concluded that the elevated disparity in Chicago is the result of inequalities in the distribution of quality health care in Chicago. Specifically, racial disparities in breast cancer mortality in Chicago result from unequal access to mammograms, mammograms of inferior quality, and inadequate access to quality treatment upon diagnosis.[2-4]

Little is known about knowledge of health disparities among minority populations themselves. A 2010 study found that 59% of adults in the U.S. were aware of racial and ethnic health disparities.[5] Although awareness of disparities was higher among black respondents, nearly half of blacks were unaware of disparities in specific health conditions that disproportionately affect them, such as infant mortality and HIV/AIDS.

Originally published in the *Journal of Community Health* 38 (2013): 766–72. © Springer Science+Business Media New York 2013. Reprinted with permission.

However, given the large breast cancer disparity in Chicago and recent local efforts to publicize and eliminate the disparity,[6] Chicago women may have a greater awareness of this local, salient health disparity. Hence, we sought to examine black women's awareness of breast cancer disparity in Chicago as well as their views of the causes of racial disparities in breast cancer. Perceptions of the causes of disparity are important because they influence support (or opposition) for specific policies to address health disparities. Prior research indicates that, consistent with the American emphasis on individual responsibility, the public views personal behaviors as the strongest influences on health.[7] In contrast, the "social determinants of health" perspective adopted by many health professionals views health disparities as resulting from factors outside of the individual, such as socioeconomic status, health policy, and the environment. These social factors in turn are believed to influence health behaviors and access to resources that protect health.[8–11] No work to date has examined views of the causes of disparity among a population living in the context of a large, well-documented, and grave health disparity. Thus, we examined black women's perceptions of the causes of breast cancer disparity and the extent to which disparity was seen as resulting from individual behaviors, such as seeking screening, or from societal factors, such as the unequal distribution of quality healthcare.

Methods

Four focus groups were conducted with adult black women ($N = 35$) in Chicago in 2011. The groups were held in community centers in predominantly black neighborhoods. We considered restricting our sample to women over age 40 as American Cancer Society guidelines recommend mammography screening beginning at age 40.[12] However, because black women are at greater risk of developing and dying from early onset breast cancer[13,14] we opted to include women under 40. Participants received $50 for their participation. All study procedures were approved by the Institutional Review Board of Northwestern University.

Focus groups were led by an experienced black female focus group moderator. Each participant provided informed consent and completed a short self-administered survey prior to the start of the focus group discussion. The survey assessed demographic characteristics, breast cancer screening history, and knowledge of racial disparities in breast cancer: "In your opinion, who is more likely to be diagnosed with breast cancer?" and "In your opinion, who is more likely to die from breast cancer?" The two disparity knowledge questions had the following response options: (1) black women, (2) white women, or (3) all women have the same chance of being diagnosed/dying from breast cancer. After the surveys were collected, group discussions began. Group discussions addressed views of breast cancer, knowledge and perceptions of breast cancer disparity, and women's sources of cancer information. A "flexible" moderator guide was used to lead the group through these topics while also pursuing unanticipated ideas that emerged in the discussion.[15]

Interview recordings were transcribed, and identifying information was removed from the transcripts. For the results described here, our analysis primarily relied on deductive strategies. First, each transcript and corresponding field notes were read in their entirety by the first author to gain a sense of the focus group content as a whole. After becoming familiar with the data, the first author reviewed participants' responses to the disparity knowledge questions. The first author divided responses according to whether participants viewed black women, white women, or neither group as being more affected by breast cancer. Next, the research assistant, who received training in qualitative data coding, independently reviewed the data and sorted the data into the same three categories. Any coding discrepancies were noted and reconciled. The two coders also independently categorized women's views of the causes of breast cancer disparity using the framework of Kim and colleagues (see table 11.1), originally developed to analyze causal explanations for coverage of health disparity in U.S. newspapers.[16] The categories succinctly capture both individual level (genetic, behavioral) and broader explanations (health care system, societal) of disparity. Catego-

TABLE 11.1 **Causal explanations for health disparities**

1. Genetic: racial and ethnic differences are due to genetic differences
2. Behavioral: racial and ethnic differences are due to differences in knowledge, attitudes, behaviors, or culture
3. Health care system: racial and ethnic differences are due to differences in access to health care, quality of care, or discrimination within health care
4. Societal: racial and ethnic differences are due to the social, physical, or environmental conditions groups live in (e.g., availability of healthy food, environmental toxins), including the availability of quality, appropriate health information

Note: Modified from Kim AE, Kumanyika S, Shive D, Igweatu U, Kim SH. 2010. "Coverage and framing of racial and ethnic health disparities in US newspapers, 1996–2005." *American Journal of Public Health.* 2010;100(suppl. 1):S224–S231.

ries were tested in initial coding and deemed to be exhaustive and mutually exclusive. Participant comments containing more than one of the four categories were coded as multi-causal by noting all relevant categories (e.g., behavioral + societal). Coding discrepancies were again noted and reconciled.

Results

Self-Administered Survey

Responses from the self-administered surveys are shown in tables 11.2 and 11.3. Almost three-quarters of the respondents reported knowing someone who had been diagnosed with breast cancer; over one-third had a family member who had been diagnosed with breast cancer. Nearly half of the participants knew someone who had died from breast cancer.

Although the majority of participants (62.9%) believed that all women have an equal chance of being diagnosed with breast cancer (table 11.3), almost one-third believed black women more likely, whereas only two believed that white women are more likely to be diagnosed. When asked who was more likely to die from breast cancer, none believed that whites were at highest risk. Responses were almost equally split between black

TABLE 11.2 **Description of sample: Age, mammogram history, and exposure to others with breast cancer ($N = 35$)**

Mean age	43 (19–76)
Ever had a mammogram?	60.0% ($N = 21$)
Ever had a mammogram? (women age $\geq$ 40, $N = 20$)	95.0% ($N = 19$)
Has anyone in your family been diagnosed with breast cancer?	34.3% ($N = 12$)
Has anyone close to you, but not in your family, such as a friend or coworker, been diagnosed with breast cancer?	71.4% ($N = 25$)
Have you known anyone who died from breast cancer?	48.6% ($N = 17$)

TABLE 11.3 **Views of racial differences in breast cancer outcomes ($N = 35$)**

In your opinion, who is more likely to be diagnosed with breast cancer?	
White women	5.7% ($N = 2$)
Black women	31.4% ($N = 11$)
All women have the same chance of being diagnosed with breast cancer	62.9% ($N = 22$)
In your opinion, who is more likely to die from breast cancer?	
White women	0% ($N = 0$)
Black women	48.6% ($N = 17$)
All women have the same chance of dying from breast cancer	51.4% ($N = 18$)

women being more likely to die from breast cancer and all women having the same chance.

Focus Group Results

The survey questions about knowledge of racial disparities were repeated during the focus group discussion. Participants typically did not distinguish between getting breast cancer (incidence) and dying of breast cancer (mortality). Additional probes were added to the focus group guide to prompt women to think about incidence and mortality separately. However, given the number of women who spoke of incidence and mortality interchangeably, we summarize all of the comments together as evidence of their views on how breast cancer *affects* black women versus white women.

None of the participants believed that breast cancer has a greater effect on white women. Several women described their view that breast cancer affects blacks and whites equally. These participants emphasized cancer's ability to strike anyone: "Cancer is an equal opportunity, evil attacker." "Anybody can get it." Other women specifically noted that cancer does not vary by race, age, or other individual characteristics: "It don't [*sic*] matter if you're black or white if you're susceptible to get it. It's just one of those things in life that happens to women." "It isn't any certain particular person who can get it, and there isn't anybody who can't get it. . . . We're all at risk, everyone. We're all women. We've got the same organs and everything, so I personally think that it's among all women." Participants who believed that all women are at equal risk of cancer often noted their fear of cancer or sadness about cancer's ability to strike at random: "I don't believe cancer has a color, an age, or anything. . . . It's just sickening, and the word cancer is sickening to me." "Cancer doesn't have any color. You can get it, anybody, any age, you can get cancer. It's really depressing."

Compared to comments about breast cancer affecting all women, comments about breast cancer having a greater impact on blacks were more numerous, longer, and contained more personal stories. Moreover, women who spoke of breast cancer's greater effect on black women often spontaneously described *why* breast cancer has a unique impact on black women.

Participants most often mentioned behavioral reasons for breast cancer disparity. According to the coding categories of Kim and colleagues, responses were coded as behavioral explanations if they referred to knowledge, attitudes, behaviors, or culture.[16] Typical behavioral explanations included black women's lack of awareness of breast cancer: "Honestly, I feel like . . . White women are more educated about it." One woman articulated the belief that women are responsible for being informed about breast cancer. She placed the blame for poorer cancer outcomes on black women, noting that black women are "our own worst enemy":

> I kind of disagree with the fact that there's not enough information. I believe that we just don't go and look for it. . . . We are our own worst enemy. You have to educate yourself in things especially things that are of some concern to you, and a lot of women don't. . . . There is plenty of information out here. You can really just ask your doctor. If you have a doctor you've been with and you're comfortable with him . . . they take an oath to give you that information, and if you don't get enough information go look it up. Do you know what I mean? So it's not that the information is not there, I believe we have just become complacent with the basic, whatever it is, and we don't go out and try to find out more. And that's what's really killing us.

Participants also noted that blacks are less aware of and do not adhere to cancer screening guidelines. "More black women die from it because they're not taught to go get their regular check-ups and mammograms, so they might have it and not know it, so it gets worse and they die of it. . . ." "I think black women [do worse] because in general we don't get our mammograms when we should." Disparities were also thought to be due to the reluctance to go to the doctor among the black community: "Black women [are more affected] because they don't go to the doctor's and get checked." The reluctance to go to the doctor was linked to a failure to care for themselves: "I think that breast cancer is now the majority in black women . . . because we haven't really been persistent to go get checked out. It's been a long while since . . . some black women have really been taking care of their bodies the way they're supposed to be. So that's why I think it's more black women than it is white women."

The failure to seek medical care or to undergo treatment for cancer was also linked to a cultural tradition of healing illness at home:

> You know, when I was a kid it was like I do not remember going to the doctor except for a school physical. Everything else was treated at home. So I think

that it's just you know awareness and the way we are raised because my mom and dad was from the south and so they had all the home remedies, and if they didn't know they were calling their sisters or brothers from the south or a cousin or somebody.

. . . A lot of times blacks think it could be self-healed. Sometimes they might go and have the surgery done and then start the treatment and then think that they are better (and quit the treatment) . . . so a lot of women just don't think they need the treatment, you know, and they eventually die from it.

Fear of cancer or fatalistic beliefs about cancer were also seen as contributing to avoidance of doctors and to worse outcomes among black women. Participants noted that because of the fear of cancer blacks do not want to know that they have cancer. "You know, we don't like to go to the doctor, especially me, and it's not just breast cancer, although that's the forum that we're holding today; it's all types of cancer that we are just afraid of because we don't know the prognosis, we don't know the treatment, and we don't care to know." "I think that it's probably more deadly to African Americans. . . . My aunt doesn't want to know. She does not want anybody to ever tell her she has cancer because to her it's a death sentence."

[. . .]

A few participants attributed black women's breast cancer outcomes to the health care system. One woman noted a reason that women may be discouraged from taking advantage of free screening:

I went to a free mammogram, and the nurse so happened to be African American, and out of all the people that were there she was the only one that seemed to be irritated because we were coming to get service. And I just . . . I kept watching that, and it was like that's the reason right there most people don't get out into the community to get these resources or take advantage of the resources.

Two other women noted that long wait times at the institutions serving poor women lead to delayed diagnosis and worse prognosis:

Sometimes (women) will be on the waiting list, and by the time it's time for them to get the mammogram checked out it's already in stage four.

When you do find something, then they'll urge you on to get a biopsy or something at County (hospital), and you wait 6 months to go and get that particular treatment, and that's 6 months that you're going untreated, whereas if you had insurance, [you could go to] U of C or something, or Northwestern, and that next week or that day they're going to try and pencil you in to get you the help that you need. But when you're poor or when you don't have insurance you can be diagnosed in March and won't make it to the mammogram until August.

One woman explicitly expressed a belief that lack of resources among black women led to preventable breast cancer death:

I don't see color, black or white, when I think of breast cancer, really. But I do notice, I could be wrong, but a lot in my reading is about more African American women that are dying because they don't have the resources or the money or the insurance or [aren't] able to see a doctor . . . and a lot of them to me are dying unnecessarily because they weren't able to get treatment and everything. So sometimes I see in the African American community unnecessary death due to breast cancer because they weren't diagnosed early enough.

None of the participants discussed either genetic or societal (i.e., availability of healthy food) explanations for racial disparities in breast cancer independent of other explanations. Several women referenced multiple types of causal explanations. For example, one participant endorsed both behavioral and health care system explanations—she believed that disparities result from an unhealthy diet and from limited access to health care. One participant named all three factors in her perceptions of disparities: behavioral (unwillingness to talk about cancer), health care (disrespectful treatment of the uninsured at health clinics), and societal factors (toxins in food).

Discussion

In this exploratory study of black women's views of local cancer disparities, over half of participants were unaware of racial disparities in breast cancer mortality. These results are similar to the 2010 survey of adults in the U.S., in which nearly half of black respondents were unaware of disparities in health conditions that disproportionately affect them.[5] Our findings are surprising given that we assessed awareness within a community facing unusually large breast cancer disparity—black women in the U.S. are 40% more likely to die of breast cancer,[17] while black women in Chicago face a 62% increased risk of breast cancer mortality.[2]

The participants who did indicate that black women with breast cancer fared worse than white women overwhelmingly placed responsibility for disparity on individual behaviors and community culture. In particular, the women linked blacks' poorer outcomes to a lack of awareness of cancer screening and to women's failure to be screened or treated for breast cancer. However, data on mammography screening rates in Illinois indicate that black women are more likely to have received a mammogram in the last 2 years than white women,[18] although national survey data may overestimate screening rates for low socioeconomic status minority women.[19] A local survey on mammography in six Chicago community areas in 2002–2003 found high rates of mammography in Chicago, with 74–90% of women over age 40 reporting receipt of mammography screening. In the most economically disadvantaged community surveyed, 77% of black women reported having received a mammogram.[20] Rates of repeat screening (i.e., receiving 2 mammograms in 3 years) were lower, with 44–62% of women reporting receipt of more than one mammogram in the previous 3 years. Thus, it appears that black women are being screened but their screening is not occurring consistently enough to ensure the best detection of cancer.

[. . .]

References

1. National Cancer Institute. Cancer health disparities fact sheet. 2008. http://www.cancer.gov/cancertopics/factsheet/cancer-health-disparities/disparities.

2. Metropolitan Chicago Breast Cancer Task Force. *Annual report back to the community.* Chicago; 2010.

3. Metropolitan Chicago Breast Cancer Task Force. *Improving quality and reducing disparities in breast cancer in metropolitan Chicago.* Chicago; 2007.

4. Whitman S, Ansell D, Orsi J, Francois T. The racial disparity in breast cancer mortality. *Journal of Community Health.* 2011;36(4):588–596.

5. Benz JK, Espinosa O, Welsh V, Fontes A. Awareness of racial and ethnic health disparities has improved only modestly over a decade. *Health Affairs (Millwood).* 2011;30(10):1860–1867.

6. Ansell D, Grabler P, Whitman S, et al. A community effort to reduce the black/white breast cancer mortality disparity in Chicago. *Cancer Causes and Control.* 2009;20(9):1681–1688.

7. Robert SA, Booske BC. US opinions on health determinants and social policy as health policy. *American Journal of Public Health.* 2011;101(9):1655–1663.

8. Link BG, Phelan J. Social conditions as fundamental causes of disease. *Journal of Health and Social Behaviour.* 1995;(extra issue):80–94.

9. Marmot M, Wilkinson R. *Social determinants of health.* Oxford: Oxford University Press; 2006.

10. Phelan JC, Link BG, Tehranifar P. Social conditions as fundamental causes of health inequalities: Theory, evidence, and policy implications. *Journal of Health and Social Behaviour.* 2010;51 (suppl.):S28–S40.

11. McKinlay JB, Marceau LD. To boldly go. *American Journal of Public Health.* 2000;90(1):25–33.

12. Smith RA, Saslow D, Sawyer KA, et al. American Cancer Society guidelines for breast cancer screening: Update 2003. *CA: A Cancer Journal for Clinicians.* 2003;53(3):141–169.

13. Shavers VL, Harlan LC, Stevens JL. Racial/ethnic variation in clinical presentation, treatment, and survival among breast cancer patients under age 35. *Cancer.* 2003;97(1):134–147.

14. Newman LA, Bunner S, Carolin K, et al. Ethnicity related differences in the survival of young breast carcinoma patients. *Cancer.* 2002;95(1):21–27.

15. Charmaz K. *Constructing grounded theory: A practical guide through qualitative analysis.* Thousand Oaks, CA: Sage; 2006.

16. Kim AE, Kumanyika S, Shive D, Igweatu U, Kim SH. Coverage and framing of racial and ethnic health disparities in US newspapers, 1996–2005. *American Journal of Public Health.* 2010;100(suppl. 1):S224–S231.

17. Siegel R, Naishadham D, Jemal A. Cancer statistics, 2012. *CA: A Cancer Journal for Clinicians.* 2012;62(1):10–29.

18. The Kaiser Family Foundation. Percent of women age 50 and older who report having had a mammogram within the last 2 years, by race/ethnicity, 2010. 2012. https://www.kff.org/statedata.

19. Peek ME, Han JH. Disparities in screening mammography: Current status, interventions and implications. *Journal of General Internal Medicine.* 2004; 19(2):184–194.

20. Whitman S, Shah AM, Silva A, Ansell D. Mammography screening in six diverse communities in Chicago—a population study. *Cancer Detection and Prevention.* 2007;31(2):166–172.

Racial/Ethnic Disparities in Hypertension Prevalence

Reconsidering the Role of Chronic Stress

Margaret T. Hicken, Hedwig Lee, Jeffrey Morenoff,
James S. House, and David R. Williams

Racial and ethnic disparities in hypertension are some of the most widely studied and consequential sources of social disparities in health in the United States.[1-3] For example, recent prevalence estimates show that roughly 40% of black adults but only 30% of white adults have hypertension.[4] In addition, the incidence of hypertension occurs at younger ages for blacks than whites.[1] These disparities are reflected in the larger burden of hypertension-related health and economic costs carried by non-white than white Americans. For example, mortality rates attributable to hypertension are roughly 15 deaths per 100,000 people for white men and women; the mortality rate for black women is 40 per 100,000 and more than 50 per 100,000 for black men.[5] Among all health conditions, hypertension accounts for the greatest portion of disparities in years of lost life.[6] Economically speaking, if black Americans had the hypertension prevalence of white Americans, about $400 million would be saved in out-of-pocket health care expenses, about $2 billion would be saved in private insurance costs, and $375 million would be saved from Medicare and Medicaid—per year.[7]

Originally published in the *American Journal of Public Health* 104, no. 1 (January 2014): 117–23, by the American Public Health Association.

Despite the tremendous amount of research devoted to clarifying the factors that generate these disparities, most studies find that they persist after adjustment for a wide range of socioeconomic, behavioral, and biomedical risk factors.[8] In fact, although disparities exist for several of these risk factors (e.g., socioeconomic status), numerous studies have shown no disparities in many others (e.g., smoking, obesity for men, lipid profile).[2] Despite substantial investment in interventions to eliminate hypertension disparities, evidence suggests that these disparities have actually grown over the past few decades, suggesting that numerous unknown factors drive disparities in hypertension.[3,9]

Chronic Stress and Racial Disparities in Hypertension

Growing evidence links chronic psychological stress to cardiovascular disease, including hypertension, and suggests that the impact of stress may be as important as other risk factors, such as cholesterol.[10] In particular, researchers argue that because of sustained effects on numerous physiological systems, the anticipation of or perseveration about (i.e., continual, perhaps involuntary, repetition of a thought) a stressor (e.g., financial or marital difficulties) is what gives chronic stress its toxic qualities.[11] Indeed, researchers have reported that the physiological (i.e., autonomic) stress effects attributable to the combination of stressors and worry are similar to the physiological effects of smoking.[12]

Many theorize that chronic stress is an important determinant of racial/ethnic disparities in health, including hypertension.[9,13] Moreover, researchers posit that perceptions of racial/ethnic discrimination (defined as chronic or acute experiences with unfair treatment or abusive behavior because of their race/ethnicity) are an important mechanism through which disparities in health, including hypertension, are produced and maintained.[10,14–16] However, empirical evidence has been mixed possibly because discrimination measures generally do not account for the anticipation or perseveration that may make this type of stressor pathogenic.[17,18]

Some have begun to examine the anticipatory and perseverative stress associated with racial and ethnic discrimination. For example, researchers recently reported that anticipation of ethnic discrimination was inversely associated with health in a Swedish sample.[19,20] In the United

States, researchers reported poorer cardiovascular outcomes, including less elasticity in large arterial vessels and higher blood pressure reactivity for those reporting higher than lower levels of anticipated racial discrimination, which the authors termed *racism-related vigilance*.[21,22]

We examined the role of racism-related vigilance in racial/ethnic disparities in hypertension prevalence in a population-based sample. We first examined whether vigilance mediated racial/ethnic disparities in hypertension prevalence. In other words, we assessed whether racial/ethnic disparities in hypertension prevalence were reduced when we accounted for racial/ethnic disparities in vigilance. In light of racial/ethnic disparities in exposure to stressors (e.g., vigilance), many researchers theorize that mediation is an important mechanism by which stress links race/ethnicity to health.[9,23-25] However, there is a dearth of empirical evidence, which may be attributable to challenges in the measurement of racially salient stress.[13,25] Second, because it may be that racism-related vigilance is salient only for non-white groups, we examined whether vigilance modified racial/ethnic disparities in hypertension prevalence. In other words, we asked whether increasing levels of vigilance were associated with wider racial/ethnic disparities in hypertension prevalence. The clinical and public health implications of this research are substantial because chronic psychological stress is increasingly recognized as an important risk factor for hypertension and for cardiovascular disease more broadly.

Methods

We used data from the Chicago Community Adult Health Study, a cross-sectional survey designed to examine the biological, social, and environmental correlates of adult physical and mental health. The study collected a multistage probability sample of 3105 adults, aged 18 years and older, living in Chicago, Illinois, stratified into 343 neighborhood clusters. Neighborhood clusters usually comprised 2 census tracts with meaningful physical and social boundaries. Study staff conducted face-to-face interviews with and took direct physical measurements from 1 respondent per household between May 2001 and March 2003, with a response rate of 71.8%.

Variables

Trained technicians obtained 3 seated blood pressure measurements about 1 minute apart with Omron oscillographic devices (Omron Healthcare Inc., Lake Forest, IL). Measurements were taken in the middle of the interview after the participant had been seated for approximately 45 to 60 minutes. We took the average of the last 2 blood pressure measurements taken or, if only 2 were recorded, the average of those 2 blood pressure measurements. We defined hypertension as having a systolic blood pressure of 140 millimeters of mercury or higher, a diastolic blood pressure of 90 millimeters of mercury or higher, a report of antihypertensive medication use in the past 12 months, or a report of being told by a physician that the respondent had hypertension, a definition consistent with the literature on cardiovascular disease from the American Heart Association.[5]

We based racism-related vigilance measures on ethnographic research describing how participants anticipated and prepared for racial discrimination.[26,27] We created a scale from responses to the following questions: In your day-to-day life, how often do you do the following things: (1) try to prepare for possible insults from other people before leaving home? (2) feel that you always have to be very careful about your appearance to get good service or avoid being harassed? and (3) try to avoid certain social situations and places? Responses were on a Likert-like scale (0 = never, 1 ≤ once/year, 2 = a few times/year, 3 = a few times/month, and 4 ≥ once/week). We reverse-coded responses and summed to create a continuous scale, with higher values representing higher levels of vigilance (Cronbach α = 0.66). We categorized respondents as non-Hispanic white (white), non-Hispanic black (black), Hispanic, and non-Hispanic other (which included American Indian, Asian, and Pacific Islander). Because the last racial category constituted only 4% of the sample and was a mixture of races, making interpretation difficult, we reported these results in the tables for completeness, but did not analyze them.

Analyses

For descriptive analyses, we estimated means with standard errors of continuous variables and percentages of categorical variables in the total sample and by race/ethnicity. We included standard errors rather than standard deviations because we used multiply imputed data. We also estimated the percentages of each response of the vigilance measure in the total sample and by race/ethnicity. We used the t test and the χ^2 test to test for differences by race/ethnicity. For our main analyses, we regressed hypertension on race/ethnicity, vigilance, their interaction, and covariates with logit models. We first regressed hypertension prevalence on race/ethnicity, with control for age, gender, and immigrant generation ($\geq$ third, second, first; model 1). We then added education ($<$ 12, 12–15, $>$ 15 years) and annual household income (logged; model 2).

To examine whether vigilance mediated racial/ethnic disparities in hypertension, we then ran a series of 3 models, as recommended in the literature.[28] In separate models, we regressed vigilance on race/ethnicity in a linear model and hypertension prevalence on vigilance in a logit model, with control for the variables in model 2, except race/ethnicity. We did not show these results in the tables, because, although 2 criteria for mediation were met (i.e., race/ethnicity was associated with vigilance, and vigilance was associated with hypertension prevalence), the third criterion was not met (the addition of vigilance to model 2 [i.e., model 3] did not attenuate the association between race/ethnicity and hypertension prevalence).

To examine whether vigilance modified racial/ethnic disparities in hypertension, we added the interaction between race/ethnicity and vigilance (model 4). In our final model, we controlled for numerous additional hypertension risk factors: body mass index (defined as weight in kilograms divided by the square of height in meters), average intensity of weekly physical activity (0 = in bed or chair or no exercise, 1 = light exercise, 2 = light–moderate exercise, 3 = moderate–heavy exercise, 4 = heavy exercise), smoking status (never, former, current), average number of alcoholic drinks per month, and diabetes status (report of being told by a physician that the respondent had diabetes). In this model, to examine the role of racism-related vigilance in the presence of perceived discrimination, we also included 2 widely used measures of perceived unfair treatment (model 5).[14] We measured major events of unfair treatment as the sum of affirmative responses to the following 4 questions: Have you ever been unfairly (1) fired or denied a promotion? (2) not hired for a job? (3) treated by the police? (4) prevented from moving into a neighborhood? We measured everyday unfair treatment on a scale created from the following questions: In your day-to-day life, how often (1) are you treated with less courtesy or respect than other people? (2) are you threatened or harassed? (3) do you receive poorer service than other people at restaurants and stores? (4) do people act as if you are not smart? (5) do people act as if they are afraid of you? Responses were on a Likert-like scale (1 = ≥ once/week, 2 = a few times/month, 3 = a few times/year, 4 = ≥ once/year, 5 = never). We reverse-coded and summed responses to create a continuous scale in which higher numbers represented reports of more frequent unfair activity.

We calculated the partial effects of vigilance for each racial/ethnic group after estimation as the product of a vigilance coefficient (i.e., the association between vigilance and hypertension prevalence for whites) and the appropriate interaction coefficient (i.e., the association between vigilance and hypertension prevalence for blacks or Hispanics, beyond the association for whites). We estimated the partial effects while holding covariates at their reference category (for categorical variables) or mean (for continuous variables).

We handled missing information on blood pressure, income, and vigilance in 2 ways, according to the amount of missing data and existence of influential outliers. First, for variables with substantial missing information, we multiply imputed blood pressure ($n = 155$) and income ($n = 501$) data with IVEware 0.2 (University of Michigan, Ann Arbor) via SAS 9.2 (SAS Institute, Cary, NC). Second, we excluded respondents with missing information on vigilance ($n = 11$) from final analyses, for a final sample size of 3094. In sensitivity analyses, we ran all models on the unimputed data set, and the results were similar to those presented (results not shown). We also included different transformations of the vigilance measure, specifically continuous measures, which we squared and cubed, and an ordinal measure of the quartiles of the distribution (data not shown, but qualitatively similar to those presented). To examine whether this vigilance measure was different than other stress measures, we included a stressful life events inventory in model 4 in sensitivity analyses. Results were nearly identical to those presented. We weighted all analyses to account for complex survey design, differential selection into the sample, nonresponse, and household size. With respect to age, race/ethnicity, and gender, the distribution of the weighted sample and the 2000 Census estimates were comparable to the City of Chicago. We conducted all analyses in Stata 11.0MP (StataCorp, College Station, TX) with both the MI and SVY suite of commands to account for the multiply imputed data and complex survey design, respectively.

Results

Descriptive statistics for hypertension prevalence and the covariates, broken down by race/ethnicity, are presented in table 12.1. Similar to national estimates, hypertension in this sample was significantly more prevalent among blacks (49%) than whites (33%) and Hispanics (32%). Vigilance was highest among blacks (mean = 3.8; SE = 0.1), followed by Hispanics (mean = 2.5; SE = 0.1) and whites (mean = 1.8; SE = 0.1). Furthermore, blacks were more likely to report the highest frequency of vigilant behaviors. For example, 14% of blacks reported preparing for insults weekly; only 2% of whites and 5% of Hispanics reported this type of vigilance.

Odds ratios (ORs) from logistic regression models for the race/ethnicity dummy variables, the vigilance scale, and interactions between race/ethnicity and vigilance are reported in table 12.2. Blacks and Hispanics had a higher likelihood of hypertension than whites, after sequential adjustment for age, gender, and immigrant generation (model 1) and then income and education (model 2).

We examined the mediating role of vigilance in the association between race/ethnicity and hypertension prevalence in 3 models, as discussed in the literature.[28] First, we examined the association between race/ethnicity and vigilance and found that, after adjustment for the covariates in model 2, blacks reported higher levels of vigilance than did whites (b = 1.51; 95% confidence interval [CI] = 1.18, 1.83). Hispanics did not differ from whites in levels of vigilance (b = 0.92; 95% CI = 0.54, 1.31). Second, we examined the association between vigilance and hypertension prevalence and found that, after adjustment for the covariates in model 2 except race/ethnicity, vigilance was associated with a greater likelihood of hypertension (OR = 1.04; 95% CI = 1.00, 1.08). Third, we added vigilance to model 2 and examined whether the disparities in hypertension prevalence were attenuated (model 3). The race/ethnicity coefficients were nearly unchanged.

We then examined the modifying role of vigilance on the association between race/ethnicity and hypertension prevalence. In model 4, we estimated this association separately for each racial/ethnic group through the introduction of interaction terms. With these interaction terms, the race/ethnicity coefficients indicated the racial/ethnic disparities in hypertension prevalence, when vigilance was zero. Blacks still showed

TABLE 12.1 **Sociodemographic and health characteristics in the total sample and by race/ethnicity: Chicago Community Adult Health Study, 2001–2003**

Characteristic	Total sample (n = 3094), % or mean ± SE	Non-Hispanic white (n = 981), % or mean ± SE	Non-Hispanic black (n = 1233), % or mean ± SE	Hispanic (n = 800), % or mean ± SE	Non-Hispanic other (n = 80), % or mean ± SE	P Black-white[a]	P Hispanic-white[b]	P Hispanic-black[c]
Hypertension[d]	38	33	49	32	26	<.001	.771	<.001
Vigilance score[e]	2.7 ± 0.1	1.8 ± 0.1	3.8 ± 0.1	2.5 ± 0.1	2.3 ± 0.3	<.001	<.001	<.001
Vigilance quartile								
1 (lowest)	37	45	27	44	37	<.001	.036	<.001
2	8	10	6	6	7			
3	20	23	17	16	32			
4	34	22	51	34	23			
Age (yr.)	42.4 ± 0.4	44.4 ± 0.8	44.1 ± 0.6	38.1 ± 0.7	37.9 ± 2.3	.783	<.001	<.001
Women	53	50	58	52	43	.007	.659	.029
Immigrant generation								
First	27	19	2	63	69	<.001	<.001	<.001
Second	14	16	1	26	17			
≥ Third	59	65	97	11	14			
Education (yr.)								
<12	23	11	24	44	4	<.001	<.001	<.001
12–15	49	44	59	45	36			
≥16	28	45	18	10	60			
Household income[f]	4.9 ± 0.3	7.0 ± 0.7	3.5 ± 0.2	3.5 ± 0.1	3.7 ± 0.4	<.001	<.001	.01
BMI, kg/m^2	28.2 ± 0.2	26.5 ± 0.2	29.6 ± 0.3	29.3 ± 0.3	25.2 ± 0.4	<.001	<.001	.424
Physical activity[g]	4.0 ± 0.0	4.1 ± 0.1	4.0 ± 0.1	4.0 ± 0.1	4.4 ± 0.2	.281	.830	.367
Alcohol use[h]	13.9 ± 0.8	17.2 ± 1.4	14.1 ± 1.4	9.5 ± 0.9	10.1 ± 2.2	.101	<.001	.004

Smoking status							
Current	25	26	31	18	19	<.001	<.001	<.001
Former	20	26	18	16	16			
Never	55	49	51	66	66			
Diabetes[i]	7	4	10	8	8	<.001	.004	.193
Everyday discrimination experiences[j]	3.7 ± 0.1	3.3 ± 0.2	4.7 ± 0.1	2.9 ± 0.2	3.4 ± 0.4	<.001	<.001	.088
Major discrimination experiences[k]	1.7 ± 0.1	1.0 ± 0.1	2.8 ± 0.1	1.3 ± 0.1	1.4 ± 0.3	<.001	.008	<.001

Note: BMI = body mass index. Results reported are percentages unless otherwise indicated. Standard deviations are not available with multiply imputed data. Results are weighted to account for complex survey design. Columns within a categorical variable sum to 100% (with some error caused by rounding).

[a]Test for difference between non-Hispanic black and non-Hispanic white.

[b]Test for difference between Hispanic and non-Hispanic white.

[c]Test for difference between Hispanic and non-Hispanic black.

[d]Defined as systolic blood pressure ≥ 140 mm Hg, diastolic blood pressure ≥ 90, report of antihypertensive medication use in the past 12 mo, or report of being told by a physician that respondent had hypertension.

[e]Range: 0 (never) to 4 (≥ once/wk).

[f]Multiple of $10,000.

[g]Range: 0 (in bed or chair or no exercise) to 4 (heavy exercise).

[h]Average drinks/mo.

[i]Report of being told by a physician that respondent had diabetes.

[j]Range: 1 (≥ once/wk) to 5 (never).

[k]Range: 0 to 4 affirmative answers.

TABLE 12.2 **Odds ratios of hypertension for race/ethnicity, vigilance, and the interaction between race/ethnicity and vigilance: Chicago Community Adult Health Study, 2001–2003**

Variable	Model 1[a] OR (95% CI)	Model 2[b] OR (95% CI)	Model 3[b] OR (95% CI)	Model 4[b] OR (95% CI)	Model 5[c] OR (95% CI)
Race/ethnicity					
Non-Hispanic white (ref.)	1.00	1.00	1.00	1.00	1.00
Non-Hispanic black	2.26 (1.74, 2.94)	1.99 (1.50, 2.63)	1.93 (1.45, 2.56)	1.53 (1.09, 2.15)	1.27 (0.89, 1.81)
Hispanic	2.03 (1.42, 2.91)	1.74 (1.19, 2.52)	1.71 (1.17, 2.48)	1.39 (0.90, 2.15)	1.10 (0.71, 1.70)
Non-Hispanic other	1.40 (0.68, 2.85)	1.49 (0.72, 3.08)	1.47 (0.71, 3.05)	1.50 (0.66, 3.41)	1.63 (0.69, 3.81)
Vigilance			1.02 (0.99, 1.06)	0.95 (0.87, 1.03)	0.94 (0.86, 1.03)
Interactions					
Non-Hispanic black * vigilance				1.10 (1.00, 1.21)	1.11 (1.00, 1.22)
Hispanic * vigilance				1.11 (1.01, 1.23)	1.12 (1.01, 1.24)
Non-Hispanic other * vigilance				1.00 (0.75, 1.35)	0.99 (0.72, 1.35)
Partial effects of vigilance[d]					
Non-Hispanic white				0.95 (0.87, 1.03)	0.94 (0.86, 1.03)
Non-Hispanic black				1.04 (1.00, 1.09)	1.04 (0.99, 1.09)
Hispanic				1.05 (0.99, 1.12)	1.06 (0.95, 1.13)

Note: CI = confidence interval; OR = odds ratio. Results are weighted to account for complex survey design.

[a]Included covariates age, gender, and immigrant generation.

[b]Added income and education to covariates in model 1.

[c]Added smoking, physical activity, alcohol use, body mass index, diabetes, everyday discrimination, and major discrimination to covariates in models 2–4.

[d]Calculated after estimation as the product of the vigilance and interaction terms.

a greater likelihood of hypertension than whites, but the difference in odds was smaller than in previous models. Hispanics no longer showed a greater likelihood of hypertension than whites. The vigilance coefficient in model 4 indicated that whites (the reference racial/ethnic category) did not show an association between vigilance and hypertension prevalence. Furthermore, as shown by the interaction terms, the association for both blacks and Hispanics was positive and statistically significantly different from that of whites. The product of the vigilance and interaction terms showed the race/ethnicity-specific associations between vigilance and hypertension prevalence (table 12.2). Vigilance had a significant and positive association with hypertension prevalence among blacks (OR = 1.04; 95% CI = 1.00, 1.09), meaning that a 1-point increase in vigilance was associated with a 4% increase in the odds of hypertension. This association was similar for Hispanics, but only reached marginal statistical significance (OR = 1.05; 95% CI = 0.99, 1.12). Vigilance was not significantly associated with hypertension prevalence for whites (OR = 0.95; 95% CI = 0.87, 1.03).

The significant interactions in model 4 between vigilance and both black and Hispanic race/ethnicity suggest that black-white and Hispanic-white disparities in hypertension varied significantly over levels of vigilance. These associations are seen more clearly in figure 12.1, which shows plots of the predicted probabilities of hypertension prevalence for blacks and whites and Hispanics and whites. As vigilance scores increased, the predicted probability of hypertension increased for blacks and Hispanics but not whites, which yielded an increased racial/ethnic disparity in hypertension prevalence.

After adjustment for hypertension risk factors and measures of discrimination (model 5), the racial/ethnic disparity in hypertension prevalence when vigilance was zero was attenuated for both blacks and Hispanics and was no longer statistically significant for blacks (OR = 1.27; 95% CI = 0.89, 1.81; table 12.2). The other coefficients in the interaction did not change markedly with further adjustment of the hypertension risk factors. These results were nearly identical to a separate model that included the hypertension risk factors but did not include the discrimination measures (results not shown).

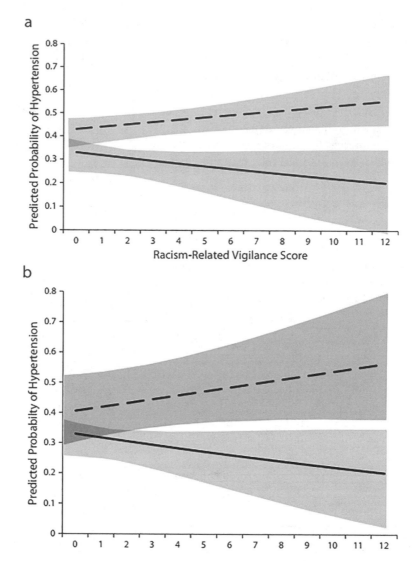

FIGURE 12.1. Association between racism-related vigilance score and predicted probability of hypertension prevalence for (*a*) non-Hispanic black vs. non-Hispanic white adults and (*b*) Hispanic vs. non-Hispanic white adults: Chicago Community Adult Health Study, 2001–2003

Note: Results weighted to account for complex survey design and adjusted for age, gender, immigrant generation, education, and annual household income. The dashed lines represent the association for (*a*) blacks and (*b*) Hispanics. The solid lines represent the association for whites. The shaded areas represent the 95% confidence interval.

Discussion

We examined the notion that a racially salient stressor contributes to racial/ethnic disparities in hypertension prevalence. Our results suggest that the stress of racism-related vigilance, with its anticipatory and perseverative qualities, is an important determinant of racial disparities in hypertension. We found that blacks reported higher levels of vigilance than both whites and Hispanics. Not only did they have the highest mean vigilance score, but they were also more likely to report weekly vigilance than were the other racial/ethnic groups. We found that vigilance was positively associated with hypertension prevalence for blacks but not whites. As vigilance increased, the black-white disparity in hypertension prevalence also increased. Although not statistically significant, our results suggested similar experiences for Hispanics. Research has shown that racial bias and discrimination are embedded in numerous domains of US society that are relevant to health, ranging from education to employment to neighborhood quality to health care access and quality.[29-33]

Although bias and discrimination are pervasive, it is the certain threat of discrimination combined with the uncertainty of exactly which situations it will occur in that is likely driving vigilant behavior. Uncertainty is derived from at least 2 sources: first, bias and discrimination are not present in every situation, and, second, the nature of modern discrimination is often subtle and ambiguous.[34] The resulting heightened vigilance reflects the reality that one can never truly relax and must always be prepared for discrimination. For example, psychologists use the term *racial microaggressions* to describe

> brief and commonplace daily verbal, behavioral, or environmental indignities, whether intentional or unintentional, that communicate hostile, derogatory, or negative racial slights and insults toward people of color.[34]

Moreover, psychologists have shown that uncertainty regarding a stressor results in vigilance about that stressor.[35]

Social scientists have documented that blacks prepare themselves daily for bias and discrimination through such behaviors as the anticipation of discrimination and the negotiation of social spaces (e.g., avoiding certain places).[27] The perseverative and anticipatory nature of vigilance sets it apart from traditional notions of perceived racial discrimination. For decades, a large scientific and lay literature has provided evidence of both the perseverative and anticipatory consequences of interpersonal and societal discrimination. In qualitative studies, social scientists often report on the way blacks continually think about the potential for discrimination.[36] It may be that racism-related vigilance is particularly toxic for blacks because it reflects living with the threat of and preparation for discrimination in the daily negotiation of situations that are common features of life in a society (e.g., shopping, banking, employment). This constant vigilance can lead to wear and tear on bodily functions.[37]

Our measure of racism-related vigilance was based on results from ethnographic work in black American samples, but our results suggest that similar mechanisms may operate for Hispanics as well. Although the mean vigilance score was lower for Hispanics than for blacks, we observed a similar positive association between vigilance and hypertension. In a recent laboratory study of Hispanic women, researchers reported greater cardiovascular reactivity in response to a stress test among participants who believed that they were working with others who held prejudiced views of non-white groups.[22] The authors concluded that the anticipation of discrimination may be an important source of stress and that "vigilance for prejudice may be a contributing factor to racial/ethnic health disparities."[22]

Our results support the notion that racism-related vigilance is an important determinant of hypertension in blacks (and perhaps Hispanics) through the continual activation of the biological stress response systems (e.g., autonomic and hypothalamic-pituitary-adrenal systems) characteristic of this type of anticipatory and perseverative stress. Researchers argue that repeated activation of the biological stress response systems results in their dysfunction, which some have termed *allostatic load*.[38] The body's inability to respond properly to further stress (acute or chronic, physical or psychological) results in the increased oxidative stress and inflammation that characterize numerous cardiovascular and cardiometabolic diseases.

We found that when vigilance is at its lowest level (zero), racial/ethnic disparities in hypertension were small—and were substantially attenuated after adjustment for hypertension risk factors. Yet, as vigilance increased, disparities increased and were not changed with adjustment for these risk factors. These results suggest that focusing only on conventional risk factors will not eliminate hypertension disparities. Furthermore, despite the focus on conventional risk factors, a recent report on *Healthy People 2010* stated that, over the previous decade, racial/ethnic disparities had not changed for 69% of the *Healthy People* outcomes monitored and had actually increased for 15% of these outcomes.[39] Our results support an argument that we need to think more broadly about the contexts that shape health disparities in hypertension.[40] Indeed, a growing body of research indicates that the conditions in which individuals live and work have an enormous impact on health before they even make contact with the health care system. Therefore, efforts to reduce these disparities

> will require expanding our focus beyond medical care and personal behaviors to the broader social and economic contexts that influence health, in part by enabling or constraining healthy behaviors.[41]

Limitations

Our sample was from a single city—Chicago—and although it was representative of the population of the city, future work is needed with other samples. Our data were also cross-sectional, so we could not determine the effect of vigilance on the risk of hypertension. Nonetheless, the data set was large and population based, and it was one of the only data sets available with objectively measured blood pressure and a measure of racism-related vigilance.

Although the Cronbach α for the vigilance measure was only marginally acceptable, this may be attributable to the scale's size: only 3 items. Furthermore, the low α provided for a conservative estimate of the association between vigilance and hypertension prevalence.

Conclusions

We carried out the first examination of racism-related vigilance and its role in hypertension disparities. We showed that racism-related vigilance is associated with hypertension, particularly for blacks and perhaps for Hispanics, but not for whites, and that this results in an increasing racial disparity in hypertension as vigilance increases. Our results compel those who seek to eliminate racial and ethnic health disparities to move beyond traditional notions of individual-level risk factors for disease to the broader social determinants that drive racism-related vigilance.

References

1. Hertz R, Unger A, Cornell J, Saundera E. Racial disparities in hypertension prevalence, awareness, and management. *Archives of Internal Medicine.* 2005;111(10):1233–1241.

2. Mensah G, Mokdad A, Ford E, Greenlunch K, Croft J. State of disparities in cardiovascular health in the United States. *Circulation.* 2005;57(3):379–380.

3. Fuchs F. Why do black Americans have higher prevalence of hypertension? An enigma still unsolved. *Hypertension.* 2011;57(3):379–380.

4. National Center for Health Statistics. *Health, United States, 2011: With special feature on socioeconomic status and health.* Hyattsville, MD; 2011.

5. Lloyd-Jones D; Adams RJ; Brown TM et al. Heart disease and stroke statistics—2010 update: A report from the American Heart Association. *Circulation.* 2010;121(7):46–215.

6. Wong MD, Shapiro MF, Boscardin WJ, Ettner SL. Contribution of major diseases to disparities in mortality. *New England Journal of Medicine.* 2002; 347(20):1585–1592.

7. Waidmann T. *Estimating the cost of racial and ethnic health disparities.* Washington, DC: Urban Institute; 2009.

8. Redmond N, Baer H, Hicks L. Health behaviors and racial disparity in blood pressure control in the National Health and Nutrition Examination Survey. *Hypertension.* 2011;57(3):383–389.

9. Geronimus AT, Bound J, Keene D, Hicken M. Black-white differences in age trajectories of hypertension prevalence among adult women and men, 1999–2002. *Ethnicity and Disease.* 2007;17(1):40–48.

10. Dimsdale J. Psychological stress and cardiovascular disease. *Journal of the American College of Cardiology.* 2008;51(12):1237–1246.

11. Brosschot J. Markers of chronic stress: Prolonged physiological activation and (un)conscious perseverative cognition. *Neuroscience and Biobehavioral Reviews.* 2010;35(1):46–50.

12. Brosschot J, Gerin W, Thayer J. The perseverative cognition hypothesis: A review of worry, prolonged stress-related physiological activation, and health. *Journal of Psychosomatic Research.* 2006;60(2):113–124.

13. Sternthal M, Slopen N, Williams D. Racial disparities in health: How much does stress really matter? *DuBois Review.* 2011;8(1):95–113.

14. White MA, Kohlmaier JR, Varnado-Sullivan P, Williamson DA. Racial/ethnic differences in weight concerns: Protective and risk factors for the development of eating disorders and obesity among adolescent females. *Eating and Weight Disorders.* 2003;8(1):20–25.

15. Harrell CJ, Burford TI, Cage BN, et al. Multiple pathways linking racism to health outcomes. *DuBois Review.* 2011;8(1):143–157.

16. Phillips B, Mannino D. Do insomnia complaints cause hypertension or cardiovascular disease? *Journal of Clinical Sleep Medicine.* 2007;3(5):489–494.

17. Krieger N. Racial and gender discrimination: Risk factors for high blood pressure? *Social Science and Medicine.* 1990;30(12):1273–1281.

18. Roberts CB, Vines AI, Kaufman JS, James SA. Cross-sectional association between perceived discrimination and hypertension in African-American men and women: The Pitt County Study. *American Journal of Epidemiology.* 2008;167(5):624–632.

19. Lindstrom M. Social capital, anticipated ethnic discrimination and self-reported psychological health: A population-based study. *Social Science and Medicine.* 2008;66(1):1–13.

20. Mohseni M, Lindstrom M. Ethnic differences in anticipated discrimination, generalised trust in other people and self-rated health: A population-based study in Sweden. *Ethnicity and Health.* 2008;13(5):417–434.

21. Clark R, Benkert RA, Flack JM. Large arterial elasticity varies as a function of gender and racism-related vigilance in black youth. *Journal of Adolescent Health.* 2006;39(4):562–569.

22. Sawyer PJ, Major B, Casad BJ, Townsend SS, Mendes WB. Discrimination and the stress response: Psychological and physiological consequences of anticipating prejudice in interethnic interactions. *American Journal of Public Health.* 2012;102(5):1020–1026.

23. Harrell SP. A multidimensional conceptualization of racism-related stress: Implications for the well-being of people of color. *American Journal of Orthopsychiatry.* 2000;70(1):42–57.

24. Schulz AJ, Kannan S, Dvonch JT, et al. Social and physical environments and disparities in risk for cardiovascular disease: The healthy environments partnership conceptual model. *Environmental Health Perspectives.* 2005;113(12): 1817–1825.

25. Turner J. Understanding health disparities: The promise of the stress process model. In *Advances in the conceptualization of the stress process* (Avison WR, ed.). New York: Springer; 2009.

26. Essed P. *Everyday racism: Reports from women of two cultures.* 1st ed. Claremont, CA: Hunter House; 1990.

27. Feagin J, Sikes M. *Living with racism: The black middle-class experience.* Boston: Beacon; 1994.

28. Baron R, Kenny D. The moderator-mediator variable distinction in social psychological research: Conceptual, strategic, and statistical considerations. *Journal of Personality and Social Psychology.* 1986;51(6):1173–1182.

29. Bertrand M, Mullainathan S. Are Emily and Greg more employable than Lakisha and Jamal? A field experiment on labor market discrimination. *American Economic Review.* 2004;94(4):991–1013.

30. Galster G. Racial steering by real estate agents: Mechanisms and motives. *Review of Black Political Economy.* 1990;19(1):39–63.

31. Williams DR, Jackson PB. Social sources of racial disparities in health. *Health Affairs (Millwood).* 2005;24(2):325–334.

32. Schulman K, Berlin J, Harless W, et al. The effect of race and sex on physicians' recommendations for cardiac catheterization. *New England Journal of Medicine.* 1999;340(8):618–626.

33. Smedley B, Stith A, Nelson A. *Confronting racial and ethnic disparities in health care.* Washington, DC: National Academies Press; 2003.

34. Sue DW, Capodilupo CM, Torino GC, et al. Racial microaggressions in everyday life: Implications for clinical practice. *American Psychologist.* 2007; 62(4):271–286.

35. Cappuccio FP, D'Elia L, Strazzullo P, Miller MA. Sleep duration and all-cause mortality: A systematic review and meta-analysis of prospective studies. *Sleep.* 2010;33(5):585–592.

36. Feagin J. The continuing significance of race—anti-black discrimination in public places. *American Sociological Review.* 1991;56(1):101–116.

37. Sapolsky R. Social status and health in humans and other animals. *Annual Review of Anthropology.* 2004;33:393–418.

38. McEwen B, Seeman T. Protective and damaging effects of mediators of stress: Elaborating and testing the concepts of allostasis and allostatic load. *Annals of the New York Academy of Sciences.* 1999;896:30–47.

39. National Center for Health Statistics. *Healthy People 2010 final review.* Hyattsville, MD: Centers for Disease Control and Prevention; 2012.

40. Braveman PA, Egerter SA, Mockenhaupt RE. Broadening the focus: The need to address the social determinants of health. *American Journal of Preventive Medicine.* 2011;40(suppl. 1):S4–S18.

41. Braveman P, Kumanyika S, Fielding J, et al. Health disparities and health equity: The issue is justice. *American Journal of Public Health.* 2011; 101(suppl. 1):S149–S155.

PART III

Separate and Unequal Health Care

The documents in this part illuminate two critical elements at the core of this *Reader*. The first is that structural violence and health care injustice have a long arc of impact. Current-day health inequities derive from long-standing political and economic practices in Chicago. One needs a historical perspective to understand that acts of structural violence cause harm over long periods of time. The second point is that observation and assessment are critical to overcoming structural violence to achieve health equity. But they are not enough; action is also necessary.

Structural violence in Chicago manifests in particular blows against particular bodies in particular neighborhoods. Many times, the structural drivers of inequity remain invisible to the general public until public action or groundbreaking studies expose them. This is particularly true concerning health care delivery in Chicago, as illustrated in figure 4.

In a 1986 *Chicago Tribune* story headlined "Poor Patients Given the Silent Treatment," Ronald Kotulak writes: "America has the best health-care system in the world—and the worst." Evidence supporting that conclusion is strong, as will be seen below.

This part of the *Reader* illustrates the structural aspects of health care inequity in Chicago and offers a glimpse of how community activism can help combat it. For many Chicagoans, race, income, and insurance affect access to care across many conditions and contribute to excess deaths, particularly in predominantly black neighborhoods. To understand this series of articles from the perspective of structural racism, we urge you to think about how these texts describe the structural conditions that

Poor patients given the silent treatment

By Ronald Kotulak
Science writer

America has the best health-care system in the industrialized world—and the worst.

Most Americans belong to a medically privileged class. When serious illness strikes, they can expect to receive sophisticated care regardless of the cost. Most of their bills are paid through private insurance, public aid or Medicare.

But an alarming number of Americans are falling through the widening cracks in the health-care system. One of every six people in this country has no form of health insurance, according to the latest surveys.

They are the medically homeless: people who have little or no access to medical care because they lack private or public medical coverage and who must make do with ever-shrinking charity from hospitals and doctors.

Like a growing stain on our national conscience, the increasing medical disenfranchisement of the poor has become a major moral dilemma.

"Perhaps the greatest ethical issue in medicine today—regardless of how little-notic-

New medicine —new ethics?

High technology has reshaped health care, but it also has created new moral dilemmas. This is the second of five reports.

ed it may be—is access to medical care," said Dr. Thomas A. Preston, a University of Washington professor and chief of cardiology at the Pacific Medical Center.

America, despite its marvelous medical achievements, is the only country in the industrialized world that doesn't provide some degree of access to medical care for all its citizens. Discouraged by a system that wants its money in advance, millions of people don't bother anymore to seek health care when they need it, experts say.

"There is growing evidence that more and more people actually are being harmed by not getting medical care," Preston said. "People are dying out there because they are not getting the care they need. There's no question

Continued on page 4

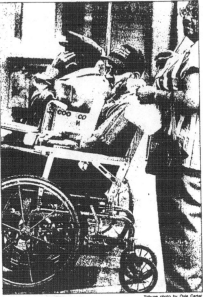

Tribune photo by Ovie Carter
Patients wait in Cook County Hospital's emergency room: A study of 467 emergency transfers from other hospitals showed that 87 percent were dumped on County because of lack of insurance.

FIGURE 4. "Poor patients given the silent treatment"
Source: Chicago Tribune. July 14, 1986.

affect health outcomes and whether they present outcomes that disproportionately disadvantage minorities.

Two important historical documents open this part. The first is a 1954 pamphlet by the Committee to End Discrimination in Chicago Medical Institutions provocatively titled, "What Color Are Your Germs?" The pamphlet outlines the systematic racism of Chicago hospitals with regard to births and deaths as well as routine medical care. The last page of the pamphlet is a map of Chicago showing the twenty-two-mile route that a sick black patient in the Altgeld Gardens neighborhood on Chicago's Far South Side would have to travel to get to Cook County Hospital, bypassing twenty-eight closer hospitals en route. The trip would take about one hour and twenty minutes. The text speaks to the racist policies created by hospitals to restrict black admissions by limiting the number of beds designated for black patients. It includes the first mention of the phenomenon later called *patient dumping*, where sick black patients were transferred to public Cook County Hospital simply because of race/racism and poverty. "Patients whose emergencies were not considered dire enough have died while being transferred to County," the pamphlet decries.

The second document is a 1967 letter from Quentin Young, a Chicago health activist and medical doctor, to the President's Advisory Commission on Civil Disorders on behalf of the Medical Committee for Human Rights. Using data collected by the City of Chicago Commission on Human Relations on black births and deaths in Chicago, Young noted that over 50% of black births and over 70% of black deaths occurred at Cook County Hospital. Just four of Chicago's many hospitals accounted for over 70% of black births. Two of these hospitals were publicly funded. One was a private African American–owned hospital. According to Young: "Data on hospital admission practices in Chicago show worsening patterns of discrimination against Negros in 1966, despite laws pledging to end this discrimination." This evidence of widespread racial discrimination by hospitals would serve to frame the narrative of health care inequality that has plagued Chicago ever since.

The next two articles feature communities taking their health into their own hands. Edwin Black's "Racism in Red Blood Cells" describes the failure of the Chicago Board of Health to notify forty-five thousand patients over seven years that they carried the sickle cell gene trait. A Board of Health official hypothesized: "The reason we didn't notify any of those 45,000 blacks was at first stupidity; and second lack of concern because it was black folks involved."

In Chicago, the Board of Health was embarrassed into beginning a notification and counseling program after the Black Panther Party began its own sickle cell screening and counseling program with the help of medical students and lab technicians. The Panthers were clear in their assessment:

Inferior medical care is an oppressive cross that black and poor people struggling in America have always been forced to bear. Nowhere is the fact more apparent than in the lack of government interest in researching or trying to cure or prevent Sickle Cell Anemia. Why is this so? We are living in a racist, exploitative society, and the victims of Sickle Cell disease are chiefly black people. At one point in time black people, as shackled slaves, were very much the asset in the building of America's economy. However, today, black people have become a liability. Because we are also struggling for liberation from this oppressive society, we, the dispossessed and economically expend-

able black community of America, now represent a great threat to Capital-
ist America. In order to protect itself from this threat, the United States rul-
ing circle has made genocide (the systematic extermination of a whole race of
people) the fascist order of the day.[1]

The Panthers were also clear in their actions:

The Illinois State Chapter of the Black Panther Party, with the aid of Lab
Technician Lois Allen Webb (who herself has the Sickle Cell Trait), began a
program for Sickle Cell screening early last year in Chicago's public schools.
Since this program started, the Black Panther Party, with help from concerned medical students and lab technicians from the Spurgeon "Jake" Win-
ters People's Free Medical Care Center, has screened children of five schools
in regular session in Chicago, and also children of five schools in the Maywood, Illinois area. Students at Farragut High School and Wright Junior College have also been tested. During the summer, Illinois Chapter members
also went through the black community with a mobile unit, giving free sickle
cell tests to the people. In all, 7,312 people in the Chicago and Maywood
black communities were tested. Out of this number of people, 614 were found
to have the Sickle Cell Trait or the actual disease itself, Sickle Cell Anemia.
It is tragic and criminal that these 614 black people had previously not known
that they were victims of the Sickle Cell disease. The black community knows
full well whom to indict for this blatant neglect of their medical needs.[1]

This direct action to improve health taken by a politicized community group foreshadowed other forms of health activism in Chicago over
the years. Other examples of activated constituencies taking direct action against health inequality and racism include a 1975 doctor's strike
at Cook County Hospital, the Committee to Save Cook County Hospital in the late 1970s, and the Trauma Care Coalition fighting for a South
Side trauma center, which we explore later in this *Reader*. Describing its
actions, the Black Panther Party said: "Sickle Cell Anemia and testing
represent one area where the people are beginning to demand that medical schools, hospitals, doctors and nurses start to become responsible to
the people they supposedly took an oath to serve."[1]

An article by John Conroy describes the creation of the Uptown People's Health Center in the Uptown neighborhood. The clinic was created
to serve the unmet health needs of the poor in the community. At its
core was a black lung screening program offering detection and health

benefits assistance to former coal miners at risk of lung damage from exposure to coal dust. Although the clinic did not survive for long, it is an example of action by a community group to address health care disparity. The black lung program outlasted the clinic, and many individuals received care as a result.

Later in this part, Robert Schiff et al. discuss the phenomenon of *patient dumping*—of mostly poor blacks and Latinos—from Chicago area hospitals to Cook County Hospital for financial reasons in the mid-1980s, despite serious delays that affected patient care and generated higher mortality rates. This was the same manifestation of structural violence in the health care system described so vividly in the pamphlet, "What Color Are Your Germs" thirty years earlier. It appeared in the targeting of uninsured minorities through routine administrative policies and agreed-on practices affecting patient outcomes.

These documents highlight two critical points: (1) Chicago's health inequities are deeply rooted in the city's patterns of neighborhood segregation and in political and economic policies that have governed life here for decades. (2) The analyses in these papers made troubling patterns of health care visible. But it is not enough simply to describe. The work of Schiff et al. and similar studies contributed to the 1986 Emergency Medical Treatment and Labor Act outlawing the practice of patient dumping. It was not sufficient to describe the practice in writing; action, in the form of lobbying for a change in public policy, was necessary to mitigate this form of structural violence.

A similar story emerges in the last selection in this part of the *Reader*, in work on *trauma deserts*. Marie Crandall et al. found that suffering a gunshot wound more than five miles from a trauma center was associated with an increased mortality rate. Underpinning this study was the well-known fact that the predominately black South Side communities of Chicago had the most gunshot wounds and were farthest from the city's trauma centers. The finding that most whites and Hispanics shot in Chicago were shot within five miles of a trauma center but that the reverse was true for blacks reinforced structural inequity in the placement of trauma centers in Chicago. This article helped propel a successful fight by community groups to pressure the University of Chicago to open an adult trauma center on its hospital campus after years of opposition (a fight depicted in some detail in part 5 of this *Reader*).

Taken as a whole, this group of articles demonstrates the remarkable power that collaboration between the academic community and community activists seeking change can generate. Today's battles for health equity in Chicago have a long historical arc, and these inequities have been stubbornly difficult to eradicate. Yet, viewed over an almost seventy-year period, some progress has been made. That progress has come, in large part, because of an activated community.

Reference

1. Will the real sickle cell program please come forward. *Black Panther*. February 5, 1972.

CHAPTER THIRTEEN

What Color Are *Your* Germs?

Committee to End Discrimination in Chicago Medical Institutions

C hicago boasts of the largest medical center in the world. But for 590,000 Negro residents—15% of the city's total population— Chicago is a dangerous town in which to fall ill. There are more than 6,000 doctors and 65 hospitals to serve the sick and injured in Chicago. But if Negro Chicagoans need a hospital—whether to treat a fever, set a broken bone, or deliver a baby—almost 50% go to one institution—Cook County Hospital.

Some go to County because it's close to their homes; some because they can't afford private hospital care. But a large percentage—patients with paid-up hospitalization policies and enough money to engage their own physicians and surgeons—go there because it's the only hospital that will accept them.

The laws of Illinois forbid a "public accommodation" to bar anyone because of race, creed, or color. Thus, if a Negro is refused service in a "Loop" hotel or restaurant, solely because of his race, he can bring suit against the owner and win. But, if a hospital turns him down for the same reason, there's nothing he can do, because hospitals are not technically "public accommodations." Despite humanitarian clauses in their charters, requiring service to all the sick, they can refuse admission, except in cases of dire emergency. Patients whose emergencies were judged not dire enough have died while being transferred to County. Many Chi-

Originally published as a pamphlet in 1954 by the Committee to End Discrimination in Chicago Medical Institutions.

cago hospitals give first aid in injury and accident cases, but patients are later transferred to County for hospitalization.

[. . .]

Overtaxed Facilities

The County Hospital has a fine medical reputation, but no hospital can give adequate medical care when severe overcrowding constantly taxes its staff and facilities. At County, the normal maternity ward of seventy-two beds has often been stretched to accommodate 115. Deliveries are sometimes made on stretchers in the open hallway, because the delivery rooms are all in use. Mothers and infants are discharged after three days, instead of the nearly six-day confinement in other Chicago maternity hospitals.

Although some private hospitals admit Negro patients, most of them maintain a rigid quota. When their "Negro beds" are filled, non-white patients are turned away. Furthermore, in most cases, patients are admitted through staff doctors. Less than ten non-governmental hospitals in Chicago have Negro attending staff physicians.

While the desperate need for nursing services has opened the doors of a number of hospitals and nurses' training schools, Negro doctors still find scant welcome on most hospital panels.

Except at County or the predominantly Negro-staffed Provident Hospital, most Negroes cannot be hospitalized unless they find white doctors willing to treat and admit them. But many white doctors, afraid of jeopardizing their own status, discourage referrals of Negro patients and sometimes even refuse to treat them.

Born in Prejudice

This problem impinges on the lives of Chicago's Negro residents from the moment of their birth. Ninety percent of all babies born at County Hospital are Negro. Although 51 other hospitals in Chicago have maternity facilities, eight had no Negro births at all, while 26 had fewer than ten. Of the 19,807 Negro children born in Chicago in 1953, approximately half were delivered at the County Hospital.

An authoritative survey conducted by the Welfare Council of Metropolitan Chicago published in May, 1954, documents segregation in Chicago's maternity hospital system.

1. In 1951 82% of Negro births were in 4 hospitals, or in the home under the supervision of the Chicago Maternity Center. Two of these hospitals were tax-supported, and two had a predominantly Negro medical staff. Of the remaining Negro births, 4 out of 5 were concentrated in 8 non-governmental hospitals, each having 100 or more Negro births.
2. 17 of 59 non-governmental Cook County hospitals had no Negro births. 24 hospitals had less than 10 Negro births. No hospitals on the far south side reported as many as 10 Negro births, yet 22% of Negro mothers lived there. 8 hospitals had but 10 to 100 Negro births.
3. Cook County Hospital is the chief resource for Negro maternity patients. In 1951 54% of 17,066 Negro births occurred there, contrasted with 2% of 65,060 white births.

The Welfare Council report concludes, regarding lack of availability of beds for Negro patients:

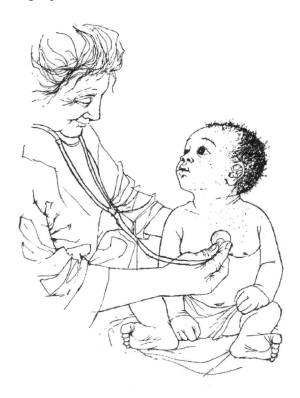

1. Voluntary hospitals and their medical staffs would need to remove intake limitations based on race, where such limitations exist, to relieve Cook County Hospital of its large load of patients (principally Negro) who are not medically indigent. Relaxation of limitations based on race would enable voluntary hospitals to use their beds more fully for the medically indigent in the event that additional funds from public or private sources are made available for this purpose.
2. Although approximately 20% of births in Cook County are Negro, maternity beds are virtually unavailable for Negros in two out of every three hospitals.
3. The almost complete lack of medical staff appointments for Negro physicians in virtually all voluntary hospitals limits the opportunity of Negroes who are private patients of Negro physicians to receive hospital maternity care under the supervision of their own private physicians.

And Babies Die

The mortality rate among Negro new-borns in Chicago is over 40% higher than for white infants.

"Most non-white infants can be saved by employing the same methods that have proved effective among the white infants," declares a report of the Chicago Board of Health. ". . . Better nutrition, improved housing, early and effective treatment of infections, proper prenatal, natal, and post-natal care should aid materially in reducing neo-natal mortality in non-white infants."

But, the report continues, ". . . If infant mortality is to be reduced materially, the greatest effort must be concentrated on those factors causing deaths immediately after birth; and this effort must be intensely continued without relaxation through the first few days of life, especially on premature infants, for it is they who constitute our greatest problem."

Negro babies can be saved. But not while hospitals continue to turn away maternity patients whose skins are dark.

Illuminating Statistics

Statistics recently released by the Chicago Board of Health on reported deaths by race and hospital for 1953 showed:

Total Negro deaths in hospitals: 3364
22 hospitals reported no Negro deaths
18 hospitals reported 5 or less Negro deaths
Cook County Hospital reported 2454 Negro deaths—71%
Provident Hospital reported 294 Negro deaths
Michael Reese Hospital reported 176 Negro deaths
Municipal Tuberculosis Sanitarium reported 27 Negro deaths
Illinois Research Hospital reported 45 Negro deaths

Thus three government supported institutions and two private hospitals had 89% of all Negro hospital deaths in 1953.

It must be kept in mind that hospitals do not report hospital admissions by race, whereas deaths, communicable diseases, and births are so reported. Therefore, these statistics are vitally important in determining a hospital's admissions policy as regards race.

[. . .]

Diagnosis: Discrimination

A Negro employee of one of the city's largest equipment manufacturing companies was suddenly taken ill with toxic, massive lobar pneumonia. His physician called for a bed at the south side hospital which has a medical cooperative agreement with the company. The resident physician refused to admit him because "all the hall beds customarily reserved for Negro patients are filled."

A few years back, a young journalist from Trinidad was struck by an automobile on Chicago's south side. He was rushed to a hospital five blocks away with a skull fracture. But the hospital refused admission. The patient died five hours after he was moved cross-town to the County Hospital by ambulance.

In February, 1954, a three year old Negro child became ill and was referred by the family physician to a nearby private hospital for hospitalization. Her mother was told at the hospital that the child was not sick enough to be hospitalized. She died the next day at home.

In October, 1953, a 15 year old Negro boy became ill and was brought by his mother to a private hospital near his home. A diagnosis of intestinal obstruction was made, and although this mother wished her son admitted and could afford hospitalization, the patient was sent to Cook

County Hospital. He was taken immediately to County Hospital, but died there four hours later.

In October, 1952, a 14 year old Negro boy was taken from the scene of an accident to a nearby private hospital. The mother, upon arriving at the hospital, was told that arrangements had already been made to have her son taken to Cook County Hospital. Hospitalization at the private hospital was not even suggested although the family carried hospitalization insurance. At Cook County Hospital the patient was admitted and treated for internal injuries and shock.

The above cases are taken from the files of the Committee to End Discrimination in Chicago Medical Institutions, and are fully documented.

A recent issue of *Today*, published by the Chicago Housing Authority, reports that ambulance service to city hospitals is now available for the 2,000 families in the Altgeld Gardens–Phillip Murray Homes. Why is this service necessary for a community on the far south side? "There have been deaths that could possibly have been prevented, and there have been near deaths that frightened the whole community because medical care was delayed," explains the newsletter. Cook County Hospital is twenty miles from the Altgeld Gardens–Phillip Murray Homes. Twenty-eight Chicago hospitals are closer.

[. . .]

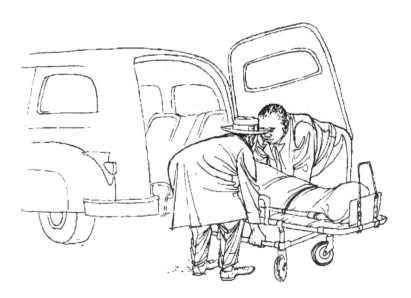

It's Up to You

These facts will no doubt astound some readers. Many Chicago residents, even doctors and hospital board members, don't realize that every sixth Chicagoan is denied adequate medical care, solely because of his color.

You and your neighbors—the citizens of Chicago—must decide if discrimination in medical services shall continue. If you really want to, you can break this undemocratic pattern and see to it that Chicago's doctors, hospitals, and clinics serve all who need them.

Here are some ways you can help:

1. *You can talk up the facts.*

Many of your friends may not know there is discrimination in Chicago's hospitals. Knowing facts is the first step in any campaign for improvement.

2. *You can write to the hospitals.*

Find out how the institutions serving your neighborhood stand on serving *all* the sick. If their policy is non-discriminatory, commend them; if it isn't, urge them to reconsider.

3. *You can take it up with your church, union, club, business or veterans organization, civic, fraternal, or educational association.*

Most of these organizations have social action committees concerned with community affairs. Their interest in democratic medical services will carry much weight with hospital and medical boards.

4. *You can discuss with your alderman, district committeeman or congressman the possibility of legal safeguards for equality of medical service.*

[. . .]

Health, like Freedom, Is Indivisible

The facts are incontrovertible. The United States Public Health Service, in its 1947 Chicago–Cook County Health Survey, recommended, "Hospital facilities and services shall be available to all patients on the basis of need and ability to pay, without regard to race, color, or creed and without segregation." What remains is for the people of Chicago to recognize that this is not exclusively a Negro health problem, but a *public* health problem. *It's up to you!*

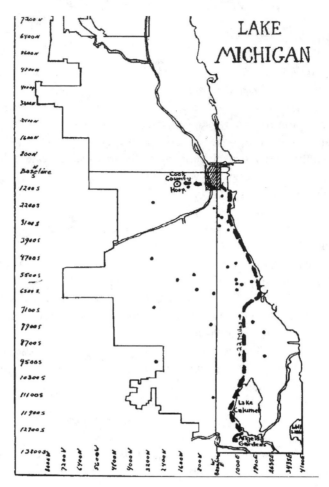

There are 28 hospitals (represented by dots on the map) closer to Altgeld Gardens than Cook County Hospital. Yet, because of discrimination practices in most of these hospitals, emergency patients ride 22 miles down to County (dotted line shows ambulance route). There is an average time delay of one hour and twenty minutes between the time the ambulance is called and the patient arrives at County. Map by Jean Stauss.

CHAPTER FOURTEEN

Letter to the President's Advisory Commission on Civil Disorders

Quentin D. Young

July 31, 1967

Hon. Otto J. Kerner, Chairman
President's Advisory Commission on Civil Disorders
Governor's Mansion
Springfield, Illinois

Dear Sir:

Mindful of the awesome responsibility you now bear, we would like to offer an example, in the field of health, of how the deprived sector of the community can become alienated through frustration of rising expectations. At the outset, it is necessary to emphasize that multiple causes doubtless combine to create the present crisis. Our presentation is limited to our own area of experience, the area of health care; if there is equivalent experience in housing, employment and education, your search for causes should be brief indeed.

The years preceding 1967 were years of promise of equality to those long cast down. The embodiment of that promise was the Civil Rights Act of 1964. The breakdown of law and order, the object of your investigation, may prove to be paradoxically linked to the breakdown of enforcement of law by responsible Federal officials. It may further be linked to the disregard of law by institutions charged with humane service to the whole community by their ethic and the Constitution. Freshly secured data on hospital admission practices in Chicago show worsening patterns of discrimination against Negros in 1966, despite laws pledging to end this discrimination. We should emphasize that we do not feel Chicago is unrepresentative of all urban centers.

On June 28, 1966, the Committee to End Discrimination in Chicago Medical Institutions lodged a formal complaint with the Surgeon General of the United States, alleging non-compliance with Title VI of the 1964 Civil Rights Act by forty-six (46) Chicago hospitals. A copy of this complaint is enclosed. This comprehensive charge, involving a majority of Chicago's hospitals, was developed on the basis of public data, that is, births and deaths by race. We must report to you that well over a year after the complaint—a fateful year for our nation—the Federal authorities responsible for law and order have not even rendered the courtesy of a response to the complainants, the form of a serious investigation of these serious charges, or, most important, the content of correcting the evil patterns described.

In June of 1966, the complainants asserted, "We feel that not only is there compelling evidence of patterns of hospital conduct not consonant with the demands of Title VI, but that this certification by Federal authorities bestows a 'seal of approval' which could well have a distinct braking effect on the development of non-discriminatory hospital practices, the object of the Civil Rights Act itself."

It is our painful duty to report to you that this dire prophecy has been proven accurate. At this writing, we have been able to secure only the birth data. In 1966 we charged twenty-one (21) of the fifty (50) hospitals with obstetrical service with discriminatory patterns. (We shall transmit the death data to you promptly when it becomes available; we have, however, no reason to expect it to differ from the new information on births that we transmit herewith.)

In enumerating particular groups of hospitals, we wish to stress that, in our view, the maldistribution in health care delivery is the fault of the entire community, not only the virtually all-white obstetrical services named. We further stress that the remedy lies in the total community plan for service to all, not in punitive measures against the worst offenders. It is the failure of leadership of the Department of Health, Education and Welfare to assert this principle, across the nation, that blocks solution of this problem.

What, then, are the patterns of hospital births by race in Chicago in the Year I of Enforcement of the 1964 Civil Rights Act? In 1966 Negro births rose from 29,053 to 29,433, while total births fell from 75,597 to 73,775. Thus, Negro births, as a per cent of total, rose from 38.4% to 39.7%.

Of the fifty (50) hospitals with obstetrical service, six (Cook County, Illinois Research and Educational, Michael Reese, Mount Sinai, Presbyterian–St. Luke's and Chicago Lying-In) delivered 21,503 Negro births (74.1% of total) in 1965 and 21,828 (74.2% of total) in 1966.

The twenty hospitals accused in the original complaint (1966 data for the twenty-first hospital is not available) and three additional hospitals now manifesting sharp drops in Negro births combine to show the following characteristics: Negro births fell from 567 in 1965 to 496 in 1966, in both instances less than 2% of the total Negro births. Yet these hospitals delivered over 50% of white births in Chicago both years, that is, 23,673 in 1965 and 22,299 in 1966. The flight of the whites to the suburbs is reflected in the overall drop in births in these hospitals of 1374. The fact that their token service to the Negro community declined at a time of rising Negro births and significantly falling white utilization of these hospitals underscores the hardening of the segregated pattern ruefully forecast in the 1966 complaint.

It is our belief that these cold numbers cruelly affect the lives of the inhabitants of our urban ghettos. These inhabitants, their rising expectations crushed, express their alienation with new figures, humans dead and millions of dollars of property loss. Our nation has broken a compact to achieve human equality. The Law has failed our disinherited. The extinction of hope may well have ignited the torch in our troubled inner city.

When your Committee commences hearings, we would be pleased to be in attendance in order to offer more information.

Sincerely yours,
Quentin D. Young, M.D.
Medical Committee for Human Rights

TABLE 14.1 **Total births and Negro births in 24* Chicago hospitals in 1965 and 1966**

	Total Births		Negro Births		Negro Numer[ator] Change
	1965	1966	1965	1966	
I. Four hospitals with small increase in Negro births (greater than 12)					
Englewood	386	364	14	46	32
Holy Cross	1,670	1,725	14	41	27
Mother Cabrini	907	880	35	67	32
Walther Memorial	881	911	21	47	26
					+117
II. Sixteen hospitals with insignificant change in Negro births					
American	437	403	3	15	12
Belmont	767	722	0	3	3
Edgewater	1,914	1,719	5	3	−2
Illinois Central	235	238	1	12	11
Loretteo	843	769	21	26	5
Lutheran Deaconess	575	559	3	5	2
Northwest	698	846	15	10	−5
Ravenswood	1,340	1,277	6	5	−1
Resurrection	1,968	1,868	0	0	0
Roseland Community	662	604	10	5	−5
South Shore	933	929	3	2	−1
St. Anne's	2,363	2,113	0	2	−2
St. Anthony	909	867	36	30	6
St. Elizabeth	1,838	1,570	76	59	−17
St. Mary	1,017	919	13	4	−9
Weiss	660	704	6	4	−2
					−5
III. Three previously undesignated hospitals showing large drop in Negro births					
Swedish Covenant	916	817	76	20	−46
Columbus	1,075	970	128	72	−56
Garfield Park	679	525	81	18	−63
					−165
Net change 1965–1966 in 24 hospitals					−53

*There is one hospital in 1965 group for which no 1966 data are available:

Central Community: 1965 total births, 498; Negro births, 2

CHAPTER FIFTEEN

Racism in Red Blood Cells

The Chicago 45,000 and the Board of Health

Edwin Black

Between 1965 and spring of this year, the Chicago Board of Health tested nearly half a million Chicago blacks for sickle cell anemia. The testing revealed 45,000 people carried the trait that could have passed the disease to their offspring. By the Board of Health's own admission, none of these people were notified of the test findings.

Sickle cell anemia is a disease primarily affecting black people. As a disease, it can debilitate and shorten life considerably. Only under continuous medical maintenance and by following a regimen of severely limiting precautions can someone stricken with the disease expect to live beyond twenty years. Even with medical care, those with the disease die before age forty-five.

Sickle cell anemia is a genetic disease, and about 9% of Chicago's black population carries the recessive trait. The trait itself is seldom dangerous. But if two people with the trait conceive offspring, a quarter of their children, on average, will be born with the fatal disease. Statistically, sickle cell anemia strikes one black person in four hundred.

In Chicago, the Board of Health has found a minimum of 45,000 people with sickle cell trait. Why weren't these people told of it?

"The sickle cell testing program originally began in 1965," recounted

From an investigative article "Racism in Red Blood Cells," by Edwin Black, originally published by *Chicago Guide* [later *Chicago Magazine*]. Copyright 1972 and 2018 Edwin Black.

Dr. Hyman Orbach, director of the Board of Health's laboratory. "We have several black people working here, and I believe we were doing blood tests on high-risk black maternity cases. At some point somebody probably said, 'Hey, we've got some extra blood left over . . . let's do a sickle cell test.'"

Laboratory records indicate blood specimens from about a thousand pregnant black women showed the disease. These women were immediately notified and given medical attention and counseling. Eighty or ninety of the pregnant women showed a positive carrier trait; but they were never told so, never asked to have their partners tested for the trait. Obviously, if both parents had the trait, they could have been counseled against further conception and on how to care for their offspring, should the children be diseased. Trait-carrying parents must take an awful gamble: For this reason, notification and proper counseling are extremely important.

Testing for sickle cell anemia was made a routine procedure in the lead-poison screenings of ghetto children, and the number of tested people increased year after year, from 38,000 in 1966 to 109,000 in 1971. But the same policy of non-notification continued. Between 465,000 and a half million were tested. Half of 1% had the disease; they were notified and given medical care. Eight to nine percent had the trait and were ignored. It's obvious that this policy could only result in keeping the disease at a constant level.

Hematologist Charles M. Shapiro explained the medical realities: "Sickle cell anemia is a change in the hemoglobin that is basically found in blacks, but also in a few other racial stocks. Essentially what happens is the hemoglobin gels to distort and destroy red blood cells. This clogs the blood vessels and causes pain. Pain because all parts of the body—from the brain to the bone—are clogged, can't get enough oxygen. Children stricken with this disease—and it's one in four hundred—are in tremendous jeopardy. Fifteen years ago, we'd expect a victim to live till age twenty. Today, with better treatment, victims live longer: We've seen some go to forty or forty-five. It varies with the medical maintenance. Victims must avoid any infections or special medical treatment that would require anesthetics. They have to avoid high altitude, running out of breath—any state of low oxygen that normal people would simply adapt to. And of course, despite all these precautions, the life expectancy will be extremely shortened.

"As for the trait," continued Dr. Shapiro, "it's basically without immediate effect. I have heard of cases of trait carriers getting into trouble with certain anesthetics and depressurized flight cabins, but these are all very rare. The big problem with carriers is when they conceive children together. And if they do have children—let's say they have four—one of them can be expected to be normal, two will be trait carriers, and one will have the disease. But that one-out-of-four figure is just a population statistic. On a family basis, it can work out to anything. A couple can have five healthy children or five defective children, and in *that* lies the disease's true devastation."

Dr. Shapiro added that once the trait is discovered, the person should be notified and counseled. The Board of Health's non-notification of 45,000 carriers, he said, "is a *big* error. There's no sense in testing the kids if you're not going to tell anyone. And as for pregnant mothers, this is horrible. Because it's crucial to tell these mothers so they can have their children tested soon after birth."

[. . .]

While the Board of Health was unable to assemble a notification and counseling procedure to accompany their sickle cell trait identification program, the job was being done through a community movement organized and sponsored by the Black Panthers. Their Chicago office began a sickle cell testing program in May of 1971, and with the permission of the Chicago Board of Education carried out a pilot program in five grammar schools. In two months the Panthers tested 2561 pupils. Two anemics and 169 carriers were found: All were informed of the results, and person-to-person counseling followed. The program operated on pennies and dimes donated by community residents and the volunteer services of doctors, lab technicians, nurses, and community workers.

The successful program expanded. The Panthers acquired a crude mobile lab and increased its staff of testing/counseling teams. Two electrophoresis devices—simple, relatively inexpensive apparatus used in protein analysis—were acquired. In the next year, over 20,000 blacks in the Chicago area were tested at rallies, in schools, in their homes. Counseling followed for the thirteen anemics and hundreds of carriers the program discovered.

In a July 27 interview, we asked Dr. Murray Brown, the Chicago Commissioner of Health, to comment on charges that the city was embarrassed by the Panther testing program and copied it under public pressure. He replied, "The Black Panthers . . . can't embarrass our program. I'd be in favor of them if they were benefitting the people. But they aren't. We were testing five years ago. . . . Now how can they talk of embarrassing us? If they had a program like ours, they could embarrass us. Are they using electrophoresis in their testing? I doubt it. Oh, they probably have some crude means of detecting the sickle cell, but the only reliable definitive test is the electrophoresis. Now you see, for the past five years our program has featured the definitive test, identification of carrier trait or disease, genetic counseling and education. We've been doing it through Urban Progress centers, the schools, through door-to-door surveys. Now have the Panthers done any of that? Have they had the counseling program we have? It's a more complex matter than just simple identification of the trait. The program's not worth a dam without counseling. They're not doing anything but prostituting medicine for political purposes."

Subsequent interviews with key Board of Health laboratory personnel, Urban Progress Center staff members, and South Side grammar school principals revealed that until May of this year, the Chicago Board of Health had done no in-school testing, there was no counseling for trait carriers, and no notification procedure. Only children with the disease were notified by letter and assigned appointments with doctors. Board of Health records verify this information.

On August 2, the Board of Health's assistant commissioner, Dr. Jack Zackler, was asked if he were aware that 45,000 sickle cell carriers identified by the Board of Health had not been counseled or even notified. "Well now, I don't know," he replied. "I guess they weren't notified. But that's only to the best of my knowledge." Dr. Zackler said he could not answer any more questions because he was tied up in an important meeting. Five minutes later Dr. Zackler called back: "That information I gave you about the notifying of carriers . . . was mistaken. I now understand that a *good* percentage of the carriers were indeed notified. I just checked." How many were notified? "I don't know that. It was done on an informal basis, and we'd have to revert back to the records for the individual patients. All I do know for certain is that a good number of them were certainly at least informed."

In a third interview that day, Dr. Zackler reaffirmed that "a good number" of the carriers were informed but not counseled, although he couldn't explain what accounted for some being told and others being ignored. Asked what means of notification was used for carriers, he admitted, "None." Notification without counseling, he said, would do "more harm than good" to the individual.

The same day Health Commissioner Brown, in another telephone interview with us, emphatically denied any statement describing a program of education and counseling for carriers prior to 1972. Disputing Dr. Zackler's earlier statement, he asserted there was no notification or counseling for those exhibiting the trait. When asked why the Board of Health—during five years of testing—had not even prepared a "see your doctor" postcard (let alone a pamphlet or letter for trait carriers), Dr. Brown answered, "Look, we didn't have the resources, and no one was interested." Later in the interview, Dr. Brown did admit to calling the 1965–72 testing an excellent program and an outstanding job. He added that "a sickle cell testing program without counseling is worthless," however, and that bad motives should not be inferred simply because carriers weren't notified: "Those with the disease were notified, and they were the ones that benefited." And Dr. Brown claimed that the city was doing the best it could with little or no finances. Neither Federal nor State funds have been made available for sickle cell testing and notification; the Board of Health has had to resort to scrabbling piecemeal funds from a variety of other programs that are only marginally related to sickle cell anemia *per se*.

Dr. Brown's situation is not really of his own making. His job involves defending a public health organization that has for years been charged to be a haven for political favorites. This present health commissioner himself has brought much needed changes and additions to the system, most notable of which are the neighborhood comprehensive care clinics—which are still far from perfect.

The decision not to notify 45,000 carriers was essentially the work of Dr. Brown's predecessors, Drs. Samuel Andelman and Morgan J. O'Connell. Dr. Andelman, reached at his Skokie Village Hall office, where he serves as health director, at first seemed to think carriers had been notified, then conceded they weren't. But, he added, "Don't you think it was wonderful that the Chicago Board of Health saw fit to make these tests in 1965, before the nation was really talking about it?" O'Connell was unavailable for comment.

[. . .]

"In a way," said one prominent Chicago research physician, the situation in Chicago is akin to the Public Health Service Tuskegee Report [which detailed how blacks were used as guinea pigs in a research project that resulted in their syphillitic deaths]. The fact remains, he told us, "that a large body of public opinion—expert public opinion within the health care profession—is persuaded, as I am, that it is no accident that these people were used for the syphillis thing, or that race is unrelated to the lack of sickle-cell programs.

"The basic information about sickle cell anemia has been available for a long time. It strains credulity to think it was accidental that the Board of Health got into a counseling program a year after the Black Panthers did. This disease is not a rarity when compared with other genetic defects that have had much research and fanfare. It is a disease that has attracted a disproportionately small amount of attention. It's only now that it's become a popular thing for the government to get involved in. It has only now become a fashionable area of research, with emerging black awareness and emerging black power.

"You better believe that if it occurred in whites, there would have been a major program mounted years and years ago."

CHAPTER SIXTEEN

The Uptown People's Health Center, Chicago, Illinois

John Conroy

A man works in the mines for 10 years in Mingo County, W. Va. Coal dust settles in his bronchial tubes. Black spots appear on his lungs, and over the years the spots grow larger. It becomes more and more difficult for the miner to breathe. His lungs aren't giving enough oxygen to his blood, and he gets flaming chest pains when he tries to do the work he once did. So he moves his family to Chicago, to a neighborhood on the north side called Uptown, where he has relatives, where he might get a job he can handle in spite of his lungs, and where welfare checks are a bit higher if things just fall apart.

His disease has been called *miner's asthma*, *silicosis*, *black lung*, and *pneumoconiosis*. It is a man-made disease, found in every coal-mining country in the world, that can be prevented but cannot be cured. It is not a new disease. It was first reported in 1813, became compensable in Britain in 1943, and, in this country, it was a 1969 Federal statute that established it as an occupational disease of coal miners.

In Chicago, however, few people seem to know the disease exists. An estimated 10,000 former coal miners from Kentucky, West Virginia, Pennsylvania, and southern Illinois live in the area, with perhaps 2,000 in Uptown. Local physicians, however, have had no training in spotting the disease, so it has been difficult for a former miner to get care and al-

Originally published in *Public Health Reports*, 94, no. 4, supp. (July–August 1979): 33–38.

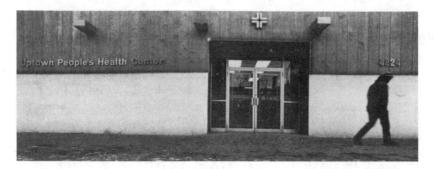

FIGURE 16.1. Opened in August 1978, the Uptown People's Health Center is located in a unique neighborhood where live former coal miners from Appalachia, American Indians, and people of many ethnic groups.

most impossible to get the certification which would allow him to receive the black lung benefits provided for in the 1969 law.

Between 1972 and 1978 almost 200 claims were filed by members of the Chicago Area Black Lung Association; only 15 members received benefits. The Commissioner of the Board of Health maintained that there was no black lung disease to speak of in Chicago even after association members and their families demonstrated at his office to call attention to their plight.

The Black Lung Association, forced to go elsewhere for help, found it in the Department of Medicine at Cook County Hospital. Money was available from the Cook County Health and Hospitals Governing Commission for a neighborhood clinic for comprehensive care if the community could show both need and desire. In the spring of 1977, association representatives went to their neighborhood coalition, collected signatures, conducted a door-to-door health survey, found a possible clinic site, and began filing the necessary forms.

Association representatives and community organizers found that the ratio of physicians to population in Uptown did not indicate that the area was medically underserved. But a closer look revealed that Uptown's physicians were serving the community's wealthier citizens and former Uptown residents now living in the suburbs.

They also found that, although there were nine hospitals in the area, most of the people served by the hospitals were not from the community. When the clinic's organizers eliminated the wealthier enclaves from the

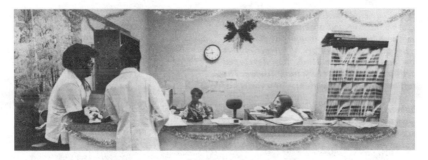

FIGURE 16.2. The center is open 40 hours, 6 days a week, including Tuesday evening and Saturday morning.

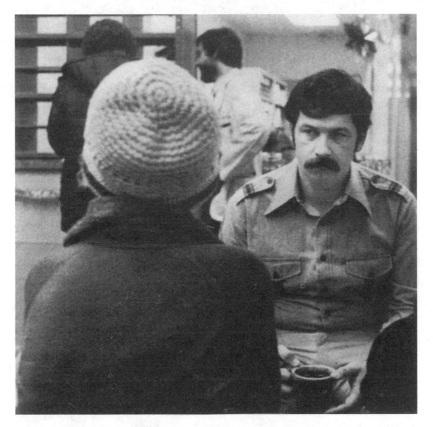

FIGURE 16.3. Health Center waiting room. More than 3,000 persons had been treated within 4 months after the clinic opened.

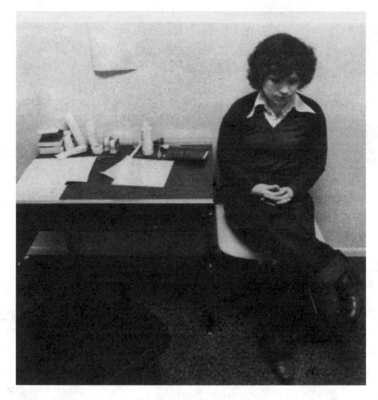

FIGURE 16.4. Pensive patient awaits test results.

Uptown statistics and concentrated on their target area, a much different picture of community health needs emerged.

Thirty percent of the people living in the area were unemployed, 55% of the families lived at poverty level, 71% had no phone, 55% no auto, and 7% no plumbing. Infant mortality was one-third higher than the city average. Alcoholism was prevalent, and deaths due to tuberculosis were twice the city average. Lead poisoning was present, and accidents were among the leading causes of death. The people surveyed complained that the neighborhood's privately owned storefront clinics, which compete for the Medicaid traffic, prescribed all kinds of pills but they never really treated the patients.

When the Chicago Board of Health learned of the community's proposal for the clinic, it objected strenuously, arguing that the proposed fa-

cility would be competing for patients with their Wilson Avenue clinic a
mile away. The neighborhood organizers maintained that there was no
competition because the need was so great.

The clinic organizers persevered, mustering busloads of people at
crucial moments in the drive, and in August 1978, the Uptown People's
Health Center opened its doors. "This was no goddamn gift of charity,"
says organizer Randy Saltz, a 30-year-old Vietnam veteran who is the
community board's man on the scene at the clinic. "Truly thousands of
people were involved in it."

The Community

Nowhere else in the world is there a place like Uptown. Blacks, whites,
Chinese, Japanese, Filipinos, Cubans, Koreans, Puerto Ricans, Mexicans, Asian Indians, Poles, Croatians, Germans, Jews, rich, and poor
live in the area.

Thousands of American Indians from 60 different tribes live there,
and Indian teenagers attend a special high school, Little Big Horn.
Twenty-one percent of the people have an Appalachian heritage; a storefront called the Southern Culture Exchange does its best to maintain
their traditions by offering classes in quilting, whittling, and cornhusk
doll–making. Thirteen thousand mental patients also live in Uptown,
and the community is swollen with halfway houses.

Uptown's most striking aspect is that the wealthy and the poor live almost side by side. Highrises along the lake and enormous mansions just
behind them house some of the wealthiest and most powerful people in
the city. A few blocks away, once-legitimate hotels are now inadequate
nursing homes. Prostitutes walk the streets four blocks from $100,000
homes, and the Aragon, formerly a famous ballroom, is a showcase for
boxing matches and rock concerts.

Wealthy homeowners, local merchants, working-class residents who
have always lived in Uptown, and young couples who bought apartment
buildings, thinking the area would someday turn middle class, have united
to form block clubs and community organizations which often do battle
with the poor. The clubs and the chamber of commerce have even considered changing the name of the community, fearing that innumerable stories about the seedy side of the area have made the word Uptown syn-

onymous with wino hotels, just released mental patients, prostitutes, and junkies. Other organizations have fought the expansion of social services in the area.

A mainstay of the poor community is the Intercommunal Survival Committee, a group which has developed a dozen projects—among them the Black Lung Association and the Uptown People's Health Center. The Survival Committee, leading the battle against an entrenched political organization, is trying to win the middle class over to its point of view. The committee feels that Uptown is one of the few neighborhoods in the city where large families with low incomes can afford to live. It argues that the lower and middle classes should recognize that each needs the other and then go on to do battle with what they perceive as the common enemies—large real estate interests and entrenched political powers.

The Health Center

Uptown People's Health Center is situated just off the corner of Lawrence and Broadway near a used book store, two furniture stores, a tavern, a candy store, and a Spanish film theater. The clinic's building was a

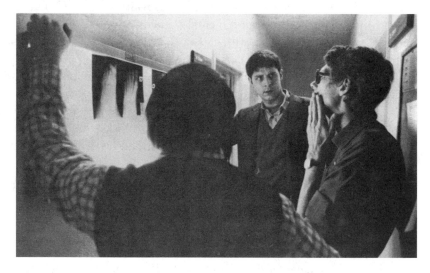

FIGURE 16.5. Dr. Roger Benson (*center*) of Cook County Hospital, attending specialist in rheumatology, confers with Dr. Ronald Shansky (*back to camera*) and Dr. Rob Brinkman (*right*).

restaurant for many years and later housed a health maintenance organization clinic which closed amid allegations of fraud. Now the space is
modern, bright, cheery, and extremely clean. It has 16 examining rooms,
a dental laboratory, a pharmacy, an X-ray room with leaded walls, a
room for proctoscopy, 2 rooms for black lung testing, 3 waiting areas,
and a staff lounge. A computer in the medical records section can produce the history of any patient who has been treated at Cook County
Hospital or any clinic associated with it.

The center is open 6 days a week, a total of 40 hours including Tuesday evening and Saturday morning. Patients, scheduled by appointment,
see the same physician each time they come. They are charged for services based on their ability to pay. The clinic's long-term goal is to have
50% of the clients able to pay in full for services. At that point, the administrators at the clinic estimate that it will be self-supporting.

The community board chose the clinic staff, interviewing 200 appli-
cants for 30 positions. They looked for people from different ethnic sectors of Uptown so that the clinic would represent all of the community.
Those chosen were Black, Latino, American Indian, East Indian, and
Appalachian. Dr. Ron Shansky, the medical director, Mary Kuttner, the
clinic administrator, and Slim Coleman, president of the community
board, have known each other for years. They are experienced in delivering health care to the poor and have similar views on how it should
be done.

"What we are trying here is to combine the best of the private sector—
the personalized care—with the best of the public sector—accountability
to the community and no economic barriers," Dr. Shansky says. He
sees the clinic as "a place where ability to pay is not the first question
asked, and where, no matter what your financial situation is, it's not going to prevent you from getting care. We're small, and we intend to stay
that way. When we reach the point where the doctors are backed up for
weeks, it's not the time for us to become a 40-doctor operation. We must
maintain the personality of the care. If Uptown needs another clinic, set
one up. Don't overload this one."

Dr. Shansky, 33, comes from the staff of Cook County Hospital,
where he is in charge of creating a model of decentralized, community-
operated, ambulatory care centers. Shansky spends 24 hours a week as
Uptown's medical director. He devotes the rest of his time to developing four other clinics and to serving as a staff doctor at the Federal jail in
downtown Chicago.

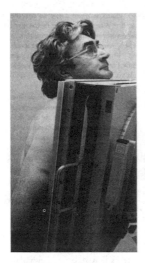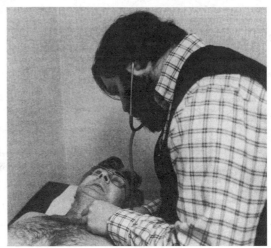

FIGURE 16.6. Dr. Shansky, medical director, examines Lawrence Zarnes, president of the Chicago Area Black Lung Association. The association helped to get the clinic started. Some 2,000 former coal miners live in Uptown area.

He wants the physicians at his clinics to be committed, to stay for a long time. He will use no trainees. One reason the Uptown Clinic got off to such a good start is that Shansky found the physicians himself and then had them apply to the National Health Service Corps, but he says the model will work with Corps-recruited physicians as well.

By the end of the first year, Shansky wants 90% of the 2-year-olds in the target area to be completely immunized, 80% of the pregnant mothers to be coming to the clinic for their first prenatal visit in the first trimester, and 90% of the women over age 18 who come for primary care to have documentation of a Pap smear. Shansky is also working on establishing privileges for the clinic's physicians at several area hospitals; the hospitals in Uptown have not welcomed the poor in the past, but Shansky has secured a promise from the Health and Hospital's Governing Commission that the Commission will guarantee all costs of the clinic's "unsponsored" patients.

By the twelfth month of operation, it was anticipated that the clinic's four physicians would be treating an average of three people per hour. By the end of the second year—because many of the patients would have been seen before—the clinic board projected that the physicians would see four patients per hour. Four months after the opening, more than 3,000 patients had been treated. Coleman, Shansky, and Kuttner were careful not to bring in more patients than they could handle, because they had had experience with clinics becoming crisis centers.

Uptown's providers spend more time with patients than physicians in other neighborhoods, usually because the health problems of the poor are often more serious than those of the middle and upper classes. The poor don't go to a physician until they are certain they cannot clear up the problem themselves.

[. . .]

No statistics are available yet on the health of the clinic's patients, but the staff indicates that the primary problems are emotional and physical ailments stemming from unemployment and poverty. Depression and hypertension are very common. Among Spanish-speaking patients, diabetes is relatively frequent, and recent immigrants from Mexico and Puerto Rico are often plagued by gum problems and darkened teeth, a condition caused by high levels of fluoride in the drinking water. A contract with a day labor agency has brought in several people hurt in industrial accidents.

The community has a relatively high incidence of tuberculosis. "Most people think those who get TB today are old winos living in men's hotels," Brinkman says. "Not so." The clinic's TB patients so far have included four children and one 20-year-old woman.

"People in this area are skeptical, even hostile with doctors," Dr. Brinkman says. "You say something to them, they might do it, they might not. It's the result of the Medicaid mills in the neighborhood, where doctors push pills on patients, don't examine them, and a premium is placed on seeing patients as quickly as possible."

Slim Coleman, president of the clinic's board, agrees. "Doctors in Uptown have not been part of the community," he says. "They're like a department store with higher prices. They're the last thing you go to when you get sick. You try home remedies, you try to find a different job, a different apartment, a different neighborhood, or maybe you cheat on your wife. You don't go to Marshall Field's when you can go to Woolworth's."

Walter Leslie Coleman, known to everyone in the neighborhood as Slim, is tall, thin, in his mid-30s, and originally from Texas. He gives the impression of being an easy-going character with a quick laugh and a remarkable ability to tell a good story. Underneath that front is a street-smart organizer with a political savvy acquired in countless battles with bureaucrats, police, aldermen, mayors, real estate tycoons, slumlords, health agencies, and businessmen. Also buried there is a Harvard education. He presides over a community board once denounced by the local alderwoman as "stacked with low-income residents."

"It *is* stacked with low-income residents," Coleman retorts, "and it will remain stacked. That's the first time I ever heard anyone plead affirmative action for the rich."

Coleman, board secretary Helen Shiller, and other members of the Intercommunal Survival Committee have been involved in many other civic projects. They have chosen officials at local schools. They have revised a local college's curriculum to cater to the community's needs for education and for full-time employment. The committee runs a food co-op and distributes toys to neighborhood kids at Christmas. Mothers affiliated with the group have paid visits to local stores to demand that shopkeepers not sell glue to children.

The health center's board is careful not to use the clinic as a political tool. "When you come in the door, you're not smacked with voter registration information or a copy of our newspaper," community board representative Randy Saltz says. "I'm concerned with health care and that this be identified as a health clinic where people can get decent care. If we get into different issues, we'll lose it."

That's not to say, however, that the clinic is isolated from the rest of the board's activities. "Somebody comes in with a cold," Saltz says, "and we try to get the providers to ask, 'Why you got a cold? You got broken windows? No heat?' Then the providers let me know, and I direct the patient to our legal department, and the next thing you know, the landlord is in court."

Board members are encouraged to visit the clinic as often as they can. "Most boards are just thrown together; they aren't strong," Coleman says. "A hospital sets up a clinic and then gets an advisory board. Well that's not the case here. This is not an advisory board; this is the board of directors."

The board has been active in outreach for the clinic and has run a dental education program in several elementary schools. Board members have also acted as advocates for patients when they have thought that a physician hasn't quite grasped a situation. "Once one of the providers told a patient, 'Go home and soak in a hot tub.' Well, the patient didn't have a hot tub," Coleman recalls. "Another time the doctor tells the mother of a kid with strep throat to keep him away from drafts and other kids. Well, the family has 10 kids, and they live in a 3-bedroom apartment where the wind blows through. We came back to the doctor and told him, 'You're just going to have to treat the whole family.'"

Not everyone shares Coleman's opinion that a good board is a strong one. One dentist resigned, in part for personal health reasons, but also because he did not share the political sympathies of the group and did not care for the board's management of activities he thought were his province. A social worker assigned to the clinic also left because her political beliefs clashed with those of the board.

It is still too early to make any predictions about the success of the clinic. A lot of equipment has yet to arrive, much of the staff have not yet been hired, and the middle-class members of the community who will have to be attracted to the clinic in order for it to become self-sufficient have not yet been solicited. Dr. Shansky, however, is confident that the model will work. "Publicly controlled care is the only source that will care for people humanely without financial impediments, that will get involved in preventive care and community education because turning a profit is not an issue," he says. "If you want to serve the poor, this is the only way to go."

CHAPTER SEVENTEEN

Transfers to a Public Hospital

A Prospective Study of 467 Patients

Robert L. Schiff, David A. Ansell, James E. Schlosser, Ahamed H. Idris, Ann Morrison, and Steven Whitman

The transfer of patients from one hospital to another is a widespread practice throughout the United States. Transfer is considered appropriate when there is a need for specialty or tertiary care that is unavailable at the transferring hospital.[1,2] Inability to pay for hospital services is also regarded by some as an acceptable reason for the transfer of patients from private to public hospitals. This has been a long-standing practice in such cities as Chicago, Oakland, Los Angeles, Dallas, Atlanta, and Washington, DC.[3–9]

In recent years there have been increases in the number of interhospital transfers of patients to public general hospitals across the United States. In Washington, DC, for example, transfers from private hospitals to District of Columbia General Hospital rose from 169 to nearly 1000 annually[8] between the years 1981 and 1984; similar increases have been noted in other cities.[10] At Cook County Hospital in Chicago, the number of interhospital transfers has risen steadily from 1,295 in 1980 to 2,906 in 1981, 4,368 in 1982, and 6,769 in 1983.

These increases in the numbers of transfers have occurred during a period of cutbacks in federal and state health care funding for the poor. Some have expressed concern that economic considerations may take

Originally published in the *New England Journal of Medicine* 314, no. 9 (1986): 552–57. Copyright © 1986, Massachusetts Medical Society.

precedence over patient well-being as a major determinant of hospital transfer policy.[4,11–12] There have also been reports that delays in treatment may be harmful to some patients.[13–15] Interhospital transfers for economic reasons cause such delays and may therefore have detrimental consequences for patients in some cases.

This report describes a prospective study of patients transferred to a public general hospital. Five hundred patients consecutively transferred to Cook County Hospital from other hospital emergency departments in the Chicago area formed the study sample. We present a demographic profile of the transferred patients and report the reason for patient transfer, whether there was admission to the intensive care unit, the length of hospital stay, patient charges, and outcome. In addition, we evaluate the stability of the patient's condition at the time of transfer and examine various aspects of the transfer process, including treatment delay caused by transfer and the informed-consent procedure. Finally, we report the costs incurred by Cook County Hospital as a result of these transfers.

Methods

The study was conducted at Cook County Hospital, Chicago's only public general hospital, which had 1342 beds, 40,076 admissions, and 242,000 emergency-department visits in 1983. Data were collected on 500 consecutive adult patients who were transferred from another hospital's emergency department to Cook County Hospital from November 20, 1983, to January 1, 1984, and subsequently admitted to the medical or surgical services. Excluded from this study were patients admitted to the obstetrical, gynecologic, or pediatric services.

The transfer process was initiated by a phone call from the transferring hospital to our emergency department. During this call, a medical or surgical resident filled out a transfer form with the name of the patient and the transferring hospital, vital signs, a brief clinical summary, and the reason for the requested transfer. The resident either accepted or rejected the transfer request. During the study period, 93% of the requests for transfer were accepted. Reasons for refusal included that hospitalization was not indicated, that the patient's condition was not sufficiently stable to permit transfer (most frequently because of possible myocardial infarction), and that there was noncompliance with transfer protocols. Neither the physicians at the transferring hospitals nor those at the Cook County Hospital were aware that this study was being conducted.

During the study period, 602 adult medical and surgical patients were transferred from other hospitals to our emergency department, and 500 were admitted. Detailed review of the hospital records identified 16 patients who did not meet our study criteria and were therefore excluded: eight because they were inpatient transfers and eight because they were not transfers to the medical or surgical service. Inpatient charts were located for 467 of the 484 patients (96%). These 467 patients constituted the study population.

Each patient was identified prospectively by daily review of the Cook County Hospital emergency-department records, transfer forms, hospital admission records, and trauma-unit admission book. Patient interviews were conducted by one of the four investigating physicians (D.A., A.I., R.S., or J.S.) or a fourth-year medical student (A.M.), usually within the first 24 hours of admission. The interview involved questions about employment, insurance status, and whether the patient had been informed of the transfer and had given consent. After discharge, data were abstracted from the transfer form, the transferring hospital's emergency-department record (photocopies of which were usually sent with the patients), the Cook County Hospital's emergency-department record, and the inpatient chart. Items that were abstracted included basic demographic data, vital signs, laboratory data, and the times and dates of all major hospital emergency-department and ward admissions and discharges of the patients. The physician investigators were not involved in the care of the study patients.

[. . .]

Results

Demographic Data

Forty-two hospitals transferred the 467 patients, sending between 1 and 36 each (median, 6). The average age of these patients was 36 years, and 78% were male. Seventy-seven percent were black, 12% Hispanic, 10% white, and 1% of other ethnic or racial origin. Eighty-one percent of the patients were unemployed, 11% worked full-time, and 8% worked part-time.

An evaluation of the medical-insurance status of 430 of the patients showed that 46% were recipients of aid from the Illinois Department of

Public Aid (this includes Medicaid), 46% had no insurance, 4% had private insurance, 3% had Medicare, and 1% had other, miscellaneous coverage. In comparison, 30% of all the 40,076 persons admitted to Cook County Hospital in 1983 had no health insurance coverage ($P < 0.0001$; figure 17.1). Nationally, only 8.2% of patients in short-term general hospitals have no insurance.[16]

The reason for transfer given to the Cook County Hospital resident in the transfer-request phone call was lack of insurance for 87% of the 245 patients for whom this information was available. The need for tertiary or specialty care was given as the reason for transfer in 4% of the cases, a lack of beds at the transferring hospital in 3%, the patient's request in 1%, and other reasons in 5%.

Resource Use and Patient Outcome

Seventy-three percent of the patients were admitted to the surgical service and 27% to the medical service. Of those admitted to the surgi-

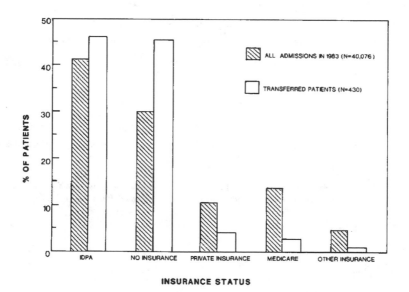

FIGURE 17.1. Distribution according to medical-insurance status of transferred patients and all patients admitted to Cook County Hospital in 1893

Note: The distributions of the two groups are significantly different (chi-square) (4) = 101.52, $P < .0001$, as are the proportions in each insurance category considered separately: Illinois Department of Public Aid (IDPA), $P < .05$; no insurance, private insurance, and Medicare, $P < .0001$; and other insurance, $P < .0001$.

cal service, the majority were admitted to the trauma (53%), orthopedic (20%), general surgical (12%), or neurosurgical services (4%). Eleven percent were admitted to other surgical services. Twenty-two percent (104) of the study patients were admitted to an intensive care unit during their hospitalization, most of these (88%) within the first 24 hours. The average length of hospital stay for the study patients was 9½ days.

Cook County Hospital uses an all-inclusive daily rate for all patient charges (e.g., room, board, physicians, laboratory, and ancillary services and supplies) of $630 per day for patients on the wards and $1500 per day for patients in the intensive care unit. The total charges for the transferred patients, based on the actual number of the intensive care and ward days, amounted to $3.35 million.

We also evaluated patient outcome. Seventeen (3.6%) of the study patients died during the hospitalization. An additional 18 (3.9%) were discharged to a chronic care facility. The proportion of transferred patients admitted to the medical service who died was 9.4% (12 of 128), whereas the proportion of non-transferred medical-service patients admitted to Cook County Hospital during the study period who died was 3.8% (43 of 1120) ($P < 0.01$). The proportion of transferred surgical patients who died was 1.5% (5 of 339), which is not significantly different from the proportion of non-transferred surgical patients (2.4%, 28 of 1149) admitted during the study period ($P > 0.10$, table 17.1).

Instability and Treatment Delay

We made a clinical assessment of the stability of the patients' condition based on the transferring hospitals' records. Of the 467 charts reviewed,

TABLE 17.1 **The proportion of transferred patients admitted to an intensive care unit (ICU) and the proportion who died according to service and stability rating**

Patient category	No. of patients	Admitted to an ICU (%)	Died (%)
All patients	467	22.3	3.6
Medical	128	14.8	9.4
Surgical	339	25.1	1.5
Stable	329	14.6	1.5
Medical	62	6.5	3.2
Surgical	267	16.5	1.1
Unstable	106	38.7	7.5
Medical	55	18.2	10.9
Surgical	51	60.8	3.9

TABLE 17.2 **Clinical features of patients in unstable condition transferred to Cook County Hospital**

Patient's study no.	Age/sex	Clinical features*
18	48/M	Pneumonia with hypoxia, PO_2 57, respiratory rate 26–33
41	46/M	Blunt head trauma with possible basilar skull fracture; was vomiting in emergency department
52	37/F	11% first- and second-degree burns of face and chest, with respiratory rate of 44
57	30/M	Blunt abdominal trauma, with falling hematocrit and syncope; required blood transfusion before transfer
88	44/M	Upper gastrointestinal bleeding, Jehovah's Witness, refusing blood transfusion; hematocrit 24%, pulse 144
138	28/M	Delirium tremens
157	26/F	Diabetic ketoacidosis, T 35.2°, ABG: pH 7.26, PO_2 106, PCO_2 26, HCO_3 11; white-cell count 17,000/mm³
161	62/M	Acute cerebrovascular accident, stuporous, BP 198/120
167	58/M	Head trauma, confusion, pupils reacting differently, T 34.1°
220	53/F	Cancer of mouth, BP 93/65, white-cell count 20,000/mm³
225	36/M	Hypertension with epistaxis, initial BP 240/170
253	28/M	Multiple trauma with probable splenic rupture, hematuria, and drop in hematocrit from 44 to 36%
290	32/M	Fell from third story, confused
368	21/M	Diabetes mellitus with T 38.3°, possible septic shoulder, white-cell count 28,500/mm³
373	42/F	Ascites, hyponatremia (serum Na 112 mmol per liter), hypoxia, ABG: pH 7.51, PO_2 76, PCO_2 22; white-cell count 13,700/mm³
426	25/M	Pelvic and radial fractures, BP 90/50
515	58/M	Confusion, fever, wet gangrene of foot
539	24/M	Acute abdomen with free air under diaphragm on x-ray films
540	57/M	Pneumonia with hypoxia, PO_2 56, respiratory rate 28
576	37/M	Hemoptysis (700 ml), hemoglobin 11.5 g per deciliter

*PO_2 denotes partial pressure of oxygen, T (temperature) expressed in degrees Celsius, ABG arterial blood gas (values expressed in millimeters of mercury), PCO_2 partial pressure of carbon dioxide, HCO_3 bicarbonate (values expressed in millimoles per liter), and BP blood pressure expressed in millimeters of mercury.

435 (93%) had sufficient information to make a determination of stability. Of these, 106 patients (24%) were classified as being in an unstable condition. Table 17.2 lists 20 randomly selected patients who were in an unstable condition with their key clinical features. In some patients, treatment was initiated before transfer, but definitive treatment was usually not begun. Examples of definitive measures not begun include emergency surgical procedures (e.g., exploratory surgery, repair of vessels or vital organs or both, and craniotomies), antibiotic therapy, and emergency invasive diagnostic tests.

The fatality ratio was 7.5% (8 of 106) among the patients in unstable condition and 1.5% (5 of 239) among those in stable condition

($P < 0.005$). Nearly 39% of the unstable patients (41 of 106) were admitted to an intensive care unit, as compared with 14.6% (48 of 329) of the stable patients ($P < 0.001$, table 17.1).

Transfer Process

The transfer process resulted in an average treatment delay of 5.1 hours (range, 1 to 18 hours; median, 4.6) after the need for hospitalization had been determined at the transferring hospital. A signed informed consent for transfer was present in only 25 (6%) of the 437 transferring-hospital records that were available for review; 21 of these were from a single hospital. Thirteen percent of the patients we interviewed reported that they were not informed in advance of their impending transfer to Cook County Hospital. Of those informed of transfer, 36% reported that they were not told why they were being transferred.

When the reason for transfer was known by the patient, it was frequently different from the reason given to the resident at Cook County Hospital during the transfer-request phone call. For example, when "no insurance" was the reason reported for transfer, there was a discrepancy between the frequency with which this reason was given during the requesting phone call (87%) and the frequency with which it was reported by the patients (64%) ($P < 0.001$).

Thirty-four percent of all patients were transferred from teaching hospitals. Thirty-five percent of the patients in an unstable condition were transferred from teaching hospitals. For 99% of the unstable patients transferred from non-teaching hospitals, there was a closer teaching hospital than Cook County Hospital.

Discussion

Reductions in federal and state funding for medical care began in earnest in 1980. Since that time, damage to the financial integrity of public hospitals and to the well-being of patients has been predicted and reported.[17-20] The marked increase in the number of patient transfers to Cook County Hospital since 1980 coincides with these cutbacks. Hospital reimbursement by the Illinois Department of Public Aid is determined by the patient's category of public aid. In Illinois, as a result of a 1983 public-aid cutback, total hospitalization was limited to $500 for those in the General Assistance category, who receive the most limited form of public aid.[21]

Most (88%) of the recipients of aid from the Illinois Department of Public Aid who were transferred to Cook County Hospital were in the General Assistance category. In fact, public-aid recipients transferred to Cook County Hospital were more likely to be receiving General Assistance than were all the public-aid recipients admitted to our hospital (38%) in 1983 ($P < 0.001$). Nearly half the patients transferred had no health insurance. Our study patients were also more likely to have had no insurance than all the patients admitted to Cook County Hospital in 1983 (figure 17.1).

The great majority of the patients (87%) were transferred because of lack of insurance. Although data on the reason for transfer were available for only 243 of the study patients (52%), our analyses suggest that this subgroup was representative of the entire study sample. Regardless of the service of admission or the stability status, the distributions of reasons for transfer were similar. The predominance of transfers made because the patient lacked insurance supports the contention that the increase in the number of transfers to Cook County Hospital and other public hospitals since 1980 has been attributable to economic reasons. Although 89% of the transferred patients were black or Hispanic, we were unable to determine whether race was a factor in the decision to transfer independent of insurance status.

A noteworthy and unexpected finding was that the proportion of the transferred medical-service patients (9.4%) who died was more than twice that of the patients who were not transferred (3.8%) during the study period ($P < 0.01$). Although this study did not attempt to determine the cause of this mortality difference, the transferred patients may have had a different case mix or been more severely ill, or some aspect of the transfer process, such as treatment delay, may have affected outcome adversely.

The absence of a difference in the mortality of transferred as compared with non-transferred surgical patients may have resulted from the preponderance of patients with trauma in the surgical group. It is well known that mortality among such patients is highest during the first three hours after injury, when 80% of deaths from trauma occur.[22] Thus, the most severely injured patients with trauma may not have survived long enough to be transferred to Cook County Hospital.

According to our criteria, 24% of our study population were in an unstable condition at the transferring hospital. It is often difficult to determine the severity of illness and the potential stability of seriously ill patients.[11,23] Objective severity-of-illness scales are available for specific types of illnesses,[24-26] but there are no scales that have been tested prospectively in a population with the diversity of conditions that ours represented. Thus, the criteria we used involved the clinical judgment of trained physicians about the urgency of immediate medical or surgical treatment.

Our requirement that all reviewing physicians agree selected against the likelihood that a patient's condition would be classified as unstable. There was uncertainty about the condition of 39 patients, and they were classified as being in a stable condition. Thus, the 106 patients we classified as being in an unstable condition may have represented an underestimation of the total number of patients in an unstable condition who were transferred to Cook County Hospital during the study. That the patients classified by us as being in an unstable condition had a significantly higher mortality rate, were significantly more likely to be admitted to an intensive care unit (table 17.1), and had significantly longer hospital stays (14.7 vs. 7.7 days; $t = 4.18$, $P < 0.001$) than those we classified as stable suggests that our rating system is valid.

For appropriately selected patients, the benefit of transfer to another facility may outweigh the risk.[1,2] The patient-transfer guidelines of the Chicago Hospital Council stipulate that patient well-being must take precedence over all other reasons for transfer.[27] The Joint Commission on Accreditation of Hospitals requires that "individuals shall be accorded impartial access to treatment or accommodations that are available or medically indicated regardless of race, creed, sex, national origin or sources of payment for care."[28] Our data suggest that these guidelines are infrequently adhered to in transfers to Cook County Hospital.

The mean treatment delay caused by the transfer process in this study was 5.1 hours. Although our study did not assess the effect of treatment delay on patient outcome directly, treatment delay has been shown to affect outcome adversely in patients with certain conditions.[13,14,29]

In addition to treatment delay, we reviewed the informed-consent process. The American Hospital Association's *Patient's Bill of Rights* states that "when medically permissible, a patient may be transferred to another facility only after he has received complete information and explanation concerning the needs for and alternatives to such transfer."[30] A disturbing number of patients reported that they were not informed of their impending transfer or were not told why they were being transferred to Cook County Hospital. For most, there was no evidence of written informed consent to the transfer.

Another important issue is the financial effect on public hospitals of economic transfers. According to Cook County Hospital data for patients with a similar distribution of insurance coverage, 84% of the $3.35 million charged to the transferred patients, or $2.81 million, was non-reimbursable. Thus, we estimate that in 1983 the non-reimbursable costs to Cook County Hospital of providing care to transferred patients was $24.1 million, or 12% of the total 1983 operating budget. This does not include the cost of care for transferred patients admitted to the obstetrical, gynecologic, or pediatric services or for inpatient transfers. Neither does it reflect the cost of care for patients referred to Cook County Hospital from other hospitals and not admitted. These non-reimbursable services represent a shift of costs from Chicago's private hospitals to a financially strapped public hospital. If our patients are representative of medical and surgical emergency-department transfers in other areas of the country, extrapolation to a national level suggests an annual cost shift of hundreds of millions of dollars from the private to the public sector. With prospects of further cutbacks in federal and state support for health care, we expect the transfer for economic reasons of patients with little or no insurance coverage to continue.

We conclude that patients are transferred to Cook County Hospital from other hospital emergency departments predominantly for economic reasons. The fact that many patients are in a medically unstable condition at the time of transfer raises serious questions about the private health sector's ability to consider the condition and well-being of patients objectively, given the strong economic incentives to transfer the uninsured. The delay in providing needed medical services as a result of the transfer process represents a serious limitation of the access to and quality of health care for the poor.

References

1. American College of Surgeons Committee on Trauma. Interhospital transfer of patients. *Bulletin of the American College of Surgeons.* 1980;65(2):13–15.

2. American College of Emergency Physicians. Guidelines for transfer of patients. *Annals of Emergency Medicine.* 1985;14(2):1221–1222.

3. Gibson G. *Emergency medical services in the Chicago area.* Chicago: University of Chicago Center for Health Administration Studies; 1970.

4. Himmelstein DU, Woolhandler S, Harnly M, et al. Patient transfers: Medical practice as social triage. *American Journal of Public Health.* 1984;74(5): 494–497.

5. Friedman E. The "dumping" dilemma: Finding what's fair. *Hospitals.* 1982; 56(18):75, 77, 80 passim.

6. Friedman E. The "dumping" dilemma: Finding what's fair. *Hospitals.* 1982; 56(18):75–84.

7. Anderson RJ, Cawley KA, Andrulis DP. The evolution of a public hospital transfer policy. *Metropolitan Hospital.* 1985;2(1).

8. Greenberg DS. Health-care thrift spurs patient-dumping. *Los Angeles Times.* November 12, 1984.

9. Roemer MI, Mera JA. "Patient-dumping" and other voluntary agency contributions to public agency problems. *Medical Care.* 1973;11(1):30–39.

10. Hospitals in cost squeeze "dump" more patients who can't pay bills. *Wall Street Journal.* March 8, 1985:27.

11. Relman AS. Economic considerations in emergency care: What are hospitals for? *New England Journal of Medicine.* 1985;312(6):372–373.

12. Wrenn K. No insurance, no admission. *New England Journal of Medicine.* 1985;312(6):373–374.

13. Stone JL, Rifai MH, Sugar O, Lang RG, Oldershaw JB, Moody RA. Subdural hematomas: I. Acute subdural hematoma: Progress in definition, clinical pathology, and therapy. *Surgical Neurology.* 1983;19(3):216–231.

14. Holmes MJ, Reyes HM. A critical review of urban pediatric trauma. *Journal of Trauma and Acute Surgery.* 1984;24(3):253–255.

15. Gentleman D, Jennett B. Hazards of inter-hospital transfer of comatose head-injured patients. *Lancet.* 1981;2(8251):853–854.

16. Coffey PA, Di Giusto J. The effects of waiting time and waiting room environment on dental patients' anxiety. *Australian Dental Journal.* 1983;28(3): 139–142.

17. US Congress Committee on Energy and Commerce. US House of Representatives. Hearings on Medicaid cutbacks on infant care. 1981.

18. Special Committee on Federal Funding of Mental Health and Other Health Services. *Health care: What happens to people when government cuts back.* Chicago: American Hospital Association; 1982.

19. Brazda J, ed. *Perspectives: Who will care for the uninsured?* Washington Report on Medicine and Health; 1982.

20. Rogers DE, Blendon RJ, Moloney TW. Who needs Medicaid? *New England Journal of Medicine.* 1982;307(1):13–18.

21. State of Illinois Department of Public Aid. *Notice to recipients of general assistance.* Springfield, IL; 1983.

22. Tortella BJ, Trunkey DD. Trauma care systems. *Trauma Quarterly.* 1984; 1:17–24.

23. Gibson G. Indices of severity for emergency medical evaluative studies: Reliability, validity, and data requirements. *International Journal of Health Services*. 1981;11(4):597–622.

24. Baker SP, O'Neill B, Haddon W Jr., Long WB. The injury severity score: A method for describing patients with multiple injuries and evaluating emergency care. *Journal of Trauma and Acute Surgery*. 1974;14(3):187–196.

25. Champion HR, Sacco WJ, Carnazzo AJ, Copes W, Fouty WJ. Trauma score. *Critical Care Medicine*. 1981;9(9):672–676.

26. Teasdale G, Jennett B. Assessment of coma and impaired consciousness: A practical scale. *Lancet*. 1974;2(7872):81–84.

27. *Guide for inter-personal transfer of patients*. Chicago: Chicago Hospital Council; 1977.

28. *Accreditation manual for hospitals*. Chicago: Joint Commission on Accreditation of Hospitals; 1984.

29. Seelig JM, Becker DP, Miller JD, Greenberg RP, Ward JD, Choi SC. Traumatic acute subdural hematoma: Major mortality reduction in comatose patients treated within four hours. *New England Journal of Medicine*. 1981;304(25): 1511–1518.

30. *A patient's bill of rights*. Chicago: American Hospital Association; 1975.

CHAPTER EIGHTEEN

Trauma Deserts

Distance from a Trauma Center, Transport Times, and Mortality from Gunshot Wounds in Chicago

Marie Crandall, Douglas Sharp, Erin Unger, David Straus, Karen Brasel, Renee Hsia, and Thomas Esposito

Traumatic injury is the leading cause of death in the United States among individuals aged 1 to 44 years.[1] Trauma centers are specialized facilities within hospitals with the expertise to care for the injured patient; resources include trauma surgeons, interventional radiology, surgical subspecialists, and immediate availability of an operating room. The development of trauma centers and trauma systems grew out of wartime experiences from the 1950s through 1970s that increasingly emphasized early and aggressive care and treatment of injured combatants. Trauma centers and organized trauma systems, including prehospital triage criteria and transport plans, have been shown to significantly decrease mortality for injured patients.[2,3]

However, not all areas of the country have equal access to trauma centers. Although 84% of Americans live within 1 hour of a trauma center, rural areas are particularly under-served.[4,5] Longer prehospital transport times likely contribute to the higher mortality rates among rural trauma patients as compared with similarly injured urban patients.[6–8]

Originally published in the *American Journal of Public Health* 103, no. 6 (June 2013): 1103–9, by the American Public Health Association.

For urban trauma patients, the relationship between transport times and outcomes is inconclusive. Feero et al. examined more than 800 urban trauma patients and found that shorter transport times were associated with improved survival.[9] Gervin and Fischer also found this association for patients with penetrating cardiac injuries.[10] Several other investigators, however, have not found a link between transport times and survival from trauma.[11–13] The largest and most recent of these studies was from Newgard et al., who used data from 10 cities and 51 trauma centers. The centers included a heterogeneous mix of urban and rural hospitals from the United States and Canada.[13] They found that prehospital transport time was not associated with increased mortality for major trauma. The disparate results from these studies may be in part attributable to the heterogeneity of injury mechanisms in the patient populations or smaller sample sizes underpowered to detect the effects of transport times.[11] The Newgard study did separately analyze patients injured by penetrating trauma (i.e., gunshot wounds [GSWs] or stab wounds), but nearly two thirds of those patients and 67% of GSW victims were within the first or second quartile of prehospital transport times (i.e., the shortest transport times). These patients also constituted only 22% of the sample size. Both of these facts may limit the generalizability of this study to areas of the country with higher rates of penetrating trauma.

The city of Chicago currently has 7 Illinois-verified level I adult trauma centers in and around the city and a mature emergency medical services (EMS) system providing care to a population of 3 million people. There are no level II centers within the city limits. (Level I and level II centers both provide 24-hour comprehensive trauma services, including trauma surgeons, radiology, and EMS; however, level II facilities do not need to have a surgical residency or ongoing research programs.) Unfortunately, Chicago also has one of the highest homicide rates in the country, ranging from 450 to 650 deaths per year from 1999 to 2009 (averaging 16 per 100,000 annually), mostly attributable to firearm-related violence.[14] As in most major cities, socioeconomically distressed neighborhoods in Chicago suffer most of the burden of firearm-related homicide; these neighborhoods, as well as the 7 trauma centers, are not evenly distributed around the city.

Urgent surgical intervention is much more frequently required for penetrating trauma than for blunt mechanisms of injury, and it is less likely that definitive care can be provided in the prehospital setting. As trauma centers are not equally distributed around the city, we hypothesized that patients who suffer GSWs in areas that are farther from trauma centers will have longer transport times and worse outcomes.

Methods

Our data source was the Illinois State Trauma Registry (ISTR), a mandatory reporting database containing information about all traumas presenting to level I and level II centers in the state. This database is maintained by the Illinois Department of Public Health; it is de-identified with respect to name and hospital, but includes other demographic information, such as gender, age, race, physiological data, mortality and discharge outcomes, and incident address information.

Patient Population

We extracted data from all patients for the years 1999 through 2009 from the registry ($n = 510,429$). The data set was restricted to Chicago by zip code and city. We also included in the data set a 1-mile perimeter around the city to incorporate spatial effects beyond the city's administrative demarcation, given that trauma center catchment areas include neighboring communities but do not necessarily adhere to published neighborhood or city boundaries ($n = 119,349$). We further limited the data set to GSWs ($n = 12,475$) by using the External Causes of Injury codes from the International Classification of Diseases, Ninth Revision[15] (e-codes 922.0–922.9, 955.0–955.7, 965.0–965.4, 968.6, 985.0–985.7, 970, and 979.4). The longitudinal trend of GSW incidence in our data set paralleled homicide data publicly available from the city of Chicago.

We mapped all incidents with available address data for the scene of the incident using ArcGIS software (Esri, Redlands, CA); more than 94% could be geocoded ($n = 11,744$). We then created maps of GSW incidence and superimposed them with a map of Chicago-area trauma centers. We calculated distance measurements as the Euclidean distance between the GSW incident and the nearest level I trauma center.

Predictors

We created a variable to denote being more than vs. less than or equal to 5 miles from a trauma center. We selected 5 miles from 1-mile increments of distance between 1 and 10 miles because it provided the best balance of minimizing geographic overlap of trauma center radii but allowed for sufficient comparison proportions. The approximately two-thirds of patients in the data set who were within this 5-mile boundary served as observational controls. We also analyzed important potential confounders, including age, gender, race, insurance status, injury severity score (ISS) greater than 16 (which is associated with higher likelihood of mortality), systolic blood pressure (SBP) in the emergency department of less than 90 millimeters of mercury, year of injury, and intent of injury. We coded insurance status as those self-paying being "uninsured" and everyone else being "insured." We determined injury intent and whether the police were involved by E-codes. Older age, male gender, non-White race, lack of insurance, and injury severity as measured by ISS and blood pressure have all been shown to predict mortality after trauma.[16-18] Insurance status is difficult to code because there is a wide spectrum between insured and uninsured, with many underinsured individuals in between. However, we have adopted a dichotomization that is consistent with current work in the trauma disparities literature.[17,19,20]

With respect to injury markers, there are many other methods to calculate injury severity (such as the Revised Trauma Score and the Trauma and Injury Severity Score), all of which have incrementally better performance than the ISS alone on mortality prediction and include anatomical and physiological markers of injury, along with demographic criteria. However, these are calculated values, some requiring use of a regression model, and they are not routinely included in all trauma data sets, including the ISTR.

We included year of injury to account for any longitudinal improvements or other changes in trauma care or systems. We included intent because firearm suicide attempts have been found to be highly lethal (over 90% fatal),[21] but firearm-related assaults seem to be less so, judging from the nonfatal firearm assault rate in the United States.

Outcomes

Outcomes of interest were mean transport times and mortality. Transport time is divided into 3 components in the ISTR: response time, scene time (i.e., time spent by EMS personnel at the scene), and travel time from the scene to the hospital. These are all actual times recorded by the EMS providers and verified in the medical record by trauma registrars.

Of the 3 components, we used travel time from the scene for our analysis because it should be the most directly correlated with distance from the scene to the closest trauma center. Response times vary irrespective of distance from the scene, because EMS personnel may or may not be in the area at any given time; although they are not all dispatched from a central location, response times are typically very brief. For this sample, 97% of response times were 10 minutes or less. Scene times for penetrating trauma are highly dependent on the ability of police to secure the scene and EMS personnel to safely evacuate the patient and are therefore not readily modifiable. Because a scene time of more than 20 minutes is a quality indicator of the American College of Surgeons Committee on Trauma, we examined this for our sample, and 95% of scene times were 20 minutes or less. Because geographic boundaries such as the Chicago River, road construction, bridges, and traffic patterns might influence transport times, we first calculated the association between transport time and distance from a trauma center.

Mortality was defined as all patients who died in the hospital, excluding those "dead on arrival" (DOAs; i.e., individuals who were pronounced dead in the emergency department without any interventions). These latter patients were excluded because we posited that they would have a lower probability of survival due to greater injury burden and that injury severity would overwhelm any smaller effect of transport times. In addition, prehospital data (e.g., vital signs and injury severity) were largely incomplete for these patients, with some data collection points having greater than 70% missing values. In addition, prehospital decision-making with respect to transporting patients in extremis may also be dependent on distance from a trauma center, introducing bias into the study.

Statistical Analysis

We calculated bivariate and multivariate analyses using Stata statistical software version 10 (StataCorp LP, College Station, TX). We estimated logistic regression models of mortality. Covariates included age, gender, race, insurance status, ISS greater than 16, SBP in the emergency department of less than 90 millimeters of mercury, year of injury, mechanism and intent of injury, and our variable of interest, being shot more than 5 miles from a trauma center. Using ArcGIS software, we then created maps of GSW mortality rates and superimposed them on a map of area trauma centers. The method used to depict mortality rates in the city was a quadrat grid of half-mile by half-mile cells symbolizing the mortality rate for GSW patients in each quadrat that contained 10 or more GSWs. We used this approach to limit small sample size or land use effects (because industrial areas have few GSWs) to optimize mortality rate mapping.

Results

Of the 11,744 GSW victims in the data set, the overwhelming majority were male (91.6%), younger than 40 (98.4%), non-White (89.9%), and victims of assault (89.9%; $p < .001$ for all). A total of 4782 patients (38.3%) were shot more than 5 miles from a trauma center (table 18.1).

Overall mortality was 18.8%, with 64% of those deaths coded as DOA or dead in the emergency department without interventions provided. Among patients who were not DOA, mortality was very high for White patients, who tended to be older ($\geq$ 50 years; 15% of White patients vs. 3% of the cohort overall; $p < .001$) and more frequently had a suicidal intent (9% vs. 3%; $p < .001$). Firearm-related suicide attempts were highly lethal; of patients surviving to the hospital, 68% ultimately died. The patients who were DOA had a much higher mean ISS (18.62 $\pm$ 18.80 vs. 9.89 $\pm$ 10.45 for other deaths) and much lower mean SBP (28.49 $\pm$ 54.39 vs. 129.47 $\pm$ 36.90; $p < .001$ for each).

Transport Times

The mean transport time was significantly higher for patients who were shot more than 5 miles away from a trauma center (16.6 $\pm$ 7.6 minutes vs. 10.3 $\pm$ 6.5 minutes; $p < .001$).

Patients shot more than 5 miles away from a trauma center were disproportionately Black ($p < .001$), were less likely to be insured ($p < .001$), had a slightly higher ISS (10.4 vs. 9.3; $p < .001$), were more likely to have suffered a primary abdominal wound (13% vs. 8%; $p < .001$), and were more frequently the victim of an assault ($p < .001$; table 18.2).

Mean transport times did not vary significantly by time of day, day of week, or month of year ($p > .05$ for all). Transport times were directly proportional to distance from a trauma center. Linear regression modeling of transport time and distance found that each additional mile increased transport time by 1.5 minutes (95% confidence interval [CI] = 1.46, 1.56; $p < .001$; $R^2 = 0.27$).

TABLE 18.1 **Patient demographics and mortality from gunshot wounds: Chicago, 1999–2009**

Variable	GSW frequency, no. (%) or mean ± SD	GSW mortality, no. (%) or mean ± SD
Total	11,744	2,204 (18.8)
Race/ethnicity		
White, non-Hispanic	495 (4.2)	125 (25.3)
Black, non-Hispanic	8,027 (68.3)	1,489 (18.5)
Hispanic	2,529 (21.6)	452 (18.5)
Other/unknown	693 (5.9)	138 (19.9)
Gender		
Female	988 (8.4)	165 (16.7)
Male	10,754 (91.6)	2,037 (18.9)
Age (yr.)		
Birth–9	109 (0.9)	26 (23.9)
10–19	3,389 (28.9)	515 (15.2)
20–29	5,274 (44.9)	1,025 (19.4)
30–39	1,815 (15.5)	369 (20.3)
40–49	750 (6.4)	157 (20.9)
50–59	260 (2.2)	62 (23.8)
60–69	89 (0.8)	20 (22.5)
≥ 70	58 (0.5)	30 (51.7)
Insurance coverage		
Insured	5,488 (47.4)	704 (12.8)
Not insured	6,086 (52.6)	1,464 (24.0)
Incident within 5 miles of trauma center		
Yes	7,736 (65.9)	1,430 (18.5)
No	4,008 (34.1)	774 (19.3)
Intent		
Unintentional	695 (5.9)	82 (3.7)
Suicide	157(1.3)	107 (4.9)
Assault	10,558 (89.9)	1,920 (87.1)
Legal intervention	85 (0.7)	17 (7.7)
Undetermined	249 (2.1)	78 (3.5)
ISS*	10.9 ± 12.8	22.3 ± 14.9
SBP, mm Hg	117.6 ± 50.5	82.0 ± 64.2

Note: GSW = gunshot wound; ISS = injury severity score; SBP = systolic blood pressure. GSW mortality is a subset of GSW frequency. Column totals should approach 100% for each variable within each column. The totals may not add to 100% because of a small amount of missing data.

*An ISS > 16 is associated with a higher likelihood of mortality.

Mortality

The strongest predictors of mortality were the 2 injury severity markers (SBP and ISS) and suicidal intent (table 18.3). Lack of insurance was also associated with a higher mortality. Being Black was associated with lower mortality in this group. Being White and having a suicidal intent markedly increased the mortality risk. There was high correlation between these 2 variables, and injury severity was much worse for the

TABLE 18.2 **Demographics of gunshot wound patients, by distance from a trauma center: Chicago, 1999–2009**

Variable	Distance ≤ 5	Distance > 5	p
Total (no.)	6,786	3,543	
Unadjusted mortality	0.070	0.087	.002[a]
Race/ethnicity (no.)			.001[b]
White, non-Hispanic	343	86	
Black, non-Hispanic	4,048	3,013	
Hispanic	1,959	279	
Other/unknown	433	165	
Gender (no. [%])			.288[b]
Female	589 (9)	286 (8)	
Male	6,192 (91)	3,257 (92)	
Age (no. [%])			.029[b]
0–19 yr.	2,142 (32)	1,027 (29)	
20–39 yr.	3,993 (59)	2,182 (62)	
40–59 yr.	575 (8)	289 (8)	
60+ yr.	73 (1)	45 (1)	
Insurance coverage (no. [%])			.001[b]
Insured	3,541 (53)	1,515 (43)	
Not insured	3,145 (47)	1,977 (57)	
Abbreviated injury scale[c] (no. [%])			.001[b]
Head	486 (13)	185 (11)	
Neck	79 (2)	42 (2)	
Chest	621 (16)	289 (16)	
Abdomen	290 (8)	222 (13)	
Other	2,816 (62)	1,257 (58)	
Intent (no. [%])			.001[b]
Unintentional	515 (8)	124 (3)	
Suicide	62 (1)	42 (1)	
Assault	6,006 (89)	3,316 (94)	
Undetermined	159 (2)	28 (1)	
Legal intervention	41 (1)	33 (1)	
SBP, mm Hg (mean)			
Overall	130.7	131.1	.494[a]
Among patients who died	83.5	79.8	.449[a]
ISS[d] (mean)			
Overall	9.3	10.4	.001[a]
Among patients who died	22.7	21.6	.335

Note: ISS = injury severity score; SBP = systolic blood pressure. The totals may not add to 100% because of a small amount of missing data.

[a]*P*-value determined by the *t*-test.

[b]*P*-value determined by the χ^2 test.

[c]Based on data from 1999 to 2003; no data from 2004 to 2009 were available.

[d]An ISS > 16 is associated with higher likelihood of mortality.

TABLE 18.3 **Adjusted odds of mortality from gunshot wounds: Chicago, 1999–2009**

Variable	OR (95% CI)	P
Male	1.1 (0.77, 1.55)	.61
Black	0.65 (0.44, 0.96)	.03
Hispanic	0.85 (0.56, 1.31)	.47
Age > 55 yr.	1.14 (0.58, 2.23)	.7
Lack of insurance	2.27 (1.86, 2.77)	<.001
ED SBP < 90	16.93 (13.72, 20.91)	<.001
ISS > 16[a]	8.06 (6.72, 9.66)	<.001
Trauma center > 5 miles away	1.23 (1.02, 1.47)	.03
Suicidal intent	8.76 (5.04, 15.24)	<.001
Suicidal intent and White	16.06 (6.52, 39.54)	<.001

Note: CI = confidence interval; ED = emergency department; ISS = injury severity score; OR = odds ratio; SBP = systolic blood pressure.

[a]An ISS > 16 is associated with higher likelihood of mortality.

group of White GSW patients with suicidal intent, which likely explains the association of increased mortality among Whites in our sample.

Unadjusted mortality was higher for patients who were shot farther than 5 miles from the nearest trauma center (8.7% vs. 7%; $p < .001$). In a multivariate model adjusting for injury severity, age, race, gender, insurance status, and intent of GSW, being shot more than 5 miles from a trauma center was independently associated with increased risk of mortality (odds ratio [OR] = 1.23; 95% CI = 1.02, 1.47; $p = .03$). To validate our model, we performed 3 additional analyses. We first compared our model using a 5-mile distance from a trauma center with a model that dichotomized patients using a 4-mile distance (46% of patients), which yielded similar results (OR = 1.19; 95% CI = 1.03, 1.27; $p = .04$). As a sensitivity analysis, we created a second regression model using SBP at the scene vs. emergency department SBP. The results were the same, but there were fewer missing values for emergency department SBP, so the latter results are reported here. Third, distance from a trauma center was independently associated with increased mortality among GSW victims, irrespective of intent. Regression modeling that limited the sample to assaults demonstrated identical results. However, regression models for suicidal intent alone had insufficient power to determine associations between transport times and outcomes. Finally, we constructed a correlation matrix, which did not demonstrate severe multicollinearity.

A GSW mortality map demonstrated higher mortality rates for individuals living outside the 5-mile boundary, despite reasonable proximity to main roadways and freeways (figure 18.1).

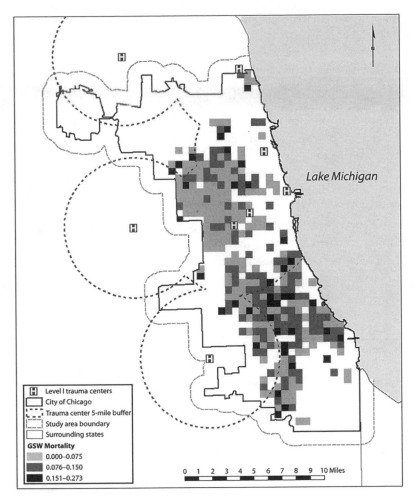

FIGURE 18.1. Density map of gunshot wound (GSW) mortality and distance from a trauma center: Chicago, 1999–2009

Source: Illinois State Trauma Registry.

Discussion

These data demonstrate an association between being shot more than 5 miles from a trauma center, longer prehospital transport times, and mortality from gunshot wounds from 1999 to 2009. Most of Chicago's gun violence occurs on its south and west sides. There are a number of trauma centers located on the west side of the city. On the south side, however, particularly the southeast side, there is no nearby trauma center to serve this high-risk population. This same population with no local access to a level I trauma care has a higher mortality rate from GSWs. The high-profile death of a young activist on the southeast side has created tremendous interest in this issue among community activists and the media.[22–24]

However, solutions are neither simple nor easy. Creation, certification, and maintenance of a trauma center in these relative "trauma deserts" could be very expensive and resource-consuming, though potentially cost-effective.[25] Another solution would be to facilitate existing local hospitals within these deserts to care for trauma patients, possibly in a level II capacity, akin to similar fresh produce initiatives in "food deserts" in the city.[26] This is a possibility because there are at least 4 hospitals in this particular area that are not trauma centers but have surgical and emergency department facilities. Lastly, trauma centers could be rebalanced on the basis of volume and proximity as opposed to capacity, including perhaps reallocating resources or forging new partnerships between academic and community centers. However, any changes to the existing system would need to be studied prospectively because a positive impact is not guaranteed. For example, some researchers have found risk-adjusted mortality to be higher at level II centers than at level I centers, although these studies were not restricted to penetrating trauma.[27,28]

This study is not without limitations. Although there was an association between distance from a trauma center and mortality, we found that injury severity, lack of insurance, and suicidal intent were much stronger predictors of mortality. Modifications of trauma systems cannot address any of these issues. In addition, given that suicidal intent predicted higher mortality but represented a small subset of our data and has very different prevention and public health implications, it might have been reasonable to exclude these patients from the analysis. However, we felt that they added value by encompassing a real-world spectrum of GSWs in which intent may not be immediately known.

Second, we excluded DOAs from the analysis; better information about these cases might have been useful. This remains a tremendous challenge in prehospital trauma research; the patients that are in extremis require intense resources, and data collection is often less rigorous, as was the case in this data set.

Third, we used a distance of 5 miles from a trauma center to compare outcomes, but this number was somewhat arbitrary given the lack of work regarding optimal trauma center proximity. However, for our particular sample, this distance yielded the optimal balance between comparison groups, and a separate model comparing patients that used a 4-mile radius did not elicit significantly different results. Fourth, systemic differences in prehospital interventions or trauma center care may partly explain mortality differences by proximity to a trauma center, but these have not been found in rigorous programmatic evaluations performed by state and local agencies. It is also possible that an as-yet-unidentified confounder exists that is correlated with both transport time and mortality that could explain these associations. Fifth, because of changes in data collection and reporting, and the problems associated with missing data in an administrative database, we were unable to completely control for anatomical location of injuries, which might have an independent effect on mortality, although overall injury severity and physiological measures of injury were taken into account.

The final question is one of generalizability. Chicago is unique in the comprehensiveness and maturity of its trauma system and the prevalence of penetrating trauma; results from this study may not be applicable to other communities. However, potential solutions to this problem could have national and global relevance. For example, designation of a new level II trauma center was employed in south Los Angeles, California, to help decrease the impact of closure of a busy level I center in 2004. Expanding the capacitance of local hospitals to act as trauma service providers may improve outcomes in Chicago, or it may be applicable to other communities with long travel distances to trauma centers or a heavy burden of penetrating trauma. As a second example, for states or communities that are beginning to implement trauma systems, such as Indiana, these data may help inform planning and infrastructure building, particularly in areas such as Gary or Hammond, which are demographically similar to Chicago.

Despite these limitations, to our knowledge this is the largest study to date looking specifically at the impact of distance from a trauma center and mortality from GSWs in a particular geographic area. To determine the effect of these results within a real-world context, an attributable risk analysis can easily be calculated for GSW patients. For example, the crude mortality for Blacks shot within 5 miles of a trauma center is 6.42%, whereas outside of 5 miles it is 8.73%; the overall mortality is 7.41%, so the percentage attributable risk is 26.05%. This would translate to 6.3 excess deaths per year for this community, and, assuming a per-patient loss of 40 quality-adjusted life years, a total of approximately 240 quality-adjusted life years. Assuming a cost-effectiveness threshold of $100,000 per quality-adjusted life year, the sum is $24 million per year, far higher than the typical annual costs of maintaining a trauma center.[29] It is unclear whether these data will affect policy or funding decisions, but they should certainly be used to inform discussions. In addition, future work should evaluate the effects of distance from a trauma center on other outcomes, such as hospital length of stay, permanent disability, and quality of life.

Gun violence remains endemic to Chicago, and GSWs account for the overwhelming majority of homicides within the city. We have demonstrated that incident proximity to a trauma center has a positive effect on survival outcomes for GSW victims. We have identified the southeast side of the city as a relative trauma desert in Chicago's regional trauma system that is associated with increased GSW mortality. We hope that the data presented will inform discussions aimed at optimizing regional trauma care in Chicago and will also aid in planning regional trauma systems in other urban settings.

References

1. Centers for Disease Control and Prevention. Scientific data, surveillance, and injury statistics. 2011. http://www.cdc.gov/injury/wisqars.

2. Nathens AB, Jurkovich GJ, Cummings P, Rivara FP, Maier RV. The effect of organized systems of trauma care on motor vehicle crash mortality. *Journal of the American Medical Association.* 2000;283(15):1990–1994.

3. MacKenzie E, Rivara F, Jurkovich G, et al. A national evaluation of the effect of trauma-center care on mortality. *New England Journal of Medicine.* 2006;4(354):366–378.

4. Centers for Disease Control and Prevention. Access to trauma care: Getting the right care at the right place at the right time. 2012. http://www.cdc.gov/traumacare/access_trauma.html [link inactive].

5. Branas CC, MacKenzie EJ, Williams JC, et al. Access to trauma centers in the United States. *Journal of the American Medical Association.* 2005;293(21): 2626–2633.

6. Gonzalez RP, Cummings G, Mulekar M, Rodning CB. Increased mortality in rural vehicular trauma: Identifying contributing factors through data linkage. *Journal of Trauma and Acute Care Surgery.* 2006;61(2):404–409.

7. Grossman DC, Kim A, Macdonald S, Klein P, Copass MK, Maier RV. Urban-rural differences in prehospital care of major trauma. *Journal of Trauma and Acute Surgery.* 1997;4(42):723–729.

8. Esposito TJ, Maier RV, Rivara FP, et al. The impact of variation in trauma care times: Urban versus rural. *Prehospital and Disaster Medicine.* 1995;10(3): 161–166; discussion 166–167.

9. Feero S, Hedges JR, Simmons E, Irwin L. Does out-of-hospital EMS time affect trauma survival? *American Journal of Emergency Medicine.* 1995;13(2): 133–135.

10. Gervin AS, Fischer RP. The importance of prompt transport in salvage of patients with penetrating heart wounds. *Journal of Trauma-Injury Infection and Critical Care.* 1982;22(6):443–448.

11. Pepe PE, Wyatt CH, Bickell WH, Bailey ML, Mattox KL. The relationship between total prehospital time and outcome in hypotensive victims of penetrating injuries. *Annals of Emergency Medicine.* 1987;16(3):293–297.

12. Petri RW, Dyer A, Lumpkin J. The effect of prehospital transport time on the mortality from traumatic injury. *Prehospital and Disaster Medicine.* 1995; 10(1):24–29.

13. Newgard CD, Schmicker RH, Hedges JR, et al. Emergency medical services intervals and survival in trauma: Assessment of the "golden hour" in a North American prospective cohort. *Annals of Emergency Medicine.* 2010;55(3): 235–246 e234.

14. CLEARpath. Crime summary. http://gis.chicagopolice.org.

15. World Health Organization. *International classification of diseases (9th revision).* Geneva: WHO; 1980.

16. Tornetta P 3rd, Mostafavi H, Riina J, et al. Morbidity and mortality in elderly trauma patients. *Journal of Trauma and Acute Surgery.* 1999;46(4):702–706.

17. Haider AH, Chang DC, Efron DT, Haut ER, Crandall M, Cornwell EE. Race and insurance status as risk factors for trauma mortality. *Archives of Surgery.* 2008;143(10):945–949.

18. Nakahara S, Yokota J. Revision of the International Classification of Diseases to include standardized descriptions of multiple injuries and injury severity. *Bulletin of the World Health Organization.* 2011;89(3):238–240.

19. Maybury RS, Bolorunduro OB, Villegas C, et al. Pedestrians struck by motor vehicles further worsen race- and insurance-based disparities in trauma outcomes: The case for inner-city pedestrian injury prevention programs. *Surgery.* 2010;148(2):202–208.

20. Salim A, Ottochian M, DuBose J, et al. Does insurance status matter at a public, level I trauma center? *Journal of Trauma and Acute Surgery.* 2010;1(68): 211–216.

21. Rhyne CE, Templer DI, Brown LG, Peters NB. Dimensions of suicide: Perceptions of lethality, time, and agony. *Suicide and Life-Threatening Behavior.* 1995;25(3):373–380.

22. In memoriam: Damien Turner. 2010. http://www.areachicago.org/p/issues/institutions-and-infrastructures/damian-turner.

23. Chicago Now. 20th Ward aldermanic candidate Rev. Andre Smith demands Damian Turner's killers to surrender. [August 17, 2010]. http://www .chicagonow.com/and-the-ordinary-people-said/2010/08/20th-ward-aldermanic -candidate-rev-andre-smith-demands-damian-turners-killers-to-surrender.

24. Health Care Now. Activists call for trauma care from University of Chicago Medical Center. [August 22, 2011]. http://www.healthcare-now.org/ activists-call-for-trauma-care-from-the-university-of-chicago-medical-center [link inactive].

25. MacKenzie EJ, Weir S, Rivara FP, et al. The value of trauma center care. *Journal of Trauma and Acute Surgery.* 2010;69(1):1–10.

26. Healthy Places. Food. 2012. http://www.healthyplaceschicago.org/food/ index.lasso [link inactive].

27. Cudnik MT, Newgard CD, Sayre MR, Steinberg SM. Level I versus level II trauma centers: An outcomes-based assessment. *Journal of Trauma and Acute Surgery.* 2009;66(5):1321–1326.

28. Demetriades D, Martin M, Salim A, Rhee P, Brown C, Chan L. The effect of trauma center designation and trauma volume on outcome in specific severe injuries. *Annals of Surgery.* 2005;242(4):512–517; discussion 517–519.

29. Rotondo MF, Bard MR, Sagraves SG, et al. What price commitment: What benefit? The cost of a saved life in a developing level I trauma center. *Journal of Trauma and Acute Surgery.* 2009;67(5):915–923.

PART IV

Communities Matter

Prior parts of this *Reader* demonstrated that place matters, witnessed by the persistent health inequalities seen among Chicago communities. Recognition that the environment has a great influence on health should come as little surprise. Communities matter. More than just places, communities are a form of social organization greater than the sum of their geographic parts. Communities have memories, and they have voices—as anyone driving down Ashland Avenue in February 2015 could attest (see figure 5).

The photograph shows a billboard featuring an African American infant beside the message: "I am an outbreak." It was part of a larger advertising campaign to promote flu shots, with other billboards placed throughout the city. This particular billboard was up for several weeks on a major avenue, just north of the Illinois Medical District.

The evocative term *outbreak* brings to mind Ebola, tuberculosis, and other feared conditions typically associated with external threats from poor countries. Juxtaposing this message with the picture inadvertently rebranded the threat to be the community itself. In this case, the billboard elicited a quick response from the community. Within days after it was erected, graffiti was painted on the image, asserting a far more positive theme: "[I am] Beautiful."

As we will see in this part of the *Reader*, public health has a long history of examining communities by measuring their deficits (e.g., their levels of poverty or rates of violence). But we know that a community's assets and strengths, sometimes described as social capital or collective efficacy, have a positive or protective effect on health. The studies in this part of our book emphasize that both ways of viewing the relationship between community and health—from the perspective of disadvantage

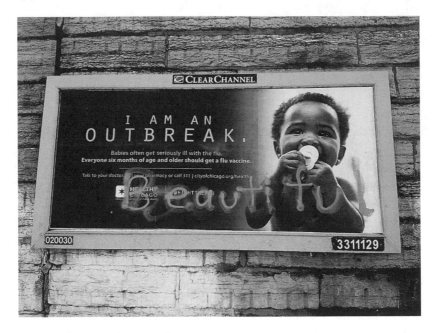

FIGURE 5. A community perspective

Source: De Maio F, Shah RC. Community response to a public health advertisement. *American Journal of Public Health*. 2016;106(11):1979.

and from the perspective of assets—offer valuable knowledge about how communities matter.

Studies in this part consider attributes such as mutual aid, social support, willingness to intervene to help others, trust, reciprocity, and civic engagement. These community-level attributes offer members protection against preventable morbidity and premature mortality, potentially buffering against the health-damaging effects of poverty and discrimination. Ruchi Gupta et al. show how positive community factors such as social capital, economic potential, and community resources protect against childhood asthma. Robert Sampson et al., in a widely cited study, measured levels of collective efficacy across Chicago communities, finding that it varied significantly between communities. Most critically, they found an association between low collective efficacy and high levels of violence. This study demonstrated that collective efficacy can, at least in part, alleviate some of the effects of concentrated disadvantage and residential instability.

Later in this part, Kimberly Lochner et al. explore the community-level association between social capital and death rates. Although similar to collective efficacy, the concept of social capital measures levels of reciprocity, trust, and civic participation. Their study found that, after adjusting for material deprivation, lower neighborhood death rates were associated with higher levels of social capital. This was a further indication that social capital—a tangible community asset—may counter the negative effects of socioeconomic deprivation.

Community disadvantages, including poverty, violence, and hardship, shorten life spans and erode quality of life. Disadvantages constrain the capacity of community resources to produce good health—and, thus, the disadvantages may negate the strengths of a community and its residents. The selections in this part point to aspects of community life in need of public attention and immediate action at all levels, including structural change.

Researchers in Chicago have grappled with how to investigate the effects of violence on health. Margo Wilson and Martin Daly show that life expectancy is most closely correlated with homicide rates, with economic inequality playing a contributing role. Their findings suggest that lowered life expectancy may contribute to risk-taking behaviors and earlier timing to life transitions. The impact that violence has on community health is also demonstrated by James Collins and Richard David, who examined the association between violent crime rates and the likelihood of low birth weight for African American mothers.

The last selection features Jan Warren-Findlow's work on the "weathering" hypothesis; how lifelong exposure to racism, discrimination, inequality, stress, and negative environment affects health, particularly for African American women. Weathering begins at an early age and continues over the life course, manifesting as susceptibility to increased chronic illness and disability. Her qualitative study confirms the value of narrative, sociocultural context, and lived experience for understanding health inequities. Warren-Findlow argues: "Without understanding the complexity of people's lives, we cannot hope to conquer effectively the health disparities experienced by lower income, underserved, and marginalized populations." Similarly, Loretta Lacey et al. relied on a qualitative approach to describe how public health interventions aimed at reducing chronic risk factors—in this case smoking—need to be tailored to fit community context in order to succeed.

These selections raise important questions: What can be done to strengthen communities and reduce disadvantage to achieve immediate and long-term health gains? What aspects of communities can be mobilized and strengthened to nurture resiliency and opportunity?

CHAPTER NINETEEN

Social Support in Smoking Cessation among Black Women in Chicago Public Housing

Loretta P. Lacey, Clara Manfredi, George Balch, Richard B. Warnecke, Karen Allen, and Constance Edwards

In the quest for a smoke-free society by the year 2000, some segments of the U.S. population lag behind. For example, smoking prevalence rates among young women with no more than high school education and low income are high, while smoking is declining in the total population.[1-3] Smoking is more prevalent among black than white women because blacks have not stopped smoking as rapidly as whites.[1-4] Existing health promotion programs that incorporate cessation have not attracted the same participation or achieved the same success among black women with low socioeconomic status (SES) as they have among black and white women whose incomes are higher.[5,6] Additionally, participation in group efforts among members of this population has been problematic.[7] Clearly, programs tailored to this segment of the population are needed.

To attract greater participation from this group of smokers, these programs must have a broader focus than cessation alone. Boyd-Franklin[8] and Trotman and Gallagher[9] document the benefits of social support groups for black women based on the sharing of their common experience and their willingness to exchange emotional, spiritual, and social assistance. Social support groups may be especially important for low-

Originally published in *Public Health Reports* 108, no. 3 (May–June 1993): 387–94.

SES urban black women because they tend to experience a type of isolation that creates fear and stress and distrust of their environment. These factors limit their chances to build or join social networks and foster dependence on smoking to reduce loneliness, reduce stress, and provide affordable pleasure.

This paper reports formative research toward a smoking cessation program that is socially support based and tailored to the needs of low-SES black women. The focus groups that we describe were originally designed to assess factors related to smoking cessation and participation in such programs. However, as the groups progressed, it became clear that there are powerful environmental factors related to smoking that inhibit participation in the kinds of programs currently offered.

We began to discover how the social environment of these women, particularly their social isolation and limited sources of social support, is inextricably linked to their smoking. It became clear that successful cessation programs must mobilize social support that will provide ways of coping with these environmental factors to enhance cessation. Cessation programs that address these larger issues will be more effective.

Background

Investigation of the factors associated with smoking among low-SES black women was prompted by the outcomes of an intervention that proved satisfactory for the general Chicago population but was less effective for low-SES black women who are residents of Chicago public housing developments. The original study[7] used a self-help manual, "Freedom from Smoking in 20 Days," and a series of televised segments on the local evening news that followed the contents of the manual. A supplement to the main intervention was introduced in public housing developments. This supplemental intervention was implemented by lay health educators, who conducted a series of specially designed classes on smoking cessation for women 18–39 years old living in the housing developments. The lay health educators had two main tasks: to promote viewing of the televised program and to elicit participation in the local smoking cessation classes that were part of the intervention.[10]

More than 600 residents, who were canvassed door-to-door in the housing developments, expressed interest in a smoking cessation program, and more than 200 pre-registered. However, maintaining continuous participation in the smoking cessation classes was problematic, and the number of actual participants was less than half that of those who preregistered.

We examined data from our baseline sample of residents in housing developments not selected for the intervention with data from a sample of the general population of female smokers in the Chicago metropolitan statistical area matched by age and divided into two groups, one black and one white. Based on this analysis, those in the public housing sample had less interest in quitting or desire to quit and were less likely to have made plans to quit compared with black or white female smokers in the general population study. Moreover, when we analyzed in detail the responses of women in the housing developments, it was evident that they did not share with other black women or with white women the same understanding about the relationship between smoking and risk of disease, especially cancer, and did not see how risks made smoking less desirable. One the other hand, it was unclear from the results exactly what value smoking held for these women.[11]

[. . .]

Method

[. . .]

We conducted eight focus groups with black women residents from three Chicago public housing developments that were not among the intervention sites for the original study. These women had sociodemographic characteristics similar to those of the women in the intervention sites. Specifically, our survey data revealed that 42% of the women in public housing had not completed high school, 66% were single parents, and all had annual household incomes of less than $13,000. By age 17, 68% had initiated smoking. Just over half (51%) smoked more than 10 cigarettes daily, and 96% smoked mentholated cigarettes. No or weak desire to quit smoking was reported by 54%.[11]

Each group session had six to eight participants and lasted about 2 hours. Discussion focused on participants' daily activities, stresses and pleasures, social environment, beliefs about smoking and health, and smoking and health behavior. The discussions followed a structured format to identify perceived benefits of smoking, barriers to cessation, and receptivity to various cessation approaches.

To ensure reliability of the findings, we used three different moderators (two black and one white), multiple observers, and immediate post-session debriefings. Observers wrote summaries of each session. In addition, audiotapes and videotapes were made of each session, and transcripts of the audiotapes were prepared and compared against each videotape for accuracy and completeness. Finally, all themes which emerged in the summaries were cross-checked against the tapes and transcripts for counter evidence.

Findings

Our synthesis of the sessions revealed a consistent theme of distinct barriers to smoking cessation that related to life circumstances and social environments of the women. Their environments as viewed through comments in the focus groups were highly stressful. Smoking seemed to provide them with relief and comfort.

Barriers to Smoking Cessation

Our synthesis of the content of the group discussions indicated seven barriers to the participants' cessation: (a) the problems of managing their lives in a highly stressful environment, (b) their isolation and the limited support systems within these environments, (c) the availability of smoking as an attainable pleasure in a milieu with very limited resources for pleasure, (d) perceived minimal health risks of smoking, (e) the commonality of smoking, (f) the scarce-to-nonexistent information about how to stop smoking, and (g) the belief that all they need is determination to quit on their own.

All of these barriers followed from social isolation and lack of support. In fact, we observed that these women were most motivated to quit when they were doing well, that is, working, attending school, and receiving positive support. When their lives left them little support or made them feel less valued, they wanted to smoke. These general feelings, however, can be best described when organized around the barriers.

MANAGING IN A HIGHLY STRESSFUL ENVIRONMENT
A consistent theme among the women in the focus groups was that smoking helps them to manage the overwhelming pressures in their lives

and to stay calm. In this context, they believed smoking offered strength for coping with the harsh realities of their life situations in communities that presented immediate and constant dangers to them and their families. These communities were unclean, had substandard housing, and offered few resources. Life there was plagued by violence and crime, often related to drug use. Although all smokers tend to emphasize the stress-management utilities of smoking as reasons for not quitting, the magnitude and nature of stressors in these communities gave stress a unique dimension. For example, one participant described vividly the extreme stress encountered daily in trying to get her daughter onto the school bus:

> My daughter use to have to get on the [school] bus. She had to walk down the stairs, stepping over the dope fiends and the junkies. And one day she walked downstairs, this guy was laying in the hallway with a needle in his neck scaring her. She ran out to the bus, she fell down, she missed the bus, she missed a couple days of school. I got to hear from the school [about her absence] you know it's bad.

Smoking was believed to bring some control when women faced so many situations over which they had minimal control. Another participant related the lack of control about the very basic issues of survival as she described an encounter with bureaucracy at the local welfare office and her response:

> To top it off, Public Aid mess me up. [She was sent to the wrong office.] . . . I got there late, and asked the gentleman, "Are you going to call my name back now?" He said, "You have to wait." So they put down "no show," then sent me a letter decreasing me for 3 months. Three months! . . . I smoked a lot on that day, do you hear me?

It was clear from watching the members of the group that "lighting up" was a natural, normatively accepted response to situations of this type. They smoked to control their reactions to uncontrollable events.

ISOLATION AND LIMITED SUPPORT SYSTEMS

The structure of these communities promoted isolation. All were located in racially and economically segregated areas of the city. Some of these women lived in housing developments considered the poorest communities in the nation. One housing complex was almost at the city limits, near a dump site. Most of the high-rise buildings had poorly functioning elevators and unsafe stairways, which limited movement outside of the home except for necessary activities. General fear for personal safety enhanced the physical and social isolation. Women in the groups believed that development of relationships and contacts beyond the immediate family were risky. Opportunities to establish close friendship networks were limited by the suspicion that relationships with persons outside the household might create additional problems in their lives. A recurring comment was that attempts to have relationships outside of their immediate families brought what was frequently described as confusion into their lives. A participant who lived in a high-rise development described why she limited outside contact to her family: "I'm not visiting too much—I'm a house person. There's too much going on down there in the streets."

Families were the most trusted source of support. For these women, family seemed focused on children, sisters, and mothers. But still, many of the participants described intense loneliness. One woman, age 23, who smoked three packs of cigarettes per day, had this vivid description of her isolation:

> I might be depressed or whatever, and I don't have anybody to talk to, and my baby . . . he'll be in his playpen. I'll just talk to him and tell him a bit of my problems. He'll just look at me, like mama I know what you are going through or, you know. . . . I just sit out there and pour all my problems out to my baby, and sometimes I feel better.

One element frequently missing in the lives of many of these women seemed to be the support that can come from a male partner. A stable relationship with a partner—whether or not he is the spouse—means one can share problems, receive emotional support, and in some cases can rely on someone to defend one's safety. But merely having a partner was not enough to reduce the overwhelming stress caused by these women's environments.

SMOKING AS AN ATTAINABLE PLEASURE
Lack of financial resources and physical and social isolation limited access to sources of pleasure. Many preferred to forgo material pleasures

for themselves to provide the basic needs for their families. One participant described her pleasure with smoking in this context:

> I have a lot of pressure on me. [She works, takes care of an aging mother, has children, and tries to keep the house together.] . . . I don't have time for me . . . so the only time I have is when I take a cigarette out of the pack and fire it. 'Cause that's the quickest thing you can do, you know, something that you want to do for yourself.

These women perceived smoking as a legal, harmless pleasure, attainable for a relatively small investment. The perceived alternatives were drugs, alcohol abuse, or losing self-control. As one participant remarked:

> I'm going to have to stop smoking because I really can't afford it, but I've got to do something. . . . I'd rather smoke than go there and shoot some drugs or smoke a pipe or something like that.

PERCEIVED MINIMAL HEALTH RISKS OF SMOKING

Although these women tended to agree about the negative effects of smoking on the health of their children, they seemed less convinced about the harmful health effects of cigarette smoking on themselves or other adults. They felt that cigarette smoking, in general, was not good, but they expressed doubts about a specific link, for example, between cancer and smoking. Few mentioned cancer as a health concern for themselves or their families.

Furthermore, they believed that the cancer that they have seen among their family members and other acquaintances was due to many other causes than smoking. In fact, they were adamant that medical scientists do not know the cause of cancer. Balshem[12] has recently described similar findings among a white working-class population. The women in Balshem's focus groups also expressed such fatalistic beliefs as "everything causes cancer" and "once it occurs, there is little that medical practitioners can do to control its course."

Surprisingly, even the actual presence of more urgent health problems that smoking aggravates did not deter these women. Several women had chronic pulmonary disease (asthma, emphysema), heart disease, or kidney disease, but they continued to smoke, apparently unaware or unaccepting of a possible relationship between smoking and these health problems. Where they perceived possible environmental effects, they attributed them to hazards in their environments. These attributions had a basis in reality, since some lived in housing developments near waste dump sites, and all lived in areas highly polluted with dust and dirt. They emphasized this situation through their description of their constant need to clean dirt from surfaces in their homes.

COMMONALITY OF SMOKING

Another barrier to cessation was the commonality of smoking in these women's social environments. A consistent theme throughout the groups was the belief that most adults smoke. These women believed that more than 75% of adults in their communities smoked cigarettes. They thought that the rate in the general population was the same.

When informed that smoking is decreasing and that less than 30% of the general adult population smokes, many of these women expressed disbelief. They seemed not to see smoking in the same negative context that it increasingly appears elsewhere. The actual prevalence within their own social groups made it difficult to avoid smokers or smoking situations and made their perceptions accurate for their effective environment.

SCARCE INFORMATION ABOUT HOW TO STOP SMOKING

Electronic media were a major source of health information often cited by the women with whom we spoke. This observation is consistent with our 1987 baseline data and has been reported by others working with similar groups.[13,14] When asked if they knew where they could go or methods they could use to help them stop smoking, nearly all reported no knowledge about such resources. The consensus was that the only way to quit smoking was to do it on their own, "cold turkey."

Another theme emerging from this discussion was that their sources of health information—electronic media—provided little guidance about smoking cessation. Although there were frequent references to smoking-related issues on television, the reports did not offer advice about or direction for smoking cessation except for the infrequent programs such as those offered in this study.

After tracking media references for 2 years, we found very little in any of the media about cessation. In our continuing work, we have found that these women may be told often by their health care providers to quit, but these recommendations do not include clear guidance on how to quit. Hence, there is minimal concrete direction to assist them.

DETERMINATION TO QUIT WITHOUT HELP

Because of a lack of specific guidance and information about the cessation process and because of social isolation, there was little awareness of the process and of the fact that many smokers relapse and have to make several attempts before successfully quitting smoking. The lack of exposure to those who have tried to quit reinforced the beliefs that only self-determination leads to smoking cessation and that those who quit must exert Herculean efforts. Pervasive smoking in the environment, the absence of social support, and the likely absence of specific constructive assistance should these women want to quit reinforced their perceptions about the high cost of trying. Besides, their reality was always to be self-reliant; to be dependent or in need of supportive help suggested vulnerability to their environment. Apparently, this ethos extended to many areas of their lives.

The operative belief was that a woman must be in control of herself to stop smoking, much as she needed control to survive at all. Impersonal sources of support in which she had little control were not compatible with this belief structure. For example, one woman recounted her failure to stop smoking. She was among those who had seen a quit-smoking manual at one of the local discount stores. When asked if she thought a manual would work, she replied:

> No, if you haven't got the will power, it's not going to work. You are just spending your money on nothing. I look at it as if they are taking my money. Because I'm not going to go along with the program [because she does not want to quit smoking]. . . . If you really want to stop smoking, you don't need a manual.

Others echoed from around the room: "It would not work because they don't want to quit."

Social Support

Smoking cessation in the face of all of these barriers requires help and perseverance, but the help must come from known and trusted sources if it is to be accepted. Traditional smoking cessation programs and the support from them seemed not to be effective even when motivation to quit is present.

Given these observations, it was surprising to observe during these sessions a consistent pattern of spontaneous formation of group support among the women as they discussed their experiences and frustration with everyday living. Most of these women did not know each other before the group sessions, yet they were remarkably accepting of each other and openly shared experiences and the accompanying sorrow, worry, and concerns. These exchanges generated supportive and empathic understanding that obviously reflected common experience and resulted in warm, nonjudgmental, and accepting interaction. As they shared personal sorrows, disappointments, joys (especially about their children), and hopes during the limited session time, each woman was accepted as having worth, human dignity, and full membership in the group.

Some examples illustrate the empathic atmosphere that emerged in each group. One young woman had just been released from the county correctional facility and shared her fear and sadness about what led to her arrest and the possibility of further incarceration:

> I was scared because I never had a record before. I was never in trouble. And I've been going to court since last year. They were getting ready to give me 6 years, and they were going to send me to Dwight [a State women's correctional facility].

She related that her incarceration followed a drug offense in which she had been both a user and pusher. Her comments revealed a trust in the members of the group, who had just discussed their fears of and anger about pushers in their communities. The trust was well founded: when she confessed to being one of those whom they had just castigated, the response was nonjudgmental, warm, and filled with expressions of relief that she did not have to be incarcerated longer.

In another group, a woman said that she always felt left out, as if she could not do anything right. She had once prepared a Tupperware party, and no one came. She felt rejected by people in general, and she did not know if group sessions (for smoking cessation) would work for her. At that point, a member of the session who had been purposely reticent and almost hostile in her interactions with the group said: "Well, you are accepted here." Others agreed. The apparent need and desire these women have to share their experiences in an empathic but neutral setting may provide a basis for interventions that might include smoking cessation as a component.

Applying Support to Smoking Cessation

Others who have studied groups with black women have reported the value of organizing the groups for social support.[8,9] Participants in our focus groups expressed enthusiasm about forming groups that might help them to stop smoking. They immediately took ownership of the idea, providing several valuable suggestions: (a) groups should be multi-purpose, allowing for other important needs to be met; (b) they do not need a professional leader, since the direction of the discussion should come from them; (c) organizers should be former smokers; and (d), most of all, they wanted the group to be a mechanism for them to give and receive emotional and social assistance.

The group appeared to be seen as a potential means of reducing the loneliness and isolation experienced in their communities. These groups were perceived as a neutral and safe environment, not unlike that found in therapy groups; the group was also seen as a potential social encounter, as recreation. The women saw these groups as providing opportunity for release from family obligations, such as the constant care of their children. Finally, the group was seen as a way to learn about life concerns from family- and household-related tasks to job training. In each group, there was considerable discussion about their desire and strong need for employment. If the support serves as a means of self-enhancement and esteem building, factors which they often associated with periods when they had stopped smoking, it may lead to cessation.

The possibility of smoking cessation occurring within groups that are formed to provide social support is promising. These groups may offer the help needed to attempt behavioral change. These participants mentioned a variety of locales and sites, some within their communities, in such places as community centers and their homes. Churches, which are often mentioned by health professionals are promising places, were not mentioned as a first choice. The strong spirituality that seemed to influence many aspects of their lives did not always translate into church affiliation or attendance. Others were interested in getting away from their communities, going even to places where people smoked to aid in building resistance. What seemed most important was the composition of the group. They wanted to be among other women to learn, share feelings, and offer and receive social and emotional support.

Conclusions

Our findings are based on a qualitative approach, and hence the limitations in interpreting this type of study data apply. Despite the methodological constraints, there are a number of relevant implications for public health programs for these populations. We observed that for women in our groups, smoking was associated with relief from the heavy burden of stress in their lives. It helped them to cope with a hostile environment and the extraordinarily difficult life situations that accentuated their lack of social support. Furthermore, it was an attainable and acceptable pleasure that had enormous value for them. These women did not see cancer as a health threat associated with smoking. Moreover, they did not see other health problems as urgent enough to motivate a change in their smoking behavior. On the other hand, smoking appeared to be intimately tied to their life experiences, and when they felt productive and supported, they appeared more likely to consider smoking cessation.

Within these groups, the women demonstrated a natural reservoir of support for one another. They shared common backgrounds as black women engaged in continuing life struggles. There was a readiness to share their common life experiences, and the sharing revealed mutual empathy and nonjudgmental support. The group context addressed many of the barriers described previously. The social isolation was lessened by the presence of sympathetic peers with limited claims on the others in the group.

If smoking cessation interventions could be introduced into such a context, the potential for support, so important in the quitting process, would be great, since there would be an environment where cessation was accepted and the experiences of relapse, slips, and so on could be shared and not judged. The challenge is to develop health promotion programs that use the participants' strengths and put the programs in the context of methods that the participants perceive as useful and acceptable.

The fact that the women enthusiastically embraced the idea of support groups and immediately wanted to assume program ownership by shaping its format gave evidence of their interest. Their responses also suggest that the need for self-reliance can be met if the women are active participants in program development and implementation as partners with the health professionals. Our experience and that of others,[7] however, suggests that attendance and participation are problematic when the program competes with the everyday concerns of living.

How then might the effort differ? Although this paper cannot offer specific answers, it does offer insights important to the development of innovative strategies by health administrators and providers. First, these women clearly indicated that smoking cessation cannot be the single focus or even the primary focus. To increase likelihood success, smoking cessation should be part of a program that has other meaningful purposes for these women. Cessation is most likely to occur in the context of programs that have some perceived relationship to improving the lives of these women. Relevance to them will focus on issues that differ from those usually associated with health promotion. These women did not see a clear relationship between smoking and major illness, even when they had an illness. Future research with black smokers should consider these barriers, and their relevance for other groups should be determined.

References

1. Novotny TE, Warner KE, Kendrick JS, Remington PL. Smoking by blacks and whites: Socioeconomic and demographic differences. *American Journal of Public Health*. 1988;78(9):1187–1189.

2. Fiore MC, Novotny TE, Pierce JP, Hatziandreu EJ, Patel KM, Davis RM. Trends in cigarette smoking in the United States: The changing influence of gender and race. *Journal of the American Medical Association*. 1989;261(1):49–55.

3. Public Health Office. The health consequences of smoking: Nicotine addiction. *A report of the surgeon general*. Rockville, MD: Office of Smoking and Health; 1988.

4. Orleans CT et al. A survey of smoking and quitting patterns among black Americans. *American Journal of Public Health*. 1989;79:176–181.

5. Gottlieb NH, Green LW. Ethnicity and lifestyle health risk: Some possible mechanisms. *American Journal of Health Promotion*. 1987;2(1):37–51.

6. Freimuth VS, Mettger W. Is there a hard-to-reach audience? *Public Health Reports*. 1990;105(3):232–238.

7. Warnecke RB, Flay BR, Kviz FJ, et al. Characteristics of participants in a televised smoking cessation intervention. *Preventive Medicine*. 1991;20(3):389–403.

8. Boyd-Franklin N. Group therapy for black women: A therapeutic support model. *American Journal of Orthopsychiatry.* 1987;57(3):394–401.

9. Trotman FK, Gallagher, AH. Group therapy with black women. In *Women's therapy groups: Paradigms of feminist treatment* (Brody CM, ed.). New York: Springer; 1987:118–131.

10. Lacey L, Tukes S, Manfredi C, Warnecke RB. Use of lay health educators for smoking cessation in a hard-to-reach urban community. *Journal of Community Health.* 1991;16(5):269–282.

11. Manfredi C, Lacey L, Warnecke R, Buis M. Smoking-related behavior, beliefs, and social environment of young black women in subsidized public housing in Chicago. *American Journal of Public Health.* 1992;82(2):267–272.

12. Balshem M. Cancer, control and causality: Talking about cancer in a working-class community. *American Ethnologist.* 1991;18(1):152–172.

13. Warnecke RB. Intervention in black populations. *Progress in Clinical and Biological Research.* 1981;53:167–183.

14. Denniston RW. Cancer knowledge, attitudes, and practices among black Americans. *Progress in Clinical and Biological Research.* 1981;53:225–235.

CHAPTER TWENTY

Life Expectancy, Economic Inequality, Homicide, and Reproductive Timing in Chicago Neighbourhoods

Margo Wilson and Martin Daly

Introduction

Psychologists, economists, and criminologists have found that young adults, poor people, and criminal offenders all tend to discount the future relatively steeply.[1-6] Such tendencies have been called "impulsivity" and "short time horizons" or, more pejoratively, impatience, myopia, lack of self-control, and incapacity to delay gratification. Behind the use of such terms lies a presumption that steep discounting is dysfunctional and that the appropriate weighting of present rewards against future investments is independent of life stage and socioeconomic circumstance.

There is an alternative view: adjustment of discount rates in relation to age and other variables is just what we should expect of an evolved psyche functioning normally.[5-11] Steep discounting may be a "rational" response to information that indicates an uncertain or low probability of surviving to reap delayed benefits, for example, and "reckless" risk taking can be optimal when the expected profits from safer courses of action are negligible.[7,8,12,13]

Originally published in the *British Medical Journal* 314 (April 26, 1997): 1271–74. Copyright © 1997, British Medical Journal Publishing Group.

Hypothesis 1

Criminal violence can be considered an outcome of steep future discounting[6] and escalation of risk in social competition.[10] This is especially true of homicide in urban parts of the United States, where a large majority of cases involve competition for status or resources among unrelated men[7,9] and even marital homicides result from sexual proprietariness in the shadow of male-male competition.[14,15] This line of reasoning suggests that criminal violence will vary in relation to local indicators of life expectancy, hence our first hypothesis: homicide rates will vary as a function of local life expectancy.

Hypothesis 2

Sensitivity to inequality is an expected feature of a psyche that adjusts risk acceptance as we envision, because those at the bottom may be especially motivated to escalate their tactics of social competition when it is clear that some "winners" are doing very well and when the expected payoffs from low risk tactics are poor.[12] This expectation accords with arguments that mortality is exacerbated by inequality itself, over and above the compromising effects of simply being poor on nutrition, access to medical care, safety, and other health promoting opportunities.[16,17] Recent papers in the *BMJ* have presented evidence that economic inequality predicts mortality in general, and moreover that it is most strongly related to "external" mortality of the sort affected by behavioural risk taking, especially homicide.[18,19] Accordingly, our second hypothesis is that economic inequality will account for additional variance in homicidal violence besides that accounted for by local life expectancy.

Previous demonstrations of the effects of inequality on homicide have focused primarily on comparisons between nations, American states, or cities.[18–21] The arguments presented above suggest that the relevant processes of social comparison might operate more locally, with the lives and deaths of people known personally being especially salient to one's mental model of life prospects. We have therefore compared neighbourhoods within a large city. This may also be a good level at which to detect the relations of interest because variables such as latitude, weather, urbanness, laws, history, and prevailing political practices complicate comparisons among larger jurisdictions.

Hypothesis 3

Finally, if low life expectancy is indeed psychologically salient in the ways we envision, it will inspire short time horizons in other domains of behavioural decision making as well. Life expectancy cues might thus affect inclinations to invest in the future through education, preventive health measures, and savings, as well as decisions about the timing of major transitions and life events. Geronimus's studies of young mothers support these ideas: although early reproduction among urban poor people is commonly viewed as an instance of social pathology and failure to exercise choice, she has shown that teenage pregnancy is often an active decision, motivated in large part by expectations about a life course more compressed in time than that of more affluent people.[22,23] Her interviewees in urban ghettoes in the United States expressly wished to become mothers and grandmothers while still young and competent because they anticipated problems of early "weathering" and poor health. Thus, our third hypothesis is that reproduction will occur earlier in the lifespan as one moves from neighbourhoods with high life expectancy to those with low life expectancy.

Data Sources

There are 77 "community areas" with relatively stable boundaries in the American city of Chicago. We used demographic data for 1988–93 for these 77 neighbourhoods (vital statistics obtained from the Illinois Department of Public Health) and population data from the 1990 Census. Following Schoen's method,[24] we used these data to compute male and female life expectancies at birth for each neighbourhood, "cause deleted" in that effects of homicide mortality were removed. We also computed sex and age specific mortality for different causes of death and age specific birth rates. We used counts of the number of households in each of 25 income intervals, derived from 1990 United States Census population and housing summary tape file 3A, to compute the Robin Hood index of income inequality (the maximum deviation of the Lorenz curve of cumulative share of total income from the straight line that would represent zero income variance)[19] for each neighbourhood.

Life Expectancy and Homicide

Neighbourhood specific, cause deleted male life expectancy at birth
(range 54.3 to 77.4 years) and homicide rates (range 1.3 to 156 per 100,000
per year) are highly correlated, confirming our first hypothesis (figure 20.1; $r = -0.88$, $P < 0.0001$).

Table 20.1 shows the bivariate correlations among homicide rates, cause
deleted life expectancies, median household income (adjusted to remove
effects of mean household size, which was correlated with median household income across the 77 neighbourhoods at $r = -0.32$), and a measure of
income inequality. All pairs of measures were highly correlated (all P values < 0.0001), but male life expectancy was more strongly related to both

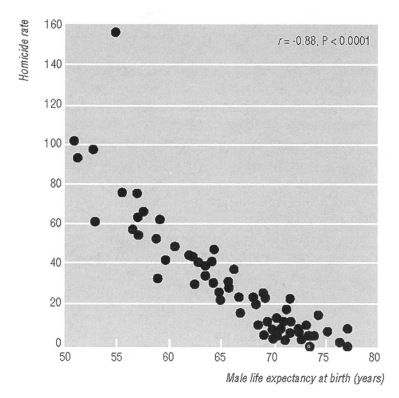

FIGURE 20.1. Neighbourhood specific homicide rates (per 100,000 population per year) in
relation to male life expectancy at birth (with effects of homicide mortality removed) for
77 community areas of Chicago, 1988–93

TABLE 20.1 **Effects of life expectancy ("cause deleted" with respect to death from homicide), income, and income inequality on homicide rates of neighbourhoods in Chicago, 1988–93: Bivariate correlations**

	Homicide rate	Life expectancy for males	Life expectancy for females	Median household income*	Robin Hood index
Homicide rate	—				
Life expectancy for males	−0.88	—			
Life expectancy for females	−0.83	0.92	—		
Median household income	−0.67	0.73	0.59	—	
Robin Hood index	0.75	−0.75	−0.66	−0.86	—

*Effects of household size partialled out.

TABLE 20.2 **Effects of life expectancy ("cause deleted" with respect to death from homicide), income, and income inequality on homicide rates of neighbourhoods in Chicago, 1988–93: Results of stepwise multiple regression predicting homicide rate of neighbourhoods from the other four variables in table 20.1**

	β	t	P-value
Variable in final equation			
Life expectancy of males	−0.74	−9.25	<.0001
Robin Hood index	0.19	2.34	.02
Variables not in final equation			
Life expectancy of females	−0.19	−1.43	.16
Median household income	0.12	1.11	.27

economic measures and the homicide rate than was female life expectancy, and male life expectancy predicted the homicide rate better than either economic measure. Stepwise multiple regression [shown in table 20.2] indicated that economic inequality adds significantly to the prediction of homicide rate that is afforded by life expectancy, supporting our second hypothesis. The adjusted median household income is apparently of less relevance than inequality, a result that is consistent with previous findings from comparisons among larger politico-geographic units,[18–21] but since the two economic measures are so highly correlated, this conclusion must be tentative.

Mortality Patterns in Best and Worst Neighbourhoods

Figure 20.2 shows age specific and sex specific death rates, distinguishing death by homicide and other "external" causes (accidents and suicides) from death by "internal" causes (all other causes—that is, by disease, broadly construed). The figure includes data only for the 10 neighbourhoods with the shortest life expectancies (panels on right) and the 10 with the longest (panels on left). Neighbourhoods with low life expectancy have higher levels of all sorts of mortality in virtually all age-sex categories; however, although the pattern of risk of death from internal causes across the lifespan is similar in the best and worst neighbourhoods, age related patterns of external mortality are quite different. These patterns support the idea that differential rates of external mortality are largely a result of differentials in risk acceptance and future discounting, especially in young adults. (Although perpetrating a homicide, rather than becoming a victim, might be thought to reflect risk ac-

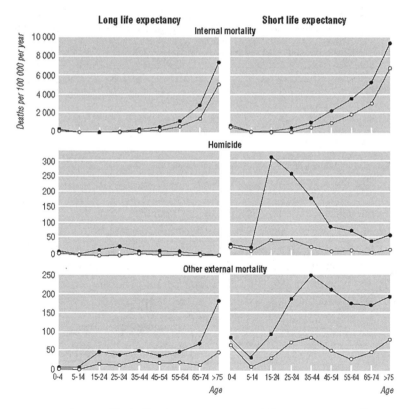

FIGURE 20.2. Age specific death rates per 100,000 population per year, according to sex (male ● female ○) and cause of death for the 10 neighbourhoods with longest life expectancy (left panels) and the 10 with the shortest life expectancy (right panels), Chicago, 1988–93

TABLE 20.3 **Age specific birth rates (per 1000 women per year) in 10 neighbourhoods with longest life expectancy, 10 with shortest life expectancy, and 10 nearest median life expectancy in Chicago, 1988–93**

	Birth rate in neighbourhoods		
Age of mother (years)	Shortest life expectancy	Median life expectancy	Longest life expectancy
10–14	9	2	1
15–19	190	86	45
20–24	224	128	90
25–29	129	103	103
30–34	83	84	89
35–39	39	43	42
40–44	9	10	7

ceptance and future discounting, the age-sex patterns for perpetrators and victims are similar,[9] largely because homicides in Chicago arise primarily from competitive interactions between male victims and killers who are drawn from the same demographic groups.)

Life Expectancy and Age Specific Birth Rates

Table 20.3 shows age specific birth rates for the 10 neighbourhoods with the highest life expectancies, the 10 with the lowest, and the 10 nearest the median. Teenage birth rates are dramatically different, but the differentials decline rapidly and have vanished by age 30. The median age of women giving birth (the "generation time") was 22.6 years in the neighbourhoods with low life expectancy, compared with 25.4 years in the intermediate neighbourhoods and 27.3 years in the neighbourhoods with long life expectancy. These differences are consistent with our third hypothesis and support Geronimus's suggestion[22,23] that the relatively high birth rates in young women in the worst neighbourhoods often reflect a distinct family planning schedule rather than a mere absence of family planning.

Effect of Life Expectancy

Life expectancy reflects not only affluence but such additional considerations as local pathogen loads, health care, and risk of violent death, and it may thus provide a more encompassing quality of life index than economic measures alone. More than just providing a useful epidemiological index, however, an "expectation" of future lifespan may be psychologically salient in its own right, although it need not be a conscious expectation. The data presented here indicate that people behave as if they have adjusted their rates of future discounting and risk acceptance thresholds in relation to local life expectancy, and that they do so in the non-violent domain of reproductive decision making as well as in the potentially violent domain of social competition.

How could such a statistical abstraction as life expectancy be a cause of anything? One possibility is that the human psyche produces what is in effect a semi-statistical apprehension of the distribution of local lifespans, based on the fates of other relevant people.[10] If a young man's grandfathers were both dead before he was born, for example, and some of his primary school classmates had already died, discounting the future could be a normal, adaptive reaction. Moreover, if much of this mortality seems to represent "bad luck" incurred more or less independently of the decedents' choices of action, then accepting more risks in the pursuit of immediate advantage would also make sense.

These inference processes are unlikely to be transparent to introspection, but they may be revealed in expressed attitudes and expectations. Ethnographic studies of urban poor people in American cities contain many articulate statements about the perceived risk of early death, the unpredictability of future resources, and the futility of long term planning.[25–28] One interesting question for psychological research is how the relevant mental models and subjective values develop and are adjusted over the lifespan.[29,30] Another is whether media representations, even fictitious ones, can affect such development in the same way as information about known relatives and neighbours. These questions may best be addressed from an evolutionary psychological perspective, which credits the mind with functional "design" for solving important problems of living in society and making decisions under uncertainty.[10,29,31,32] Such an approach has already shed considerable light on detailed aspects of sex differences and age effects.[5,9]

Feedback Effects

The regression analysis in table 20.1 and our emphasis on life expectancy as a predictive variable must not be taken to imply that economic inequality plays only a secondary role. Considerable evidence indicates that such inequality is itself a major determinant of life expectancy variation,[17] so the more basic (and remediable) causes of violence and other manifestations of steep future discounting are socioeconomic and structural. How our proposal differs from some other accounts is in suggesting that inequality has its effects not only by virtue of non-adaptive or maladaptive stress effects but also by inspiring a "rational" escalation of costly tactics of social competition.[7–10,33] This consideration complicates causal analysis, because it implies that the distribution of age specific mortality is more than an outcome variable, having feedback effects on its own causal factors and hence on itself. [. . .]

The number of likely feedback loops among the phenomena of interest is daunting. If many people react to a local socioecological milieu by discounting the future and lowering their thresholds for risk and violence, the behavioural consequences are likely to worsen the very problems that provoke them, as well as contributing to fear, distrust, and perhaps even economic inequality itself. Living where any resources that one accumulates are apt to be expropriated will also exacerbate these tendencies. Wilkinson has proposed that the behavioural and health effects of unequal resource distributions reflect breakdowns in social and community relations, a proposition that we do not dispute. But exactly how the correlated phenomena of poverty, inequality, injustice, and exogenous threats to life and well-being affect the perceptions, motives, and actions of individuals remains to be elucidated. The causal links are several and multidirectional, but we cannot let that deter us from trying to disentangle them.

References

1. Gottfredson MR, Hirschi T. *A general theory of crime.* Stanford, CA: Stanford University Press; 1990.

2. Green L, Fry AF, Myerson J. Discounting of delayed rewards: A life-span comparison. *Psychological Science.* 1994;5(1):33.

3. Lawrance E. Poverty and the rate of time preference: Evidence from panel data. *Journal of Political Economy.* 1991;99:54–77.

4. Loewenstein G, Elster J. *Choice over time.* New York: Sage; 1992.

5. Rogers A. Evolution of time preference by natural selection. *American Economic Review.* 1994;84:460–481.

6. Wilson J, Herrnstein R. *Crime and human nature.* New York: Simon & Schuster; 1985.

7. Wilson M, Daly M. Competitiveness, risk-taking and violence: The young male syndrome. *Ethology and Sociobiology.* 1985;6:59–73.

8. Daly M, Wilson M. *Homicide.* Hawthorne, NY: Aldine de Gruyter; 1988.

9. Daly M, Wilson M. Killing the competition. *Human Nature.* 1990;1:83–109.

10. Daly M, Wilson M. Crime and conflict: Homicide in evolutionary psychological perspective. *Crime and Justice.* 1997;22:51–100.

11. Charlton BG. What is the ultimate cause of socio-economic inequalities in health? An explanation in terms of evolutionary psychology. *Journal of the Royal Society of Medicine.* 1997;89(1):3–8.

12. Rubin PH, Paul CW. An evolutionary model of taste for risk. *Economic Inquiry.* 1979;17(4):585–596.

13. Kacelnik A, Bateson M. Risky theories—the effects of variance on foraging decisions. *American Zoologist.* 1996;36(4):402–434.

14. Wilson M, Daly M. Who kills whom in spouse killings? On the exceptional sex ratio of spousal homicides in the United States. *Criminology.* 1992;30(2):189–215.

15. Barkow J, Cosmides L, Tooby J, Wilson MI, Daly M. The man who mistook his wife for a chattel. In *The adapted mind* (Barkow J, Cosmides L, Tooby J, eds.). New York: Oxford; 1992:289–322.

16. Wilkinson RG. Income distribution and life expectancy. *British Medical Journal.* 1992;304(6820):165–168.

17. Wilkinson RG. *Unhealthy societies: The afflictions of inequality.* London: Routledge; 1996.

18. Kaplan GA, Pamuk ER, Lynch JW, Cohen RD, Balfour JL. Inequality in income and mortality in the United States: Analysis of mortality and potential pathways. *British Medical Journal.* 1996;312(7037):999–1003.

19. Kennedy BP, Kawachi I, Prothrow-Stith D. Income distribution and mortality: Cross sectional ecological study of the Robin Hood index in the United States. *British Medical Journal.* 1996;312(7037):1004–1007.

20. Krahn H, Hartnagel T, Gartrell J. Income inequality and homicide rates: Cross-national data and criminological theories. *Criminology.* 1986;24(2): 269–295.

21. Hsieh CC, Pugh MD. Poverty, income inequality and violent crime: A meta-analysis of recent aggregate data studies. *Criminal Justice Review.* 1993; 18(2):182–202.

22. Geronimus AT. The weathering hypothesis and the health of African-American women and infants: Evidence and speculations. *Ethnicity and Disease.* 1992;2(3):207–221.

23. Geronimus AT. What teen mothers know. *Human Nature.* 1996;7(4): 323–352.

24. Schoen R. Calculating life tables by estimating Chiang's *a* from observed rates. *Demography.* 1978;15(4):625–635.

25. Hagedorn J. *People and folks*. Chicago: Lake View; 1988.

26. Jankowski MS. *Islands in the street*. Berkeley: University of California Press; 1992.

27. Waldman L. *My neighborhood: The words and pictures of inner-city children*. Chicago: Hyde Park Foundation; 1993.

28. Wilson WJ. *The truly disadvantaged: The inner city, the underclass, and public policy*. Chicago: University of Chicago Press; 1987.

29. Hill E, Ross LT, Low BS. The role of future unpredictability in human risk-taking. *Human Nature*. 1997;8(4):287–325.

30. Nisbett RE, Cohen D. *Culture of honor: The psychology of violence in the South*. Boulder, CO: Westview; 1996.

31. Barkow J, Cosmides L, Tooby J, eds. *The adapted mind*. New York: Oxford; 1992.

32. Gigerenzer G, Goldstein DG. Reasoning the fast and frugal way: Models of bounded rationality. *Psychological Review*. 1996;103(4):650–669.

33. Frank RH. *Choosing the right pond*. New York: Oxford; 1985.

CHAPTER TWENTY-ONE

Neighborhoods and Violent Crime

A Multilevel Study of Collective Efficacy

Robert J. Sampson, Stephen W. Raudenbush, and Felton Earls

For most of this century, social scientists have observed marked variations in rates of criminal violence across neighborhoods of U.S. cities. Violence has been associated with the low socioeconomic status (SES) and residential instability of neighborhoods. Although the geographical concentration of violence and its connection with neighborhood composition are well established, the question remains: Why? What is it, for example, about the concentration of poverty that accounts for its association with rates of violence? What are the social processes that might explain or mediate this relation?[1–3] In this article, we report results from a study designed to address these questions about crime and communities.

Our basic premise is that social and organizational characteristics of neighborhoods explain variations in crime rates that are not solely attributable to the aggregated demographic characteristics of individuals. We propose that the differential ability of neighborhoods to realize the common values of residents and maintain effective social controls is a major source of neighborhood variation in violence.[4–7] Although social control is often a response to deviant behavior, it should not be equated with formal regulation or forced conformity by institutions such as the police and courts. Rather, social control refers generally to the capacity

Originally published in *Science* 277 (August 15, 1997): 918–24. Reprinted with permission from the American Association for the Advancement of Science.

of a group to regulate its members according to desired principles—to realize collective, as opposed to forced, goals.[8] One central goal is the desire of community residents to live in safe and orderly environments that are free of predatory crime, especially interpersonal violence.

In contrast to formally or externally induced actions (for example, a police crackdown), we focus on the effectiveness of informal mechanisms by which residents themselves achieve public order. Examples of informal social control include the monitoring of spontaneous play groups among children, a willingness to intervene to prevent acts such as truancy and street-corner "hanging" by teenage peer groups, and the confrontation of persons who are exploiting or disturbing public space.[7,9-11,a] Even among adults, violence regularly arises in public disputes, in the context of illegal markets (for example, prostitution and drugs), and in the company of peers.[12,13] The capacity of residents to control group level processes and visible signs of social disorder is thus a key mechanism influencing opportunities for interpersonal crime in a neighborhood.

Informal social control also generalizes to broader issues of import to the well-being of neighborhoods. In particular, the differential ability of communities to extract resources and respond to cuts in public services (such as police patrols, fire stations, garbage collection, and housing code enforcement) looms large when we consider the known link between public signs of disorder (such as vacant housing, burned out buildings, vandalism, and litter) and more serious crime.[14]

Thus conceived, neighborhoods differentially activate informal social control. It is for this reason that we see an analogy between individual efficacy and neighborhood efficacy: both are activated processes that seek to achieve an intended effect. At the neighborhood level, however, the willingness of local residents to intervene for the common good depends in large part on conditions of mutual trust and solidarity among neighbors.[15,16] Indeed, one is unlikely to intervene in a neighborhood context in which the rules are unclear and people mistrust or fear one another. It follows that socially cohesive neighborhoods will prove the most fertile contexts for the realization of informal social control. In sum, it is the linkage of mutual trust and the willingness to intervene for the common good that defines the neighborhood context of collective efficacy. Just as individuals vary in their capacity for efficacious action, so too do neighborhoods vary in their capacity to achieve common goals. And just as individual self-efficacy is situated rather than global (one has self-efficacy relative to a particular task or type of task),[17] in this paper we view neighborhood efficacy as existing relative to the tasks of supervising children and maintaining public order. It follows that the collective efficacy of residents is a critical means by which urban neighborhoods inhibit the occurrence of personal violence, without regard to the demographic composition of the population.

What Influences Collective Efficacy?

As with individual efficacy, collective efficacy does not exist in a vacuum. It is embedded in structural contexts and a wider political economy that stratifies places of residence by key social characteristics.[18] Consider the destabilizing potential of rapid population change on neighborhood social organization. A high rate of residential mobility, especially in areas of decreasing population, fosters institutional disruption and weakened social controls over collective life. A major reason is that the formation of social ties takes time. Financial investment also provides homeowners with a vested interest in supporting the commonweal of neighborhood life. We thus hypothesize that residential tenure and homeownership promote collective efforts to maintain social control.[19,20]

Consider next patterns of resource distribution and racial segregation in the United States. Recent decades have witnessed an increasing geographical concentration of lower income residents, especially minority groups and female-headed families. This neighborhood concentration stems in part from macroeconomic changes related to the deindustrialization of central cities, along with the out-migration of middle-class residents.[21] In addition, the greater the race and class segregation in a metropolitan area, the smaller the number of neighborhoods absorbing economic shocks and the more severe the resulting concentration of poverty will be.[22,23] Economic stratification by race and place thus fuels the neighborhood concentration of cumulative forms of disadvantage, intensifying the social isolation of lower income, minority, and single-parent residents from key resources supporting collective social control.[1,24,25]

Perhaps more salient is the influence of racial and economic exclusion on perceived powerlessness. Social science research has demonstrated, at the individual level, the direct role of SES in promoting a sense of control, efficacy, and even biological health itself.[26] An analogous process may work at the community level. The alienation, exploitation, and dependency wrought by resource deprivation act as a centrifugal force that stymies collective efficacy. Even if personal ties are strong in areas of concentrated disadvantage, they may be weakly tethered to collective actions.

We therefore test the hypothesis that concentrated disadvantage decreases and residential stability increases collective efficacy. In turn, we assess whether collective efficacy explains the association of neighborhood disadvantage and residential instability with rates of interpersonal violence. It is our hypothesis that collective efficacy mediates a substantial portion of the effects of neighborhood stratification.

Research Design

This article examines data from the Project on Human Development in Chicago Neighborhoods (PHDCN). Applying a spatial definition of neighborhood—a collection of people and institutions occupying a subsection of a larger community—we combined 847 census tracts in the city of Chicago to create 343 "neighborhood clusters" (NCs). The overriding consideration in formation of NCs was that they should be as ecologically meaningful as possible, composed of geographically contiguous census tracts, and internally homogeneous on key census indicators. We settled on an ecological unit of about 8000 people, which is smaller than the 77 established community areas in Chicago (the average size is almost 40,000 people) but large enough to approximate local neighborhoods. Geographic boundaries (for example, railroad tracks, parks, and freeways) and knowledge of Chicago's neighborhoods guided this process.[b]

The extensive racial, ethnic, and social-class diversity of Chicago's population was a major criterion in its selection as a research site. At present, whites, blacks, and Latinos each represent about a third of the city's population. Table 21.1 classifies the 343 NCs according to race or ethnicity and a trichotomized measure of SES from the 1990 census.[c] Although there are no low-SES white neighborhoods and no high-SES Latino neighborhoods, there are black neighborhoods in all three cells of SES, and many heterogeneous neighborhoods vary in SES. Table 21.1 at once thus confirms the racial and ethnic segregation and yet rejects the common stereotype that minority neighborhoods in the United States are homogeneous.

To gain a complete picture of the city's neighborhoods, 8,782 Chicago residents representing all 343 NCs were interviewed in their homes

TABLE 21.1 **Racial and ethnic composition by SES strata: Distribution of 343 Chicago NCs in the PHDCN design**

	SES		
Race or ethnicity	Low	Medium	High
≥ 75% black	77	37	11
≥ 75% white	0	5	69
≥ 75% Latino	12	9	0
≥ 20% Latino and ≥ 20% white	6	40	12
≥ 20% Latino and ≥ 20% black	9	4	0
≥ 20% black and ≥ 20% white	2	4	11
NCs not classified	8	15	12
Total	114	114	115

as part of the community survey (CS). The CS was designed to yield a representative sample of households within each NC, with sample sizes large enough to create reliable NC measures.[d] Henceforth, we refer to NCs as "neighborhoods," keeping in mind that other operational definitions might have been used.

Measures

"Informal social control" was represented by a five-item Likert-type scale. Residents were asked about the likelihood ("Would you say it is very likely, likely, neither likely nor unlikely, unlikely, or very unlikely?") that their neighbors could be counted on to intervene in various ways if (i) children were skipping school and hanging out on a street corner, (ii) children were spray-painting graffiti on a local building, (iii) children were showing disrespect to an adult, (iv) a fight broke out in front of their house, and (v) the fire station closest to their home was threatened with budget cuts. "Social cohesion and trust" were also represented by five conceptually related items. Respondents were asked how strongly they agreed (on a five-point scale) that "people around here are willing to help their neighbors," "this is a close-knit neighborhood," "people in this neighborhood can be trusted," "people in this neighborhood generally don't get along with each other," and "people in this neighborhood do not share the same values" (the last two statements were reverse coded).

Responses to the five-point Likert scales were aggregated to the neighborhood level as initial measures. Social cohesion and informal social control were closely associated across neighborhoods ($r = 0.80$, $P < 0.001$), which suggests that the two measures were tapping aspects of the same latent construct. Because we also expected that the willingness and intention to intervene on behalf of the neighborhood would be enhanced under conditions of mutual trust and cohesion, we combined the two scales into a summary measure labeled collective efficacy.[e]

The measurement of violence was achieved in three ways. First, respondents were asked how often each of the following had occurred in the neighborhood during the past 6 months: (i) a fight in which a weapon was used, (ii) a violent argument between neighbors, (iii) a gang fight, (iv) a sexual assault or rape, and (v) a robbery or mugging. The scale construction for perceived neighborhood violence mirrored that for social control and cohesion. Second, to assess personal victimization, each respondent was asked: "While you have lived in this neighborhood, has anyone ever used violence, such as in a mugging, fight, or sexual assault, against you or any member of your household anywhere in your neighborhood?"[f] Third, we tested both survey measures against independently recorded incidents of homicide aggregated to the NC level.[g] Homicide is one of the most reliably measured crimes by the police and does not suffer the reporting limitations associated with other violent crimes, such as assault and rape.

Ten variables were constructed from the 1990 decennial census of the population to reflect neighborhood differences in poverty, race and ethnicity, immigration, the labor market, age composition, family structure, homeownership, and residential stability (see table 21.2). The census was independent of the PHDCN CS; moreover, the census data were collected 5 years earlier, which permitted temporal sequencing. To assess whether a smaller number of linear combinations of census characteristics describe the structure of the 343 Chicago neighborhoods, we conducted a factor analysis.[h]

Consistent with theories and research on U.S. cities, the poverty-related variables given in table 21.2 are highly associated and load on the same factor. With an eigenvalue greater than 5, the first factor is dominated by high loadings (> 0.85) for poverty, receipt of public assistance, unemployment, female headed-families, and density of children, followed by, to a lesser extent, percentage of black residents. Hence, the predominant interpretation revolves around concentrated disadvantage—African Americans, children, and single-parent families are differentially found in neighborhoods with high concentrations of poverty.[27]

TABLE 21.2 **Oblique rotated factor pattern (loadings $\geq$ .60) in 343 Chicago neighborhoods**

Variable	Factor loading
Concentrated disadvantage	
Below the poverty line	0.93
On public assistance	0.94
Female-headed families	0.93
Unemployed	0.86
Less than age 18	0.94
Black	0.60
Immigration concentration	
Latino	0.88
Foreign born	0.70
Residential stability	
Same house as 1985	0.77
Owner-occupied house	0.86

Note: Data are from the 1990 census.

To represent this dimension parsimoniously, we calculated a factor regression score that weighted each variable by its factor loading.

The second dimension captures areas of the city undergoing immigration, especially from Mexico. The two variables that define this dimension are the percentage of Latinos (approximately 70% of Latinos in Chicago are of Mexican descent) and the percentage of foreign-born persons. Similar to the procedures for concentrated disadvantage, a weighted factor score was created to reflect immigrant concentration. Because it describes neighborhoods of ethnic and linguistic heterogeneity, there is reason to believe that immigrant concentration may impede the capacity of residents to realize common values and to achieve informal social controls, which in turn explains an increased risk of violence.[1-7,9-11]

The third factor score is dominated by two variables with high (> 0.75) loadings: the percentage of persons living in the same house as 5 years earlier and the percentage of owner-occupied homes. The clear emergence of a residential stability factor is consistent with much past research.[19,20]

Analytic Models

The internal consistency of a person measure will depend on the intercorrelation among items and the number of items in a scale. The internal consistency of a neighborhood measure will depend in part on these factors, but it will hinge more on the degree of intersubjective agreement among informants in their ratings of the neighborhood in which they share membership and on the sample size of informants per neighborhood.[28] To study reliability, we therefore formulated a hierarchical statistical model representing item variation within persons, person variation within neighborhoods, and variation between neighborhoods. Complicating the analysis is the problem of missing data: inevitably, some persons will fail to respond to some questions in an interview. We present our hierarchical model as a series of nested models, one for each level in the hierarchy.[29]

Level 1 Model

Within each person, Y_{ijk}, the ith response of person j in neighborhood k, depends on the person's latent perception of collective efficacy plus error:

(1)
$$Y_{ijk} = \pi_{jk} + \sum_{p=1}^{9} \alpha_p D_{pijk} + e_{ijk}.$$

Here D_{pijk} is an indicator variable taking on a value of unity if response i is to item p in the 10-item scale intended to measure collective efficacy and zero if response i is to some other item. Thus, α_p represents the "difficulty" of item p, and π_{jk} is the "true score" for person jk and is adjusted for the difficulty level of the items to which that person responded.[i] The errors of measurement, e_{ijk}, are assumed to be independent and homoscedastic (that is, to have equal standard deviations).

Level 2 Model

Across informants within neighborhoods, the latent true scores vary randomly around the neighborhood mean:

(2)
$$\pi_{jk} = \eta_k + r_{jk}, r_{jk} \sim N(0, \tau_\pi).$$

Here η_k is the neighborhood mean collective efficacy, and random effects r_{jk} associated with each person are independently, normally distributed with variance τ_π, that is, the "within-neighborhood variance."

Level 3 Model

Across neighborhoods, each neighborhood's mean collective efficacy η_k varies randomly about a grand mean:

(3) $$\eta_k = \gamma + \mu_k, \mu_k \sim N(O, \tau_n),$$

where γ is the grand mean collective efficacy, μ_k is a normally distributed random effect associated with neighborhood k, and τ_n is the between-neighborhood variance. According to this setup, the object of measurement is η_k. The degree of intersubjective agreement among raters is the intra neighborhood correlation, $\rho = \tau_n/(\tau_n + \tau_\pi)$. The reliability of measurement of η_k depends primarily on ρ and on the sample size per neighborhood. The entire three-level model is estimated simultaneously via maximum likelihood.[28]

The results showed that 21% of the variation in perceptions of collective efficacy lies between the 343 neighborhoods.[j] The reliability with which neighborhoods can be distinguished on collective efficacy ranges between 0.80 for neighborhoods with a sample size of 20 raters to 0.91 for neighborhoods with a sample size of 50 raters.

Controlling Response Biases

Suppose, however, that informant responses to the collective efficacy questions vary systematically within neighborhoods as a function of demographic background (such as age, gender, SES, and ethnicity), as well as homeownership, marital status, and so on. Then variation across neighborhoods in the composition of the sample of respondents along these lines could masquerade as variation in collective efficacy. To control for such possible biases, we expanded the level 2 model (eq. 2) by incorporating 11 characteristics of respondents as covariates. [. . .]

Association between Neighborhood Social Composition and Collective Efficacy

The theory described above led us to expect that neighborhood concentrated disadvantage (con. dis.) and immigrant concentration (imm. con.) would be negatively linked to neighborhood collective efficacy and residential stability would be positively related to collective efficacy, net of the contributions of the 11 covariates defined in the previous paragraph. To test this hypothesis, we expanded the level 3 model. [...]

We found some effects of personal background (table 21.3): high SES, homeownership, and age were associated with elevated levels of collective efficacy, whereas high mobility was negatively associated with collective efficacy. Gender, ethnicity, and years in neighborhood were not associated with collective efficacy.

At the neighborhood level, when these personal background effects were controlled, concentrated disadvantage and immigrant concentration were significantly negatively associated with collective efficacy, whereas residential stability was significantly positively associated with collective efficacy (for metric coefficients and t ratios, see table 21.3). The standardized regression coefficients were -0.58 for concentrated disadvantage, -0.13 for immigrant concentration, and 0.25 for residential stability, explaining over 70% of the variability across the 343 NCs.

TABLE 21.3 **Correlates of collective efficacy**

Variable	Coefficient	SE	t-ratio
Intercept	3.523	0.013	263.20
Person-level predictors			
Female	-0.012	0.015	-0.76
Married	-0.005	0.021	-0.25
Separated or divorced	-0.045	0.026	-1.72
Single	-0.026	0.024	-1.05
Homeowner	0.122	0.020	6.04
Latino	0.042	0.028	1.52
Black	-0.029	0.030	-0.98
Mobility	-0.025	0.007	-3.71
Age	2.09×10^{-3}	0.60×10^{-3}	3.47
Years in neighborhood	0.64×10^{-3}	0.82×10^{-3}	0.78
SES	3.53×10^{-2}	0.76×10^{-2}	4.64
Neighborhood-level predictors			
Concentrated disadvantage	-0.172	0.016	-10.74
Immigrant concentration	-0.037	0.014	-2.66
Residential stability	0.074	0.130	5.61
Variance component			
Within neighborhoods	0.320		
Between neighborhoods	0.026		
Percentage of variance explained			
Within neighborhoods	3.2		
Between neighborhoods	70.3		

Collective Efficacy as a Mediator of Social Composition

Past research has consistently reported links between neighborhood social composition and crime. We assessed the relation of social composition to neighborhood levels of violence, violent victimization, and homicide rates, and asked whether collective efficacy partially mediated these
relations.

Perceived Violence

Using a model that paralleled that for collective efficacy, we found that
reports of neighborhood violence depended to some degree on personal
background. Higher levels of violence were reported by those who were
separated or divorced (as compared with those who were single or married), by whites and blacks (as opposed to Latinos), by younger respondents, and by those with longer tenure in their current neighborhood. Gender, homeownership, mobility, and SES were not significantly associated
with responses within neighborhoods. When these personal background
characteristics were controlled, the concentrations of disadvantage ($t =$
13.30) and immigrants ($t = 2.44$) were positively associated with the level of
violence (see table 21.4, model 1). The corresponding standardized regression coefficients are 0.75 and 0.11. Also, as hypothesized, residential stability was negatively associated with the level of violence ($t = -6.95$), corresponding to a standardized regression coefficient of -0.28. The model
accounted for 70.5% of the variation in violence between neighborhoods.

Next, collective efficacy was added as a predictor in the level 3 model
(table 21.4, model 2). The analysis built in a correction for errors of measurement in this predictor.[k] We found collective efficacy to be negatively
related to violence ($t = -5.95$), net of all other effects, and to correspond
to a standardized coefficient of -0.45. Hence, after social composition
was controlled, collective efficacy was strongly negatively associated
with violence. Moreover, the coefficients for social composition were
substantially smaller than they had been without a control for collective efficacy. The coefficient for concentrated disadvantage, although
still statistically significant, was 0.171 (as compared with 0.277). The difference between these coefficients (0.277 − 0.171 = 0.106) was significant ($t = 5.30$). Similarly, the coefficients for immigrant concentration
and for residential stability were also significantly reduced: The coeffi-

TABLE 21.4 **Neighborhood correlates of perceived neighborhood violence, violent victimization, and 1995 homicide events**

Variable	Model 1: Social composition			Model 2: Social composition and collective efficacy		
	Coefficient	SE	t	Coefficient	SE	t
Perceived neighborhood violence*						
Concentrated disadvantage	0.277	0.021	13.30	0.171	0.024	7.24
Immigrant concentration	0.041	0.017	2.44	0.018	0.016	1.12
Residential stability	−0.102	0.015	−6.95	−0.056	0.016	−3.49
Collective efficacy				−0.618	0.104	−5.95
Violent victimization†						
Concentrated disadvantage	0.258	0.045	5.71	0.085	0.054	1.58
Immigrant concentration	0.141	0.046	3.06	0.098	0.044	2.20
Residential stability	−0.143	0.050	−2.84	−0.031	0.051	−0.60
Collective efficacy				−1.190	0.240	−4.96
1995 homicide events‡						
Concentrated disadvantage	0.727	0.049	14.91	0.491	0.064	7.65
Immigrant concentration	−0.022	0.051	−0.43	−0.073	0.050	−1.45
Residential stability	0.093	0.042	2.18	0.208	0.046	4.52
Collective efficacy				−1.471	0.261	−5.64

*Estimates of neighborhood-level coefficients control for gender, marital status, homeownership, ethnicity, mobility, age, years in neighborhood, and SES of those interviewed. Model 1 accounts for 70.5% of the variation between neighborhoods in perceived violence, whereas model 2 accounts for 77.8% of the variation.

†Neighborhood-level coefficients are adjusted for the same person-level covariates listed in the first note. Model 1 accounts for 12.3% of the variation between neighborhoods in violent victimization, whereas model 2 accounts for 44.4%.

‡Model 1 accounts for 56.1% of the variation between neighborhoods in homicide rates, whereas model 2 accounts for 61.7% of the variation.

cient for immigrant concentration, originally 0.041, was now 0.018, a difference of 0.023 ($t = 2.42$); the coefficient for residential stability, which had been −0.102, was now −0.056, a difference of −0.046 ($t = −4.18$). The immigrant concentration coefficient was no longer statistically different from zero. As hypothesized, then, collective efficacy appeared to partially mediate widely cited relations between neighborhood social composition and violence. The model accounted for more than 75% of the variation between neighborhoods in levels of violence.

Violent Victimization

Violent victimization was assessed by a single binary item ($Y_{jk} = 1$ if victimized by violence in the neighborhood and $Y_{jk} = 0$ if not). The latent outcome was the logarithmic odds of victimization π_{jk}. The structural model for predicting π_{jk} had the same form as before.[1] Social composition, as hypothesized, predicted criminal victimization, with positive coefficients for concentrated disadvantage and immigrant concentration and a negative coefficient for residential stability (table 21.4, model 1). The relative odds of victimization associated with a 2-SD elevation in the predictor were 1.67, 1.33, and 0.750, respectively. These estimates controlled for background characteristics associated with the risk of victimization. When added to the model, collective efficacy was negatively associated with victimization (table 21.4, model 2). A 2-SD elevation in collective efficacy was associated with a relative odds ratio of about 0.70, which indicated a reduction of 30% in the odds of victimization. Moreover, after collective efficacy was controlled, the coefficients associated with concentrated disadvantage and residential stability diminished to nonsignificance, and the coefficient for immigrant concentration was also reduced.

Homicide

To assess the sensitivity of the findings when the measure of crime was completely independent of the survey, we examined 1995 homicide counts (Y_k is the number of homicides in neighborhood k in 1995). A natural model for the expected number of homicides in neighborhood k is $E(Y_k) = N_k\lambda_k$, where λ_k is the homicide rate per 100,000 people in neighborhood k and N_k is the population size of neighborhood k as given by the 1990 Census (hundreds of thousands). [. . .]

Although concentrated disadvantage was strongly positively related to homicide, immigrant concentration was unrelated to homicide, and residential stability was weakly positively related to homicide (table 21.4, model 1). However, when social composition was controlled, collective efficacy was negatively related to homicide (table 21.4, model 2). A 2-SD elevation in collective efficacy was associated with a 39.7% reduction in the expected homicide rate. Moreover, when collective efficacy was controlled, the coefficient for concentrated disadvantage was substantially diminished, which indicates that collective efficacy can be viewed as partially mediating the association between concentrated disadvantage and homicide.[m]

Control for Prior Homicide

Results so far were mainly cross-sectional, which raised the question of the possible confounding effect of prior crime. For example, residents in neighborhoods with high levels of violence might be afraid to engage in acts of social control.[14] We therefore reestimated all models controlling for prior homicide: the 3-year average homicide rate in 1988, 1989, and 1990. Prior homicide was negatively related ($P < 0.01$) to collective efficacy in 1995 ($r = -0.55$) and positively related ($P < 0.01$) to all three measures of violence in 1995, including a direct association ($t = 5.64$) with homicide (table 21.5). However, even after prior homicide was controlled, the coefficient for collective efficacy remained statistically significant and substantially negative in all three models.

Further Tests

Although the results have been consistent, there are still potential threats to the validity of our analysis. One question pertains to discriminant validity: How do we know that it is collective efficacy at work rather than some other correlated social process?[30] To assess competing and analytically distinct factors suggested by prior theory,[4,7] we examined the measure of collective efficacy alongside three other scales derived from the CS of the PHDCN: neighborhood services, friendship and kinship ties, and organizational participation.[n] On the basis of the results in tables 21.3–21.5 and also to achieve parsimony, we constructed a violent crime scale at the neighborhood level that summed standardized indicators of the three major outcomes: perceived violence, violent victimization, and homicide rate.

Consistent with expectations, collective efficacy was significantly ($p < 0.01$) and positively related to friendship and kinship ties ($r = 0.49$), organizational participation ($r = 0.45$), and neighborhood services ($r = 0.21$). Nonetheless, when we controlled for these correlated factors in a multivariate regression, along with prior homicide, concentrated disadvantage, immigrant concentration, and residential stability, by far the largest predictor of the violent crime rate was collective efficacy (standardized coefficient $= -0.53$, $t = -8.59$). Collective efficacy thus retained discriminant validity when compared with theoretically relevant, competing social processes. Moreover, these results suggested that dense personal ties, organizations, and local services by themselves are not sufficient; reductions in violence appear to be more directly attributable to informal social control and cohesion among residents.[o]

A second threat stems from the association of racial composition with concentrated disadvantage, as shown in table 21.2. Our interpreta-

TABLE 21.5 **Predictors of neighborhood-level violence, victimization, and homicide in 1995, with prior homicide controlled**

Variable	Violence as outcome			Victimization as outcome			Homicide in 1995 as outcome		
	Coefficient	SE	t	Coefficient	SE	t	Coefficient	SE	t
Intercept	3.772	0.379	9.95	−2.015	0.042	−49.24	3.071	0.050	62.01
Concentrated disadvantage	0.157	0.025	6.38	0.073	0.060	1.22	0.175	0.072	2.42
Immigrant concentration	0.020	0.016	1.25	0.098	0.045	2.20	−0.034	0.044	−0.77
Residential stability	−0.054	0.016	−3.39	−0.029	0.052	−0.56	0.229	0.043	5.38
Collective efficacy	−0.594	0.108	−5.53	−1.176	0.251	−4.69	−1.107	0.272	−4.07
Prior homicide	0.018	0.014	1.27	0.017	0.049	0.34	0.397	0.070	5.64
Variance									
Between-neighborhood variance	0.030			0.091			0.207		
Percentage of variance explained between neighborhoods	78.0			43.8			73.0		

Note: For violence and victimization as outcomes, the coefficients reported in this table were adjusted for 11 person-level covariates (see table 21.3), but the latter coefficients are omitted for simplicity of presentation.

tion was that African Americans, largely because of housing discrimination, are differentially exposed to neighborhood conditions of extreme poverty.[22,23] Nonetheless, a counterhypothesis is that the percentage of black residents and not disadvantage accounts for lower levels of collective efficacy and, consequently, higher violence. Our second set of tests therefore replicated the key models within the 125 NCs where the population was more than 75% black (see the first row of table 21.1), effectively removing race as a potential confound. Concentrated poverty and residential stability each had significant associations with collective efficacy in these predominantly black areas ($t = -5.60$ and $t = 2.50$, respectively). Collective efficacy continued to explain variations in violence across black NCs, mediating the prior effect of concentrated disadvantage. Even when prior homicide, neighborhood services, friendship and kinship ties, and organizational participation were controlled, the only significant predictor of the violent crime scale in black NCs was collective efficacy ($t = -4.80$). These tests suggested that concentrated disadvantage more than race per se is the driving structural force at play.

Discussion and Implications

The results imply that collective efficacy is an important construct that can be measured reliably at the neighborhood level by means of survey research strategies. In the past, sample surveys have primarily considered individual-level relations. However, surveys that merge a cluster sample design with questions tapping collective properties lend themselves to the additional consideration of neighborhood phenomena.

Together, three dimensions of neighborhood stratification—concentrated disadvantage, immigration concentration, and residential stability—explained 70% of the neighborhood variation in collective efficacy. Collective efficacy in turn mediated a substantial portion of the association of residential stability and disadvantage with multiple measures of violence, which is consistent with a major theme in neighborhood theories of social organization.[1-7] After adjustment for measurement error, individual differences in neighborhood composition, prior violence, and other potentially confounding social processes, the combined measure of informal social control and cohesion and trust remained a robust predictor of lower rates of violence.

There are, however, several limitations of the present study. Despite the use of decennial census data and prior crime as lagged predictors, the basic analysis was cross-sectional in design; causal effects were not proven. Indicators of informal control and social cohesion were not observed directly but rather inferred from informant reports. Beyond the scope of the present study, other dimensions of neighborhood efficacy (such as political ties) may be important, too. Our analysis was limited also to one city and did not go beyond its official boundaries into a wider region.

Finally, the image of local residents working collectively to solve their own problems is not the whole picture. As shown, what happens within neighborhoods is in part shaped by socioeconomic and housing factors linked to the wider political economy. In addition to encouraging communities to mobilize against violence through "self-help" strategies of informal social control, perhaps reinforced by partnerships with agencies of formal social control (community policing), strategies to address the social and ecological changes that beset many inner-city communities need to be considered. Recognizing that collective efficacy matters does not imply that inequalities at the neighborhood level can be neglected.

Notes

a. A key finding from past research is that many delinquent gangs emerge from unsupervised spontaneous peer groups [F. Thrasher, *The Gang: A Study of 1,313 Gangs in Chicago* (Univ. of Chicago Press, Chicago, IL, 1963); C. Shaw and H. McKay, *Juvenile Delinquency and Urban Areas* (Univ. of Chicago Press, Chicago, IL, 1969), pp. 176–185; J. F. Short Jr. and F. Strodtbeck, *Group Process and Gang Delinquency* (Univ. of Chicago Press, Chicago, IL, 1965)].

b. Cluster-analyses of census data also helped to guide the construction of internally homogeneous NCs with respect to racial and ethnic mix, SES, housing density, and family organization. Random-effect analyses of variance produced intracluster correlation coefficients to assess the degree to which this goal had been achieved; analyses revealed that the clustering was successful in producing relative homogeneity within NCs.

c. For purposes of selecting a longitudinal cohort sample, SES was defined with the use of a scale from the 1990 Census that included NC-level indicators of poverty, public assistance, income, and education. Race and ethnicity were also measured with the use of the 1990 census, which defined race in five broad categories: "white," "black," "American Indian, Eskimo, or Aleut," "Asian or Pacific

Islander," and "other." We use the census labels of "white" and "black" to refer to persons of European American and African American background, respectively. We use the term "Latino" to denote anyone of Latin American descent as determined from the separate census category of "Hispanic origin." "Hispanic" is more properly used to describe persons of Spanish descent (i.e., from Spain), although the terms are commonly used interchangeably.

d. The sampling design of the CS was complex. For purposes of a longitudinal study, residents in 80 of the 343 NCs were oversampled. Within these 80 NCs, a simple random sample of census blocks was selected, and a systematic random sample of dwelling units within those blocks was selected. Within each dwelling unit, all persons over 18 were listed, and a respondent was sampled at random with the aim of obtaining a sample of 50 households within each NC. In each of the remaining NCs ($n = 263$), nine census blocks were selected with probability proportional to population size, three dwelling units were selected at random within each block, and an adult respondent was randomly selected from a list of all adults in the dwelling unit. The aim was to obtain a sample of 20 in these 263 NCs. Despite these differences in sampling design, the selected dwelling units constituted a representative and approximately self-weighting sample of dwelling units within every NC ($n = 343$). ABT Associates (Cambridge, MA) carried out the data collection with the cooperation of research staff at PHDCN, achieving a final response rate of 75%.

e. "Don't know" responses were recoded to the middle category of "neither likely nor unlikely" (informal social control) or "neither agree nor disagree" (social cohesion). Most respondents answered all 10 items included in the combined measure; for those respondents, the scale score was the average of the responses. However, anyone responding to at least one item provided data for the analysis; a person specific standard error of measurement was calculated on the basis of a simple linear item-response model that took into account the number and difficulty of the items to which each resident responded. The analyses reported here were based on the 7729 cases having sufficient data for all models estimated.

f. Respondents were also asked whether the incident occurred during the 6 months before the interview; about 40% replied affirmatively. Because violence is a rare outcome, we use the total violent victimization measure in the main analysis. However, in additional analyses, we examined a summary of the prevalence of personal and household victimizations (ranging from 0 to four) restricted to this 6-month window. This test yielded results very similar to those based on the binary measure of total violence.

g. The original data measured the address location of all homicide incidents known to the Chicago police (regardless of arrests) during the months of the community survey.

h. The alpha-scoring method was chosen because we are analyzing the universe of NCs in Chicago and are interested in maximizing the reliability of measures [H. F. Kaiser and J. Caffry, *Psychometrika* 30, 1 (1965)]. We also estimated an oblique factor rotation, allowing the extracted dimensions to covary. A principal components analysis with varimax rotation nonetheless yielded substantively identical results.

i. Although the vast majority of respondents answered all items in the collective efficacy scale, the measurement model makes full use of the data provided by those whose responses were incomplete. There is one less indicator, D_{pijk}, than the number of items to identify the intercept.

j. This degree of intersubjective agreement is similar to that found in a recent national survey of teachers that assessed organizational climate in U.S. high schools.

k. The analysis of collective efficacy and violence as outcomes uses a three-level model in which the level 1 model describes the sources of measurement error for each of these outcomes. The level 2 and level 3 models together describe the joint distribution of the "true scores" within and between neighborhoods. Given the joint distribution of these outcomes, it is then possible to describe the conditional distribution of violence given "true" collective efficacy and all other predictors, thus automatically adjusting for any errors of measurement of collective efficacy. See S. Raudenbush and R. J. Sampson (paper presented at the conference "Alternative Models for Educational Data," National Institute of Statistical Sciences Research Triangle Park, NC, 16 October 1996) for the necessary derivations. This work is an extension of that of C. Clogg, E. Petkova, and A. Haritou [*Am. J. Sociol.* 100, 1261 (1995)] and P. Allison (ibid., p. 1294). Note that census blocks were not included as a "level" in the analysis. Thus, person-level and block-level variance are confounded. However, this confounding has no effect on standard errors reported in this manuscript. If explanatory variables had been measured at the level of the census block, it would have been important to represent blocks as an additional level in the model.

l. The resulting model is a logistic regression model with random effects of neighborhoods. This model was estimated first with penalized quasi-likelihood as described by N. E. Breslow and D. G. Clayton [*J. Am. Stat. Assoc.* 88, 9 (1993)]. The doubly iterative algorithm used is described by S. W. Raudenbush ["Posterior modal estimation for hierarchical generalized linear models with applications to dichotomous and count data" (Longitudinal and Multilevel Methods Project, Michigan State Univ., East Lansing, MI, 1993)]. Then, using those results to model the marginal covariation of the errors, we estimated a population-average model with robust standard errors [S. Zeger, K. Liang, P. Albert, *Biometrics* 44, 1049 (1988)]. Results were similar. The results based on the population-average model with robust standard errors are reported here.

m. Although the zero-order correlation of residential stability with homicide was insignificant, the partial coefficient in table 21.4 is significantly positive. Recall from table 21.3 that stability is positively linked to collective efficacy. But higher stability without the expected greater collective efficacy is not a positive neighborhood quality according to the homicide data.

n. "Neighborhood services" is a nine-item scale of local activities and programs (for example, the presence of a block group, a tenant association, a crime prevention program, and a family health service) combined with a six-item inventory of services for youth (a neighborhood youth center, recreational programs, after-school programs, mentoring aid counseling services, mental health services, and a crisis intervention program). "Friendship and kinship ties" is a scale that measures the number of friends and relatives that respondents report are living in the neighborhood. "Organizational participation" measures actual involvement by residents in (i) local religionist organizations; (ii) neighborhood watch programs; (iii) block group, tenant association, or community council; (iv) business or civic groups; (v) ethnic or nationality clubs; and (vi) local political organizations.

o. Similar results were obtained when we controlled for a measure of social interaction (the extent to which neighbors had parties together, watched each other's homes, visited in each other's homes, exchanged favors, and asked advice about personal matters) that was positively associated with collective efficacy. Again the direct effect of collective efficacy remained, suggesting that social interaction, like friendship and kinship ties, is linked to reduced violence through its association with increased levels of collective efficacy.

References

1. Sampson RJ, Lauritsen J. *Understanding and preventing violence: Social influences.* Vol. 3. Washington, DC: National Academy Press; 1994.

2. Short JF. *Poverty, ethnicity, and violent crime.* Boulder, CO: Westview Press; 1997.

3. Mayer SE, Jencks C. Growing up in poor neighborhoods: How much does it matter? *Science.* 1989;243(4897):1441–1445.

4. Kornhauser RR. *Social sources of delinquency: An appraisal of analytic models.* Chicago: University of Chicago Press; 1978.

5. Bursik RJ. Social disorganization and theories of crime and delinquency. *Criminology.* 1988;26(4):519–551.

6. Elliott DS, Wilson JW, Huizinga D, Sampson RJ, Elliott A, Rankin B. The effects of neighborhood disadvantage on adolescent development. *Journal of Research in Crime and Delinquency.* 1996;33(4):389–426.

7. Sampson RJ, Groves WB. Community structure and crime: Testing social-disorganization theory. *American Journal of Sociology.* 1989;94(4):774–802.

8. Janowitz M. Sociological theory and social control. *American Journal of Sociology.* 1975;81(1):82–108.

9. Maccoby EE, Johnson JP, Church RM. Community integration and the social control of juvenile delinquency. *Journal of Social Issues.* 1958;14(3):38–51.

10. Taylor R, Gottfredson S, Brower S. Block crime and fear: Defensible space, local social ties, and territorial functioning. *Journal of Research in Crime and Delinquency.* 1983;21(4):303–331.

11. Hacker JC, Ho K, Ross CU. The willingness to intervene: Differing community characteristics. *Social Problems.* 1974;21(3):328–344.

12. Reiss AJ, Roth J. *Understanding and preventing violence.* Washington, DC: National Academy Press; 1993.

13. Reiss AJ. *Criminal careers and "career criminals."* Washington, DC: National Academy Press; 1986.

14. Skogan W. *Disorder and decline: Crime and the spiral of decay in American neighborhoods.* Berkeley: University of California Press; 1990.

15. Coleman JS. *Foundations of social theory.* Cambridge, MA: Harvard University Press; 1990.

16. Putnam RD. *Making democracy work.* Princeton, NJ: Princeton University Press; 1993.

17. Bandura A. *Social foundations of thought and action: A social cognitive theory.* Englewood Cliffs, NJ: Prentice-Hall; 1986.

18. Logan J, Molotch H. *Urban fortunes: The political economy of place.* Berkeley: University of California Press; 1987.

19. Kasarda J, Janowitz M. Community attachment in mass society. *American Sociological Review.* 1974;39(3):328–339.

20. Sampson RJ. Local friendship ties and community attachment in mass society: A multilevel systemic model. *American Sociological Review.* 1988;53(5): 766–779.

21. Wilson WJ. *The truly disadvantaged: The inner city, the underclass, and public policy.* Chicago: University of Chicago Press; 1987.

22. Massey DS, Denton NA. *American apartheid: Segregation and the making of the underclass.* Cambridge, MA: Harvard University Press; 1993.

23. Massey DS. American apartheid: Segregation and the making of the underclass. *American Journal of Sociology.* 1990;96(2):329–357.

24. Brooks-Gunn J, Duncan G, Kato P, Sealand N. Do neighborhoods influence child and adolescent behavior? *American Journal of Sociology.* 1993;99(2): 353–395.

25. Furstenberg Jr. FF, Cook TD, Eccles J, Elder GH, Sameroff A. *Managing to make it: Urban families and adolescent success.* Chicago: University of Chicago Press; 1998.

26. Williams DR, Collins C. US socioeconomic and racial differences in health: Patterns and explanations. *Annual Review of Sociology.* 1995;21:349–386.

27. Land KC, McCall PL, Cohen LE. Structural covariates of homicide rates: Are there any invariances across time and space? *American Journal of Sociology.* 1990;95(4):922–963.

28. Raudenbush SW, Rowvan B, Kang SJ. A multilevel, multivariate model

for studying school climate in secondary schools with estimation via the EM algorithm. *Journal of Educational Statistics.* 1991;16(4):295–330.

29. Lindley DV, Smith AFM. Bayes estimates for the linear model. *Journal of the Royal Statistical Society, Series B (Methodological).* 1972;34(1):1–41.

30. Cook TD, Shagle SC, Degirmencioglu SM. Capturing social process for testing mediational models of neighborhood effects. In *Neighborhood poverty: Context and consequences for children* (Brooks-Gunn J, Duncan G, Aber JL, eds.). New York: Sage; 1997.

CHAPTER TWENTY-TWO

Urban Violence and African American Pregnancy Outcome

An Ecologic Study

James W. Collins Jr. and Richard J. David

Introduction

Numerous studies have shown that differences in individual risk factors, including maternal sociodemographic characteristics and prenatal utilization, fail to explain why African American race is an independent predictor of poor pregnancy outcome.[1-5] However, individual attributes do not account for the geographic polarization of the races.[6-8] Few studies have addressed the extent to which residential segregation affects the health of pregnant African American women.[4,9-12] Over 45 years ago, Yankauer reported that the infant mortality in New York City rose as the percentage of non-white births increased.[9] In a more recent analysis of 176 U.S. cities, LaVeist found a positive association between the degree of African American:white segregation and the infant mortality rate among African Americans.[10] This association was independent of poverty prevalence.

An unmeasured ecologic variable, such as chronic exposure to urban violence, may play a key role in explaining the racial disparity in pregnancy outcome. Urban violence is likely to exert different effects on

Originally published in *Ethnicity & Disease* 7 (1997): 184–90. Ethnicity & Disease © 1997. Collins et al. Reprinted with permission. All rights reserved.

health as a neighborhood (compared to an individual) risk factor. Haan et al. found a complex mixture of environmental factors, including high crime rates, and explained the association between social class and mortality in a cohort of adults.[13] There are limited available data on the community effects of individual violent acts on pregnancy outcome, and none include Americans.[14-16] Zapata et al. reported that among otherwise healthy women in Chile, residence in violent neighborhoods was associated with an increased risk of pregnancy complicatons.[14] Ascherio and co-investigators found a negative effect of the Gulf War on infant mortality rates in Iraq,[15] with the association being strongest in the most violent areas.

A better understanding of the relationship between place of residence and pregnancy outcome is needed to focus policy recommendations that address the long-standing racial disparity in infant outcome. We hypothesized that residence in violent communities is an independent risk factor for adverse pregnancy outcome among African American women in Chicago.

Methods

We used a dataset of Illinois vital records, United States Census income information, and Chicago Police Department violent crime rates to examine the birth outcomes of all liveborn singleton infants born to African American mothers in Chicago during 1983. To control for socioeconomic status, only infants with mothers who resided in very low-income census tracts (median family income < $10,000/year) were eligible for study. Thus, census tract income was used as an integral group variable;[8] it affected all women in the study. The vast majority of low-income census tracts in Chicago are homogeneous with respect to race and family income.[17] A categorical violence variable was created using 1983 Chicago police district violent crime rates (number of murders, rapes, robberies, and aggravated assaults per 1,000 residents). The median violent crime rate (VCR) was 11/1,000. *A priori* the VCR was categorized into 4 strata: < 11/1,000, 11–20/1,000, 21–30/1,000 and > 30/1,000. Median community VCR was evaluated as a contextual group variable;[8] each affected a proportion of mothers in the study. There were 24 police districts.

Within each VCR stratum, we calculated the proportion (per 100 live births) of low birth weight (< 2500 g), small-for-gestational age (weight for gestational age < 10th percentile), and preterm (gestational age derived from last menstrual period < 260 days). As a first step in exploring the possible role of other variables as mediators of the violence effect, we looked for difference in the prevalence of various demographic and prenatal variables. We used trimester of initiation listed in the viral records as the sole proxy of prenatal care adequacy.[18] [...]

Multivariate logistic regression analyses were used in an attempt to better estimate the independent association of community violence and African American pregnancy outcome. Only covariates univariately associated with birth weight were put into logistic models. The adjusted ORs for violence were calculated by taking the antilogarithm of the beta coefficient from each respective model.[19]

Results

The study population consisted for 7,592 African American infants who resided in very low (median family income < $10,000/yr) income census tracts. Twenty-two percent (N = 1,676) lived in police districts with VCR in excess of 30/1,000. Four percent (N = 316) lived in districts with VCR < 11/1,000. Sixteen percent of infants born to mothers who resided in the most violent (VCR > 30/1,000) communities and 12% of infants with mothers who lived in the least violent (VCR < 11/1,000) communities were low birth weight (LBW); OR = 1.5 (1.0–2.1). The proportion of small-for-gestational-age (SGA) infants was substantially elevated among mothers who resided in the most violent communities compared to those who lived in the safest areas; 7% and 3%, respectively, OR = 2.6 (1.5–2.1). VCR were not significantly associated with prematurity (table 22.1).

TABLE 22.1 **African American pregnancy outcome in very low income (median family income** < **$10,000/year) communities according to violent crime rates: Chicago, 1983**

	Violent crime rate (per 1000 residents)			
Outcome variable	< 11 (N = 316)	11–20 (N = 4547)	21–30 (N = 1054)	> 30 (N = 1676)
% Low birth weight	12	14	13	16
% Small-for-gestational age	3	6	7	7
% Premature	22	24	23	25

TABLE 22.2 **Distribution of individual risk factors by community violent crime rates: Chicago, 1983**

Variable	Violent crime rate (per 1000 residents)			
	< 11 (N = 316)	11–20 (N = 4547)	21–30 (N = 1054)	> 30 (N = 1676)
Maternal age				
< 20 years	33	35	33	37
Maternal education				
< 12 years	43	55	49	57
Maternal marital status				
Unmarried	76	84	81	85
Parity*				
High parity	30	32	29	32
Prenatal care†				
Inadequate	42	38	35	42

*Parity was defined as high in third or higher-numbered births to women under 25 years of age and fourth or higher-numbered births to women 25–29 years of age.

†Prenatal care was defined as inadequate when initiated after the first trimester.

Within each VCR stratum, there were marginal differences in maternal age, parity, marital status, and trimester of prenatal care initiation (table 22.2). Mothers who resided in the most violent areas were more likely to have < 12 years of formal education than mothers who lived in the least violent areas, $p < 0.01$.

Table 22.3 shows the proportion of LBW infants according to maternal age, education, marital status, parity, and trimester of prenatal care usage. While the odds ratios for maternal residence in the most violent communities fluctuated, the majority were greater than 1.0. In each VCR stratum, the proportion of LBW infants tended to decline as maternal risk status improved.

Table 22.4 shows the proportion of SGA infants according to measured sociodemographic variables. The percentage of SGA infants rose as community VCR increased, regardless of maternal risk status. In the highest VCR stratum, traditional risk factors (with the exception of maternal education) were minimally associated with SGA rates. We found no consistent association between VCR and gestation length (table 22.5). In all VCR strata, maternal risk status tended to be associated with prematurity rates.

We next fitted logistic regression models. Controlling for maternal age, education, marital status, parity, and prenatal care eliminated the

TABLE 22.3 **The proportion of low birth weight African American infants by violence and individual risk status: Chicago, 1983**

Variable	Violent crime rate (per 1000 residents)				
	< 11 (N = 316)	11–20 (N = 4547)	21–30 (N = 1054)	> 30 (N = 1676)	Highest:Lowest OR (95% CI)
Maternal age (years)					
< 20 years	10	13	12	16	1.8 (0.9–3.5)
20–35	13	14	14	17	1.4 (0.9–2.1)
Maternal education (years)					
< 12 years	18	15	15	18	1.2 (0.8–1.9)
12	11	13	13	14	1.4 (0.7–2.6)
> 12	7	11	11	12	1.7 (0.6–4.7)
Marital status					
Unmarried	14	14	13	18	1.3 (0.9–1.9)
Married	4	12	12	10	2.7 (0.8–9.1)
Parity*					
High parity	17	16	14	18	1.1 (0.6–1.9)
Low parity	11	13	12	16	1.4 (0.8–2.8)
Primiparity	8	13	12	15	2.2 (1.0–4.6)
Prenatal care†					
Inadequate	12	15	15	18	1.5 (0.9–2.4)
Adequate	12	13	12	15	1.4 (0.8–2.2)

*Parity was defined as high in third or higher-numbered births to women under 25 years of age and fourth or higher-numbered births to women 25–29 years of age.

†Prenatal care was defined as inadequate when initiated after the first trimester.

increased LBW risk experienced by those who resided in violent areas; adjusted OR = 1.5 (1.1–2.1).

Discussion

To our knowledge, the present study is the first to document the impact of urban violence on African American pregnancy outcome. The association of VCR and LBW rates abates when maternal sociodemographic characteristics and trimester of prenatal care initiation usage are controlled in a multivariable logistic regression model. In contrast, our stratified and logistic regression analyses show that known individual risk factors do not fully account for the relationship between VCR and SGA rates. We conclude that urban violence is associated with intrauterine growth retardation among infants born to African American women.

The National Advisory Commission on Civil Disorders (commonly

TABLE 22.4 **The proportion of SGA African American infants by violence and individual risk status: Chicago, 1983**

	Violent crime rate (per 1000 residents)				
Variable	< 11 (N = 316)	11–20 (N = 4547)	21–30 (N = 1054)	> 30 (N = 1676)	Highest:Lowest OR (95% CI)
Maternal age (years)					
< 20 years	4	5	6	6	1.6 (0.6–4.2)
20–35	2	6	8	8	3.5 (1.2–12.5)
Maternal education (years)					
≤12 years	3	6	7	7	4.6 (2.2–9.4)
>12	*	3	6	4	
Marital status					
Unmarried	4	6	7	7	2.6 (1.3–5.1)
Married	*	6	8	7	
Parity[†]					
High parity	4	7	7	8	2.0 (0.7–5.8)
Low/primiparity	2	5	7	6	3.0 (1.2–7.4)
Prenatal care[‡]					
Inadequate	2	5	9	8	3.8 (1.2–12.5)
Adequate	3	6	6	6	1.9 (0.8–4.2)

*Undefined, < 3 SGA infants.
†Parity was defined as high in third or higher-numbered births to women under 25 years of age and fourth or higher-numbered births to women 25–29 years of age.
‡Prenatal care was defined as inadequate when initiated after the first trimester.

called the Kerner Commission) noted in the 1968 that segregation and poverty had created a destructive environment in the racial ghetto.[7] This residential pattern maintains an urban underclass that is defined more by race than income. Regardless of African Americans' economic status, they rarely reside in white areas; while whites, no matter how poor, rarely live in African American ghettos.[20] Thus, it has been very difficult to untangle the effects of race, class, and place of residence on pregnancy outcome. In a seminal study, Polednak found that residential segregation was the most important risk factor for African American infant mortality independent of median family income and poverty prevalence.[6] In an attempt to study the effect of place of residence, we examined the pregnancy outcome of a rather homogenous group of African American mothers who resided in very low-income neighborhoods.[4] Similar to prior investigations that focused on living conditions in certain Third World countries, the present study provides evidence that chronic community-wide strain due to residence in high-crime neighborhoods in the United States is indeed linked to poor birth outcome.

TABLE 22.5 **The proportion of preterm African American infants by violence and individual risk status: Chicago, 1983**

Variable	Violent crime rate (per 1000 residents)				
	< 11 (N = 316)	11–20 (N = 4547)	21–30 (N = 1054)	> 30 (N = 1676)	Highest:Lowest OR (95% CI)
Maternal age (years)					
< 20 years	19	26	24	28	1.7 (1.0–3.1)
≥ 20	23	22	24	23	1.0 (0.7–1.5)
Maternal education (years)					
< 12 years	23	25	24	29	1.4 (0.9–2.2)
12	24	21	22	24	1.0 (0.6–1.6)
> 12	16	21	18	14	0.8 (0.4–1.8)
Marital status					
Unmarried	24	24	23	27	1.2 (0.9–1.7)
Married	17	19	19	14	0.7 (0.4–1.5)
Parity*					
High parity	28	24	24	28	1.0 (0.6–1.7)
Low	21	23	23	24	1.2 (0.7–1.9)
Primiparity	16	24	20	24	1.6 (0.9–3.0)
Prenatal care†					
Inadequate	28	26	23	26	1.0 (0.6–1.6)
Adequate	17	22	22	25	1.6 (1.0–2.5)

*Parity was defined as high in third or higher-numbered births to women under 25 years of age and fourth or higher-numbered births to women 25–29 years of age.

†Prenatal care was defined as inadequate when initiated after the first trimester.

Our data suggest that in urban ghettos, the effect of violence on SGA rates outweighs the benefits of early initiation of prenatal care. We suspect that chronic stress from exposure to urban violence provokes a range of emotions and physiologic responses, which result in placental insufficiency and consequent infant weight-for-gestation length less than the tenth percentile,[21–23] a condition associated with an increased morbidity and mortality risk. Alternatively, violence may be a proxy for other conditions that adversely affect health. Women exposed to high levels of urban violence may be more likely to smoke cigarettes and/or use illicit drugs, in part to cope with stress, which could lead to placental insufficiency and altered fetal growth. In addition, other community-level variables such as dense housing, gang activity, and unemployment rates may underlie the association between urban VCR and SGA rates.

The cumulative evidence is that psychosocial factors, particularly acute stressors, are associated with an increased risk of preterm delivery.[23] However, we found no consistent relationship between urban violence and prematurity risk. This may be a Type II error related to the small number of infants with very low-income mothers from relatively safe neighborhoods. It may also signal a difference between acute and chronic stress. The latter may be more likely to hinder intrauterine growth than gestation length. Further research is required to better address this possibility.

[...]

References

1. Wegman ME. Annual summary of vital statistics—1992. *Pediatrics.* 1993; 92(6):743–754.

2. Kleinman JC, Kessel SS. Racial differences in low birth weight: Trends and risk factors. *New England Journal of Medicine.* 1987;317(12):749–753.

3. Schoendorf KC, Hogue CJ, Kleinman JC, Rowley D. Mortality among infants of black as compared with white college-educated parents. *New England Journal of Medicine.* 1992;326(23):1522–1526.

4. Collins JW Jr., David RJ. The differential effect of traditional risk factors on infant birthweight among blacks and whites in Chicago. *American Journal of Public Health.* 1990;80(6):679–681.

5. Murray JL, Bernfield M. The differential effect of prenatal care on the incidence of low birth weight among blacks and whites in a prepaid health care plan. *New England Journal of Medicine.* 1988;319(21):1385–1391.

6. Polednak AP. Black-white differences in infant mortality in 38 standard metropolitan statistical areas. *American Journal of Public Health.* 1991;81(11): 1480–1482.

7. US Commission on Civil Disorders. *Reports of the National Advisory Commission on Civil Disorders.* New York: Bantam; 1968.

8. Susser M. The logic in ecological: 1. The logic of analysis. *American Journal of Public Health.* 1994;84(5):825–829.

9. Yankauer A. The relationship of fetal and infant mortality to residential segregation. *American Sociological Review.* 1950;15(5):644–648.

10. LaVeist TA. Linking residential segregation to the infant mortality race disparity in U.S. cities. *Sociology and Social Research.* 1989;73(2):90–94.

11. Polednak AP. Trends in US urban black infant mortality, by degree of residential segregation. *American Journal of Public Health.* 1996;86(5):723–726.

12. Collins JW, Herman AA, David RJ. Very low birth-weight infants and income incongruity among African-American and white parents in Chicago. *American Journal of Public Health.* 1997;86(3):414–417.

13. Haan M, Kaplan GA, Camacho T. Poverty and health: Prospective evi-

dence from the Alameda County Study. *American Journal of Epidemiology.* 1987;125(6):989–998.

14. Zapata BC, Rebolledo A, Atalah E, Newman B, King MC. The influence of social and political violence on the risk of pregnancy complications. *American Journal of Public Health.* 1992;82(5):685–690.

15. Ascherio A, Chase R, Cote T, et al. Effect of the Gulf War on infant and child mortality in Iraq. *New England Journal of Medicine.* 1992;327(13):931–936.

16. Savitz DA, Thang NM, Swenson IE, Stone EM. Vietnamese infant and childhood mortality in relation to the Vietnam War. *American Journal of Public Health.* 1993;83(8):1134–1138.

17. Collins JW Jr., Shay DK. Prevalence of low birth weight among Hispanic infants with United States–born and foreign-born mothers: The effect of urban poverty. *American Journal of Epidemiology.* 1994;139(2):184–192.

18. McDermott J, Drews C, Green D, Berg C. Evaluation of prenatal care information on birth certificates. *Paediatric and Perinatal Epidemiology.* 1997; 11(1):105–121.

19. Statistical Package for the Social Sciences. *SPSS user's guide.* 3rd ed. Chicago: SPSS; 1990.

20. US Bureau of the Census. *Statistical abstract of the United States.* 110th ed. Washington, DC: US Government Printing Office; 1990.

21. McLean DE, Hatfield-Timajchy K, Wingo PA, Floyd RL. Psychosocial measurement: Implications for the study of preterm delivery in black women. *American Journal of Preventive Medicine.* 1993;9(6 suppl.):39–81.

22. Istvan J. Stress, anxiety, and birth outcomes: A critical review of the evidence. *Psychological Bulletin.* 1986;100(3):331–348.

23. Newton RW, Hunt LP. Psychosocial stress in pregnancy and its relation to low birth weight. *British Medical Journal (Clinical Research Edition).* 1984;288(6425):1191–1194.

CHAPTER TWENTY-THREE

Social Capital and Neighborhood Mortality Rates in Chicago

Kimberly A. Lochner, Ichiro Kawachi, Robert T. Brennan,
and Stephen L. Buka

Introduction

There is growing interest in identifying neighborhood-level influences on health.[1] A series of studies have suggested that residents of poor neighborhoods have higher rates of premature mortality compared to residents of more affluent neighborhoods.[2-5] Moreover, the poorer health status of disadvantaged neighborhoods is not entirely explained by the characteristics of individuals living in them.[6] In other words, there appear to be distinct features of *places* that make a difference to health, as opposed to the characteristics of people. For example, studies have shown that the number of supermarkets is lower[7] and the number of liquor stores higher in lower income areas.[8] In turn the availability of services and amenities (recreational spaces, commercial stores) can facilitate or constrain a person's ability to engage in healthy behaviors (such as taking up regular exercise or buying fresh foods). However, these physical characteristics are not the only features of neighborhoods that potentially affect health. Neighborhoods also matter because of the nature of their social organization. One such characteristic is the *social capital* of a neighborhood.

Originally published in *Social Science & Medicine* 56 (2003): 1797–805. Copyright © 2003, Elsevier.

Social capital has been defined as features of social structure—such as trust, norms, and networks—that facilitate collective action for mutual benefit.[9,10] It is a resource that resides in the relationships that people have with each other, and that individuals within a social structure (such as a neighborhood) can draw upon to achieve certain actions.[11,12] Social capital has been used to account for schooling and educational attainment[13] as well as for the smooth functioning of democracies and civic institutions.[10] However, the benefits of social capital as it applies to health have only recently been examined. For example, studies linking social capital to health have examined mortality,[14] violent crime,[15] self-rated health status,[11,16] and binge drinking.[4]

[...]

[...] Sampson et al.[15] examined what they termed "collective efficacy" as a determinant of neighborhood variation in violence, including homicide rates in Chicago neighborhoods. Their collective efficacy scale was comprised of two sub-scales, social cohesion and informal social control, which overlap with the concept of social capital.[17] The index of collective efficacy was significantly inversely associated with reports of neighborhood violence and violent victimization as well as homicide rates. For example, a two standard deviation (SD) elevation in collective efficacy was associated with a 39.7% reduction in the expected homicide rate.

[...]

[...] The purpose of the present study was to replicate the previously demonstrated state-level relationships between social capital and health at the level of neighborhoods. We set out to test the ecological association between neighborhood-level social capital and mortality rates, taking advantage of the community survey data collected as part of the Project on Human Development in Chicago Neighborhoods.

Methods

Social Capital Indicators

Indicators of neighborhood social capital were obtained from the 1995 Community Survey of the Project on Human Development in Chicago Neighborhoods (PHDCN). Neighborhood-level data for the city of Chicago were gathered in 1995 as part of the PHDCN and combined with 1990 US census data. Applying a spatial definition of neighborhood, the PHDCN combined all 847 census tracts in Chicago to create 343 ecologically meaningful and homogeneous "neighborhood clusters" (NCs), using geographic boundaries and knowledge of traditional Chicago neighborhoods. Each NC included about 8000 residents. The PHDCN community survey was conducted as a clustered random household survey of all NCs. The selected sample constituted a representative and approximately self-weighting sample of dwelling units within each of the 343 NCs. The overall response rate of the survey was 75%.[15]

Following our previous studies[11,14] we assessed social capital by three indicators: residents' perceptions of reciprocity and trust, as well as associational membership. Perceptions of reciprocity were assessed as the proportion of residents in each NC answering strongly agree/agree to the question that "people around here are willing to help their neighbors." Perceptions of trust were measured by the proportion of residents in each NC answering strongly agree/agree to the question that "people in this neighborhood can be trusted." Survey respondents were asked about membership in a variety of voluntary associations, including religious organizations, neighborhood associations, business or civic groups, neighborhood ethnic or nationality clubs, as well as neighborhood/local political organizations. From these responses, we constructed a measure of the average per capita associational membership in each NC.

Neighborhood All-Cause and Cause-Specific Mortality

Counts of all-cause and cause-specific deaths in each NC by sex and race (white and black) for persons 45–64 years were obtained from the 1994, 1995, and 1996 Illinois Department of Public Health mortality file. In addition to all cause mortality, we examined the following major causes of death defined by *International Classification of Diseases*, 9th revision (ICD-9): heart disease (codes 390–398, 402, 404–429), malignant neoplasms (cancers) (codes 140–208) and "other" causes. The "other" cause category excluded deaths from heart disease and cancer as well as "external" causes of death (codes E800–949 and E950–978). The latter categories were excluded because the association between social capital indicators and external causes of death, such as homicide at the neighborhood level, have been reported in a previous publication.[15] Sex-, race-, and age-specific population counts for each NC were obtained from the 1990 decennial census of population and housing.[18]

We limited mortality to 45–64 years of age because we were interested in examining premature mortality at mid-life. The racial categories "white" and "black" refer to those used for statistical reporting by all Federal agencies and may include people of Hispanic origin.[18]

Neighborhood Material Deprivation

We sought a neighborhood-level index of economic disadvantage as a potential confound in the relation between social capital and mortality rates. Using data from the 1990 census we derived an aggregate measure of neighborhood economic disadvantage, calculated for each NC as the first principal component of the proportion of residents: (1) below the poverty line; (2) on public assistance; and (3) unemployed. This scale was standardized at the NC level to mean = 0 and SD = 1.

Research Design and Data Analysis

We estimated a hierarchical generalized linear model (HGLM) with a log link function to examine the association between social capital and death rates at the NC level. The outcome, represented by Y_{ij}, is the observed death count for an NC for persons 45–64 years in each sex-race group i of NC_j. In addition, the HGLM used in these analyses allows each NC to have a unique "exposure," which is represented by n_{ij}.[19] In this case, n_{ij} represents the number of residents, 45–64 years of age, in an NC in each of the four sex (male, female) by race (white, black) categories (Level 1). The NC level independent variables included the social capital indicators—trust, reciprocity, and associational membership—and neighborhood deprivation (Level 2).

Level 1 model:

$$\log(\text{NC death rate}) = \beta_{1j}(\text{white male}) + \beta_{2j}(\text{white female}) + \beta_{3j}(\text{black male}) + \beta_{4j}(\text{black female}).$$

Level 2 model:

$$\beta_1 = \Upsilon_{10} + \Upsilon_{11} \text{ (social capital)} + \Upsilon_{12} \text{ (deprivation)} + \mu_1,$$

$$\beta_2 = \Upsilon_{20} + \Upsilon_{21} \text{ (social capital)} + \Upsilon_{22} \text{ (deprivation)} + \mu_2,$$

$$\beta_3 = \Upsilon_{30} + \Upsilon_{31} \text{ (social capital)} + \Upsilon_{32} \text{ (deprivation)} + \mu_3,$$

$$\beta_4 = \Upsilon_{40} + \Upsilon_{41} \text{ (social capital)} + \Upsilon_{42} \text{ (deprivation)} + \mu_4.$$

[. . .]

For each of the four causes of death outcomes, we calculated three separate models, each of which included one of the three social capital indicators along with the composite measure of neighborhood deprivation. The NC independent variables were centered at their grand mean. All analyses were conducted using the statistical software package Hierarchical Linear Modeling.[19]

Results

The PHDCN community survey included household interviews from 343 NCs. One NC was missing key social and economic information and was dropped from the analysis. In the remaining 342 Chicago NCs, 70% of respondents agreed that people were willing to help their neighbors, and 56% agreed that people in their neighborhood could be trusted, while the average per resident number of associational membership was < 1.0 (table 23.1). The three indicators of NC social capital—reciprocity, trust, and civic participation—were positively correlated with each other. The strongest correlation was between reciprocity and trust ($r = 0.78$, $p < 0.0001$), while civic participation was correlated with both reciprocity and trust at approximately 0.40 ($p < 0.0001$). All three social capi-

TABLE 23.1 **Mean neighborhood death rates for persons 45–64 years of age; indicators of neighborhood social capital and deprivation in Chicago neighborhoods**

	Mean death rate						
	White men	White women	Black men	Black women	Mean	SD	Range
Neighborhood death rates[a]							
All causes	1,371	695	2,487	1,124			
Heart disease	460	164	711	328			
Cancer	285	262	581	341			
Other causes	440	189	790	333			
Neighborhood social capital indicators							
Reciprocity					0.70	0.17	0.25–1.00
Trust					0.56	0.22	0.10–1.00
Civic participation					0.80	0.27	0.05–1.88
Neighborhood deprivation[b]					0.00	1.00	−1.38–3.91

Note: Neighborhoods refers to "neighborhood clusters" or NCs.

[a]Posterior means per 100,000.

[b]Composite measure of % poverty, % public assistance, % unemployed. Standardized to mean = 0 and SD = 1.

tal indicators were negatively correlated with neighborhood deprivation: trust ($r = -0.61, p < 0.0001$); reciprocity ($r = -0.46, p < 0.0001$); and civic participation ($r = -0.31, p < 0.0001$).

All-Cause Mortality

Adjusted for neighborhood deprivation, the three indicators of social capital showed inverse relationships to death rates from all causes (table 23.2). The results were most consistent for whites with reciprocity, trust, and civic participation all showing significant associations for both men and women. For blacks, civic participation was significantly associated with total death rates for both black women and men, while trust showed marginally significant associations for black women and men, and reciprocity showed significant associations only for black men. As expected, neighborhood deprivation showed significant direct associations with all-cause death rates for whites and blacks as well as men and women. The association between per capita civic participation and all-cause death rates are shown in figure 23.1.

TABLE 23.2 **Estimated regression coefficients from a Poisson model predicting all-cause death rates for persons 45–64 years in 342 Chicago neighborhoods**

	White women		White men		Black women		Black men	
	Estimated coefficient	SE	Estimated coefficient	SE	Estimated coefficient	SE	Estimated coefficient	SE
Intercept	−4.81		−4.16		−4.54		−3.76	
Reciprocity	−0.72***	0.18	−0.40*	0.17	−0.20	0.14	−0.38*	0.16
Neighborhood deprivation	0.32***	0.05	0.33***	0.05	0.08**	0.03	0.10**	0.03
Intercept	−4.81		−4.16		−4.55		−3.76	
Trust	−0.40**	0.13	−0.44***	0.12	−0.29*	0.14	−0.29	0.16
Neighborhood deprivation	0.33***	0.05	0.29***	0.05	0.06*	0.03	0.09**	0.03
Intercept	−4.81		−4.17		−4.53		−3.75	
Civic participation	−0.30**	0.10	−0.49***	0.10	−0.21*	0.09	−0.39**	0.11
Neighborhood deprivation	0.37**	0.05	0.32***	0.04	0.07**	0.02	0.09**	0.03

Note: Coefficients are on the log scale. Neighborhoods refers to "neighborhood clusters" or NCs. Independent variables are centered at their mean.

*$p \leq .05$; **$p \leq .01$; ***$p \leq .0005$

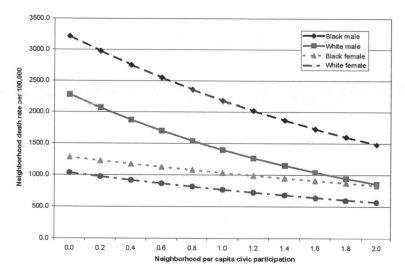

FIGURE 23.1. Predicted all-cause death rates for persons 45–64 years by level of neighborhood per capita civic participation, adjusted for mean level of neighborhood deprivation, in 342 Chicago neighborhoods

Heart Disease Mortality

Table 23.3 shows the association of social capital to heart disease mortality at the NC level. Adjusted for neighborhood deprivation, for white men and women, higher levels of reciprocity, trust, or civic participation were all associated with lower death rates from heart disease. However, there was no relationship between social capital and heart disease mortality for black men and women. Again neighborhood deprivation showed significant direct associations for all groups.

Cancer Mortality

Overall, adjusted for neighborhood poverty, the social capital indicators were not associated with cancer death rates. However, there were a few exceptions. For example, higher levels of trust were modestly associated with higher cancer death rates for white men, but were associated with lower cancer death rates for black women (data not shown).

TABLE 23.3 **Estimated regression coefficients from a Poisson model predicting heart disease death rates for persons 45–64 years in 342 Chicago neighborhoods**

	White women		White men		Black women		Black men	
	Estimated coefficient	SE	Estimated coefficient	SE	Estimated coefficient	SE	Estimated coefficient	SE
Intercept	−6.16		−5.17		−5.83		−5.09	
Reciprocity	−0.54	0.28	−0.50*	0.21	0.02	0.24	−0.27	0.19
Neighborhood deprivation	0.46***	0.08	0.38***	0.06	0.15***	0.04	0.20***	0.04
Intercept	−6.16		−5.17		−5.84		−5.11	
Trust	−0.48*	0.21	−0.56**	0.16	−0.18	0.24	−0.25	0.19
Neighborhood deprivation	0.43***	0.09	0.32***	0.06	0.14**	0.05	0.19***	0.04
Intercept	−6.18		−5.18		−5.82		−5.09	
Civic participation	−0.56**	0.17	−0.45**	0.13	−0.12	0.15	−0.10	0.11
Neighborhood deprivation	0.45***	0.08	0.38***	0.05	0.14**	0.04	0.20***	0.04

Note: Coefficients are on the log scale. Neighborhoods refers to "neighborhood clusters" or NCs. Independent variables are centered at their mean.

*$p \leq .05$; **$p \leq .01$; ***$p \leq .0005$

TABLE 23.4 **Estimated regression coefficients from a Poisson model predicting death rates for persons 45–64 years from "other" causes in 342 Chicago neighborhoods**

	White women		White men		Black women		Black men	
	Estimated coefficient	SE	Estimated coefficient	SE	Estimated coefficient	SE	Estimated coefficient	SE
Intercept	−6.07		−5.26		−5.84		−4.95	
Reciprocity	−1.43***	0.30	−0.80**	0.26	−0.40	0.24	−0.85***	0.23
Neighborhood deprivation	0.47***	0.07	0.40***	0.08	0.15**	0.05	0.10	0.05
Intercept	−6.05		−5.28		−5.85		−4.96	
Trust	−0.86***	0.23	−0.94***	0.20	−0.25	0.22	−0.60**	0.21
Neighborhood deprivation	0.47***	0.08	0.30***	0.08	0.15**	0.05	0.10	0.05
Intercept	−6.06		−5.28		−5.82		−4.92	
Civic participation	−0.58**	0.17	−0.77***	0.14	−0.35*	0.15	−0.68***	0.17
Neighborhood deprivation	0.57***	0.07	0.41***	0.07	0.14**	0.04	0.11	0.06

Note: Coefficients are on the log scale. Neighborhoods refers to "neighborhood clusters" or NCs. Independent variables are centered at their mean.

*$p \leq .05$; **$p \leq .01$; ***$p \leq .0005$

Mortality from "Other" Causes

Higher levels of reciprocity, trust, and civic participation were associated with lower death rates from "other" causes for all race-sex groups (table 23.4). However, the associations among black women were again the weakest, with civic participation being the only social capital indicator to reach statistical significance at $p < 0.05$. For whites as well as black women, as levels of neighborhood deprivation increased, so did the death rate. However, for black men, neighborhood deprivation was not associated with death rates from these "other" causes.

Discussion

The present analysis extends the existing literature on social capital and health to the level of neighborhoods. We operationalized social capital using three indicators. Civic participation taps into formal networks, while reciprocity and trust are consequences of both formal and informal networks.[20] Overall for whites, we found that higher levels of NC social capital were associated with lower NC death rates from all causes, heart disease, and "other" causes (which excluded homicide, suicide, and all injuries), after adjustment for neighborhood deprivation. However, for blacks, particularly black women, the association between social capital and mortality rates was less consistent. Although the social capital indicators, in general, were inversely associated with mortality rates for blacks, the associations often were not statistically significant.

The data are cross-sectional, hence we cannot exclude reverse causation that is the possibility that higher death rates led to erosion of trust and other indicators of social capital. In addition, although we controlled for deprivation at the NC level, we did not control for individual-level socioeconomic indicators (e.g., household income or educational attainment) and cannot exclude the possibility that individual characteristics account for the observed relationships at the grouped level. In other words, we cannot exclude the possibility that any apparent contextual effect of NC level variables were, in fact, due to the characteristics of individuals residing in them.[21] Also there may be other omitted neighborhood level factors, such as residential isolation, which could account for the association between social capital and mortality rates. [. . .]

This study also extends the findings from a previous report from the
PHDCN[15] that demonstrated an association between indicators of collective efficacy and homicide rates at the NC level. In criminology, social capital (and its related construct, *collective efficacy*) is believed to
operate through the willingness of neighbors to intervene in situations
that might lead to crime. Although the mechanisms underlying the link
between social capital and health outcomes have not been established,
neighborhood social capital might similarly promote health through the
maintenance of healthy norms—for example, neighbors exercising informal social control over "deviant" behaviors such as underage smoking
and binge drinking, as well as the collective efficacy of residents to organize and pass local ordinances (such as those banning smoking in public
areas). Another important potential mechanism through which neighborhood social capital may operate is via the provision of mutual aid
and social support. A great deal of evidence from epidemiology suggests
that social support is an important determinant of longevity and quality of life.[22]

The reasons for the generally null associations between social capital and cancer mortality in this analysis are not clear. In general, studies have not been able to find neighborhood characteristics that explain
variations in cancer rates. This may reflect the long induction period
between exposure and cancer onset, which increases the potential for
null associations via exposure misclassification. This is generally true
for the association between social class and cancer as well (where the
link is much weaker than for heart disease and other outcomes). By contrast, the induction time between residential exposure and heart disease
(as well as other outcomes, such as deaths due to traumatic causes) is
believed to be much shorter, which may explain why we found a cross-
sectional association with community-level social capital. In addition,
the less consistent association between social capital and death rates for
black men and women raises additional questions. [. . .]

[. . .]

References

1. Macintyre S, Ellaway A. Ecological approaches: Rediscovering the role
of the physical and social environment. In *Social epidemiology* (Berkman LP,
Kawachi I, eds.). New York: Oxford University Press; 2000.

2. Haan M, Kaplan GA, Camacho T. Poverty and health: Prospective evi-

dence from the Alameda County Study. *American Journal of Epidemiology.* 1987;125(6):989–998.

3. Anderson RT, Sorlie P, Backlund E, Johnson N, Kaplan GA. Mortality effects of community socioeconomic status. *Epidemiology.* 1997;8(1):42–47.

4. Weitzman ER, Kawachi I. Giving means receiving: The protective effect of social capital on binge drinking on college campuses. *American Journal of Public Health.* 2000;90(12):1936–1939.

5. Cubbin C, LeClere FB, Smith GS. Socioeconomic status and injury mortality: Individual and neighbourhood determinants. *Journal of Epidemiology and Community Health.* 2000;54(7):517–524.

6. Macintyre S, Maciver S, Sooman A. Area, class and health: Should we be focusing on places or people? *Journal of Social Policy.* 1993;22(2):213–234.

7. Weinberg Z, Epstein M. *No place to shop.* Washington, DC: Public Voice for Food and Health Policy; 1996.

8. LaVeist TA, Wallace JM. Health risk and inequitable distribution of liquor stores in African American neighborhood. *Social Science and Medicine.* 2000; 51(4):613–617.

9. Coleman JS. *Foundations of social theory.* Cambridge, MA: Harvard University Press; 1990.

10. Putnam RD. *Making democracy work.* Princeton, NJ: Princeton University Press; 1993.

11. Kawachi I, Kennedy BP, Glass R. Social capital and self-rated health: A contextual analysis. *American Journal of Public Health.* 1999;89(8):1187–1193.

12. Veenstra V. Social capital and health. *Canadian Journal of Policy Research.* 2001;2(1):72–81.

13. Coleman JS. Social capital in the creation of human capital. *American Journal of Sociology.* 1988;94(suppl.):S95–S120.

14. Kawachi I, Kennedy BP, Lochner K, Prothrow-Stith D. Social capital, income inequality, and mortality. *American Journal of Public Health.* 1997;87(9): 1491–1498.

15. Sampson RJ, Raudenbush SW, Earls F. Neighborhoods and violent crime: A multilevel study of collective efficacy. *Science.* 1997;277(5328):918–924.

16. Veenstra G. Social capital, SES and health: An individual-level analysis. *Social Science and Medicine.* 2000;50(5):619–629.

17. Lochner K, Kawachi I, Kennedy BP. Social capital: A guide to its measurement. *Health and Place.* 1999;5(4):259–270.

18. Geolytics Inc. *CensusCD+Maps, Version 2.1.* 1999.

19. Raudenbush SW, Bryk AS, et al. *HLM 5: Hierarchical linear and nonlinear modeling.* Skokie, IL: Scientific Software International; 2000.

20. Putnam RD. Social capital: Measurement and consequences. *Isuma.* 2001;2(1):41–51.

21. Kawachi I, Berkman LF. Social cohesion, social capital, and health. In

Social epidemiology (Kawachi I, Berkman LF, eds.). New York: Oxford University Press; 2000.

22. Berkman LF, Glass T. Social integration, social networks, social support, and health. In *Social epidemiology* (Kawachi I, Berkman LF, eds.). New York: Oxford University Press; 2000:137–173.

CHAPTER TWENTY-FOUR

Weathering

Stress and Heart Disease in African American
Women Living in Chicago

Jan Warren-Findlow

It is well established that individual factors such as lifestyle behaviors and genetics play a significant role in explaining one's health and health risks. Ecological factors in the form of neighborhood socioeconomic status and physical environment characteristics have recently been shown to have a strong correlation with group prevalence of morbidity and mortality.[1] These lifestyle and ecological risk factors are disproportionately distributed in low socioeconomic subgroups. African American women are at high risk for heart disease and other chronic illnesses both because of lifestyle behaviors (such as being sedentary and smoking) and because of their environment. In this article, I describe individual African American women's narratives of stress as the cause of, and as a contributor to, early stage heart disease. I examine their stories through the lens of the socioeconomic, cultural, and environmental context in which these women live. I begin by discussing the weathering conceptual framework with respect to the early onset of chronic illness in African American women and the effects of neighborhood and physical environment particularly in relation to Chicago, where this sample resides. I then present the women's narratives of chronic stress and envi-

Originally published in *Qualitative Health Research* 16, no. 2 (February 2006): 221–37. Copyright © 2006, SAGE Publications.

ronmental hazards that correspond to the hypothesized mechanisms of the weathering framework.

Background

Weathering Conceptual Framework

African American women are at risk for early onset of heart disease and its resulting complications.[2,3] One theory that explains this early onset is that the cumulative stress and health disparities that African American women experience throughout their lives results in negative health outcomes that accelerate aging.[4] Geronimus has called this conceptual framework weathering and contends that from the time female African Americans are in utero until their deaths, their exposure to institutionalized racism and pollutants, obligations to family and kinship networks, and deprivation causes early onset of chronic illness and increases their risk of early disability and mortality. African American women residing in high-poverty, urban areas are more likely to have chronic illnesses in their 20s and 30s and have the same risk of dying by age 45 as white women do by age 65.[5] Early onset of chronic illness increases a woman's overall risk of disability and, more specifically, disability at an earlier age. Weathering looks beyond the individual aspects of poverty or lifestyle to encompass institutional inequalities as well as racism and gender discrimination.

The weathering framework hypothesizes that early first childbirth in African American women is better both for the mother and the child, as teen mothers have had less exposure to hazards and have not yet experienced the onset of chronic illness, and children are less likely to be of low birthweight. This is in contrast to European American mothers, who have healthier babies when they delay childbearing until their mid- to late 20s. Research to support the concept of weathering has examined women's age at first birth, incidence of low-birthweight babies, and neonatal mortality, and found that younger age at first birth is associated with a lower risk of low-birthweight babies and neonatal mortality in disadvantaged women.[6–8] A related study that examined African American women's age at first birth and its association with longevity[9] also supports the weathering hypothesis, as disadvantaged women who delayed childbirth had higher mortality rates than those who became mothers before age 25.

Among the mechanisms that contribute to weathering is "persistent psychosocial stress."[4] Cited examples are frequent socioeconomic crises, excessive family and kin obligations, and disruption of the family unit. Another hypothesized weathering mechanism is one's exposure to hazards in residential or work surroundings; these can be social hazards (such as crime) or environmental ones (such as pollution). This environmental mechanism is supported by research on neighborhood and physical environment effects on health.[10–13]

The weathering framework acknowledges that how African American women respond to their situation can exacerbate their health.[4] Continual striving to overcome inequality and barriers can worsen a woman's health, not improve it. A related theory, the Sojourner syndrome,[14] hypothesizes that it is African American women's coping response to the inequalities they experience that increases their health risks.

Sojourner syndrome is named after Sojourner Truth, a former slave who traveled the United States preaching for women's rights for black women. In a speech made famous by her query "Ain't I a woman?,"[14] she described the many hardships and challenges experienced by black women within a society governed by racial and gender oppression. The Sojourner syndrome is the female version of John Henryism,[15] wherein black women become more susceptible to disease and illness because of their constant exertion to stay strong, work hard, be head of the household and often primary wage earner, fulfill responsibilities, and overcome obstacles that they encounter in their social and physical environment. Thus, there are two forces operating negatively on women's health, the chronic stress and their coping response to that stress.

Neighborhood and Environment

There is growing recognition that neighborhood socioeconomic status plays a significant role in health and might increase the chronic stress experienced by African American women. Low socioeconomic status has been linked to higher rates of all-cause mortality, chronic disease morbidity, and low-birthweight babies in African Americans.[12] Neighborhood has been defined geographically and is generally operationalized as a census tract.[10,16] Within census tracts, individual- and group-level measures such as home ownership, median income, percentage of population with a college degree,[17] residential stability,[18] percentage of affluent families, and percentage of residents who are unemployed have been analyzed as predictors of health outcomes.

Individuals living in socioeconomically disadvantaged neighborhoods have been found to have significantly higher risk for coronary heart disease than those living in the most advantaged neighborhoods even after controlling for individual income, education, and occupation.[17] In an analysis of 23 local areas across the United States, researchers[4] found that African Americans living in lower income urban neighborhoods had the fewest years of active life expectancy after age 16. Blacks living in economically better areas had greater life expectancy but only slightly better functional status. In comparison to the other areas, African American women from the south side of Chicago had the highest poverty rate of the communities studied and the shortest overall life expectancy (age 55). Other social factors can also influence heart disease. Older African American women experienced higher rates of heart disease mortality in census tracts with high female-headship rates, independent of individual socioeconomic and health risk factors.[19]

Similarly, race-based residential segregation has been associated with entrenched poverty, low educational attainment, and high rates of unemployment. Williams and Collins[13] have hypothesized that racial residential segregation is an institutional mechanism of racism and a fundamental cause of racial disparities in health.[12,13] [. . .]

Chicago

Chicago, where this study is conducted, reflects many of the characteristics of racially segregated and lower income neighborhoods that have been previously studied. Chicago has a diverse population that is approximately one-third white, one-third black, and one-third Hispanic.[20] Chicago continues to be highly segregated; of the 50 metropolitan areas in the United States with the largest black populations, Chicago ranks third in the level of segregation experienced by blacks.[21] The average black person living in Chicago resides in a neighborhood that is 73% black, down from 83% in 1980 and 78% in 1990.

Socioeconomically, however, blacks in Chicago are experiencing a widening income gap in relation to whites. Chicago ranks fifth among urban areas with large black populations in terms of median income gap between blacks and whites.[22] The average white person in Chicago earned a median income of almost US$60,000, whereas the average black person earned only $33,000. In 1990, the income disparity between blacks and whites was only about $24,000.

Crime and violence are ongoing features of black neighborhoods in Chicago. According to national crime statistics from 2003, Chicago was the "homicide capital" of the United States,[23] with the highest per capita homicide rate among large metropolitan cities. More than 40% of these fatalities are gang related and are attributed to increasing tensions among gangs and disputes over drug transactions and turfs.[24] In the past 5 years, street gangs in Chicago have been responsible for more than 1,300 killings,[23] with many of these fatalities occurring in predominantly black neighborhoods.

National health status indicators show that health disparities between blacks and whites are narrowing; however, the reverse is true in Chicago.[25] There, African Americans' health improved on 14 health status indicators analyzed from 1990 to 1998 (mortality rates from seven causes, including heart disease, four birth-related outcomes, and incidence of tuberculosis and syphilis); however, only four indicators actually had a narrowing of the black:white rate ratio. The remaining indicators, including heart disease mortality rates, showed widening black:white rate ratios. Thus, national statistics obscure the health problems facing blacks in Chicago and the difficulties facing health care and public health professionals.

For the reasons I have cited, African Americans residing in Chicago face many challenges: worsening health in relation to whites, reduced income and high unemployment, segregation and discrimination, and worsening crime and violence. In this article, I describe the role of stress in relation to heart disease as reported by African American women living in Chicago. Their narratives and their individual and neighborhood socioeconomic and demographic data are examined with regard to the weathering conceptual framework and its hypothesized processes.

Method

This analysis is part of a larger dissertation project that examined explanatory models of early stage heart disease in older black women. A modified version of Kleinman's[26] explanatory model of illness framework formed the basis for the interview guide. Women were also asked some basic demographic questions. Characteristics of their neighborhood, defined as a census tract, were determined using publicly available U.S. Census 2000 data.

Recruitment

This is a purposeful sample selected for in-depth study of early stage heart disease in African American women. Women were recruited by nurses and cardiologists from a large, urban hospital that serves a lower income and minority population. Eligible women were black, age 50 or older, with nonobstructive coronary artery disease.

The study met ethical review board standards as determined by the appropriate university. Consent to participate was obtained on a minimum of three occasions. First, verbal and written consent was obtained by physicians and nurses who approached eligible women; the women filled out a flyer with their names and contact information if they were interested in participating; the flyers were then passed on to me. Verbal consent to participate was obtained again when I telephoned women to explain the study and to schedule an interview; last, written consent was obtained at the first interview. Either women read the consent form themselves, or I offered to read it to them (about half the woman chose this latter option). The consent form was written at the ninth grade reading level. Women were given US$20 cash at the completion of each interview.

Study Participants

The sample consists of 12 women ranging in age from 50 to 73, all of whom self-described as being black or African American. The participants described various forms of heart disease that were being managed through medication and lifestyle change over the course of the study.

Most of the women were born and raised in the southern United States (Alabama, Arkansas, Mississippi, Missouri, and Tennessee) and migrated north as children or young wives. Three women were currently married and living with their spouse, 3 reported living alone, 3 lived with and were raising small children, and the others lived with adult children and grandchildren. More than half of the sample had not finished high school, and half earned less than US$10,000 per year.

All women were currently receiving specialist care for their heart problem. All had some form of health insurance. Most received health care through either Public Aid or Medicare, or else by qualifying for disability supplements. Only 2 women had private insurance. In addition to their heart disease, participants self-reported having between three and eight other chronic illnesses or health conditions: arthritis, asthma, cancer (breast, cervical, and ovarian), depression or "nerves," diabetes, gastroesophageal reflux disease (GERD), hypertension, stroke, sleep apnea, high cholesterol, or overweight or obesity. Women reported taking between 4 and 25 different medications. Two thirds of participants were taking prescribed antidepressants, antianxiety medications, or "nerve pills."

Data Generation

Interviews were conducted between August 2002 and May 2004: Two women were interviewed once, 5 were interviewed twice, and the rest were interviewed three times. All interviews were conducted face-to-face in participants' homes. Interviews ranged in length from 45 to 90 minutes. I conducted and audiotaped all the interviews, wrote field notes, and kept a reflexive journal on my research experience. Interviews were transcribed verbatim.

Data Analysis

I used Atlas/Ti software to store all interview texts, field notes, codes and code definitions, and categories. Data collection and analysis occurred simultaneously as described in grounded theory methods.[27,28] Analysis began with in-depth reading of the transcripts. After multiple readings, I coded the text on a line-by-line basis. I attached codes to whole sentences or paragraphs to avoid fragmentation of meaning. Codes were defined and refined and then sorted into categories. The original purpose of the study was to describe women's explanatory models of heart disease for a dissertation project. That analysis revealed that women perceived that stress was the principal cause of their heart disease and that stress coping was their primary form of self-care. Ongoing stressful incidents were a pervasive theme throughout their narratives that compelled a deeper analysis. The categories of stress that subsequently emerged were concurrent with the mechanisms of weathering. Census data were included to provide additional contextual background on women's neighborhood environments.

Data Presentation

I have not corrected the participants' grammar, nor have I edited or changed any words in the comments reported here. In the quoted text

passages in this article, my verbal and nonverbal words of encouragement have been removed for readability (e.g., "right" and "uh-huh").
Many women often inserted "you know" into their sentences. These
phrases are often removed for readability; however, I wish to acknowledge that these "you knows" have been interpreted as participants' requests for understanding.[29] My comments are enclosed in < > that signal
explanatory remarks about sounds or physical movements, or references
to previous statements.

Field Description

I had not previously been to any of the participants' neighborhoods despite having lived and worked as an adult in the Chicago area for the
past 20 years. Although blacks often leave their predominantly black
neighborhoods to go to work or seek services, most whites rarely need to
enter black neighborhoods in Chicago. Most of the time, I was the only
white person on the street except for some construction workers or City
employees working on a water main. I did not feel unsafe, just noticeably white, and the participants were aware that I stuck out. One woman,
who had forgotten about our interview, peered out her window and said
to her daughter "Who is that white lady out there?" Most women either
subtly or directly acknowledged that I was white and assumed I did not
know black culture or lifestyles. In the manner of the "expert" participant, they often volunteered comments and explanations to educate me.

With the exception of 2 women who lived in subsidized housing, the
rest of the women lived in what are typical older Chicago neighborhoods: residential blocks containing a mixture of single family homes
(such as the classic Chicago-style brick bungalow), brick or graystone
two- and three-flat buildings, and slightly larger apartment buildings.
Larger apartment buildings all had security gates and buzzers. There
were older model cars parked out front and occasionally young black
men talking in groups outside. In some neighborhoods, older people sat
out on their front porches, talking to each other and generally keeping
an eye on things.

Commercial areas on the major streets around the participants' neighborhoods were also typically Chicagoan, albeit businesses associated
with a somewhat lower income population (no upscale coffee shops).
One commercial strip contained the following businesses: currency ex-

changes (where people cash checks, wire funds, pay utility bills, and get auto licenses), storefronts selling cell phones, convenience stores selling lottery tickets, small branch banks, and storefronts promising instant tax refunds are intermingled with fast food chain restaurants such as White Castle and Taco Bell, and unfranchised chicken-and-rib shacks, a discount shoe store, and shoeshine and shoe repair shops. There were some businesses that catered specifically to the African American community, such as hair salons specializing in hair braiding and extensions and stores selling African cloth.

Findings

Neighborhood Data

The socioeconomic picture of participants' neighborhoods is determined from Census 2000 data.[30] The 12 women in the study live in nine different census tracts, mostly clustered on the South and West sides of Chicago. All nine of these census tracts contain populations that are more than 91 to 99% African American. These figures indicate that the participants' neighborhoods are more segregated than the reported average figures for blacks living in Chicago.[21,22]

The median household income for participants' census tracts ranges from US$10,175 to $53,221, with four census tracts having median incomes below the $33,000 reported for blacks in Chicago. Seven women in the sample lived in those four census tracts. Only the 3 married women reported incomes greater than the median for blacks in Chicago. Although most of the women in this study would be classified as lower income, they did not live in "ghettos."

With respect to crime, of the 12 neighborhoods with the highest homicide rates in the city,[24] 10 of the 12 participants lived in one these dangerous neighborhoods. These neighborhoods are geographically large and composed of many census tracts.

The neighborhood with the lowest income in the sample, based on U.S. Bureau of the Census[20] data, had more than 50% of the population in this census tract living below the poverty level. Most of the available housing stock in that census tract is owned and run by the Chicago Housing Authority (CHA). This public housing complex is made up of four different housing projects all slated for one of the largest redevelopment projects in the city. In addition, there are some HUD (Housing and Urban Development) senior buildings that are open only to adults aged 55 and older who are disabled. One participant lived in a CHA town home, and another lived in a HUD senior building.

Mechanisms of Weathering

The weathering hypothesis describes the cumulative effect of exposure to inequality, stress, and negative environmental situations on African American women. The mechanisms of weathering have two characteristics: First, they begin at an early age; and, second, they are persistent and continue throughout one's lifetime. Weathering manifests as early onset of chronic illness. This was evident with several of the participants who related to me that they started having hypertension in their early 20s. Some noted that the onset coincided with pregnancies. Women also tended to leave the workforce because of disability; for some, this occurred as early as their 40s.

STRESS AND A "BAD HEART"

Women described many stressful situations, and stress was an ongoing theme throughout their lives. Women perceived that stress was the primary cause of their heart problem, which they termed "bad heart." Women often talked about stress or being "stressed out." Related ways of expressing stress were "nerves," as in "I have bad nerves" or "my nerves are on edge." Women who expressed having bad nerves took "nerve pills" (antidepressants or antianxiety medications). Two-thirds of the women were taking some form of prescription medicine for depression or nerves. Stress and nerves are intertwined with depression, as one woman explained to me:

> Well okay when I'm like that I get, I'm tense. I'm like, it's a feeling I have, uh uh a depression I have, and I feel like <sigh>, it's somethin' gonna happen, that's the kind of feelin' I have. That somethin' is gonna happen, and I don't know what it is. That's the kind of feelin' I have. And it's like I wanna cry sometimes.

Seven women described being depressed, but only 5 used the terms *depression* or *depressed*. The other 2 describe the affect of being depressed: sadness, needing or wanting to cry, not wanting to go anywhere or do anything, or "I get all down and out." All of these women also talk about stress and often within the same context as depression. These concepts are not distinguishable based on the data collected, so they are combined for purposes of this article.

Stress was viewed as something that caused bad heart, worsened bad heart, or could cause a heart attack. As one woman explains, "I think stress is what's killin' a lotta people." Stress affects bad heart directly. As one woman notes, "But um, the main thing that causes um chest pain, is when I'm stressed out."

Race and gender were also acknowledged as causes of stress. Women acknowledged that men and women responded differently to problems.

> But I guess that's because women worry a little bit more and have a little bit more pressure than men do. Men can walk over things and women got to stop and think and women's try to relieve it to help you.

One acknowledged cultural aspect of stress was that black girls are raised to be strong. Thus "being a strong woman" is an important coping mechanism for dealing with the many challenges these women faced.

FAMILY DISRUPTION

Most women experienced incidences of family disruption when they were younger, although they did not generally associate these episodes with their heart health. Most of these women began having children as early as age 16 or 17, soon after their marriages. Ten of the 12 women had children; they gave birth to between 2 and 12 children. Half the sample were separated, divorced or widowed while their children were still school age, forcing them to become heads of the household. Four women have been separated from their husbands for decades. The oldest participant in the study described her marital status in this way:

> We were married about, I guess in all, . . .'nough to git all them children. Eight children and then he decide I wasn't good enough . . . he wouldn't give me a divorce. But he jumped up and he married someone else but it wasn't, it wasn't legal. But he never really did divorce me 'cause I went downtown to the, to the court house and find out.

Two women lost their mothers at a young age and assumed the responsibility of raising much younger siblings. One woman, who did not have children, was one of 15 siblings. She and her husband raised her 7 younger siblings after her parents died. Another woman lost her mother when she was only 12. She then looked after 8 siblings and 5 step-siblings until her father married her to an older man when she was 17. Family disruptions from early loss of a parent or abandonment or death of a husband were a common theme. Women often acknowledged that parents died from heart attacks or heart-related illnesses.

Women also told stories of caregiving for ill or aging parents. This sometimes caused participants to leave the workforce and transition into full-time home care workers. Most women worked at relatively low-wage jobs and often with few benefits: sewing drapes, sorting mail for the postal service, working for the city health department, home care worker, factory worker, certified nursing assistant, housekeeper, day care worker, special education teacher, hotel cook, and anesthesiology technician. Only 2 women worked until retirement and received pension benefits.

ECONOMIC AND FINANCIAL HARDSHIP

Finances were a concern for most of the women in the study. For some, the inability to pay their basic monthly living expenses was a problem. Others had to choose between riding the bus using a senior citizen discount card or paying $4.25 for parking. One participant was forced to quit working and go on disability when she was diagnosed with cervical cancer more than 3 years ago. Around the same time, she lost her voucher for federally subsidized housing and briefly became homeless. She now lives with, and is financially dependent on, one of her sons. Her story describes the "one paycheck away from homelessness" type of stress that she believes caused her heart disease.

> Now I'm just scramblin' for a livin', you know. I just get this disability, which is nothing. I worked all my life and I don't even get enough disability for my needs. Just, even just to survive. You know it's, it's killin' me because when I worked I paid my bills and I had excess money. I don't have anything. And that's a hardship, that's a lot on you.

In a later interview, she relates the trauma of her son's being shot. She had to deal not only with the stress and emotional consequences of almost losing her son but also with the resulting financial difficulties. Without her son's income, her phone was shut off, she was almost evicted, and she had to pay several hundred dollars to retrieve the family car from the police impound lot, where it was being held for evidence.

Institutional Stress. Almost all the women in this sample are dependent on city, state, or federal government "safety net" services for some portion of their health care, income, food, and/or housing. Dealing with institutions, particularly government agencies, can be highly stressful. In addition to Department of Children and Family Services (DCFS), the police (who are not to be trusted), and the justice system, there is also Social Security and TANF (Temporary Assistance for Needy Families, which controls food stamps), utility companies, and the CHA.

One 51-year-old participant, who receives disability benefits, notified Social Security that she would be working part-time at a local school, but when she was laid off a few months later and went to get her full benefits reinstated, she encountered resistance, misinformation, and disrespect:

> They was acting as though that this money and the food stamps was coming out of their pockets. This is what I, uh, you picked up from them. They telling me that they can't do this, they can't do that. But I was on disability. And I said, "You all told that once I stopped working that was it." So it's and it was very stressful 'cause when I went to Social Security and talked to this lady, she talked real smart and snotty with me. . . . I kind of got upset with her, I'm not gonna lie. . . . I just looked at her and I told her, I said, "Well, you know what, you need to know how to talk to people." . . . I said, "You don't see me going all off on you. I expect the same from you."

The gap in income she experienced between the loss of her job and the delay in reinstating her disability benefits caused this woman significant financial hardship. She fell behind on her gas bill, and the utility company turned off her gas in the middle of winter. Reinstating her gas service required a $350 deposit plus late fees, which she ultimately borrowed from a friend. In her efforts to battle the system for the benefits to which she is legally entitled, she must also stand up to bureaucrats and disrespectful attitudes.

[. . .]

ENVIRONMENTAL HAZARDS

Housing Displacement. In addition to her caregiving stress, this same participant lives in one of the city-run housing projects that are scheduled for redevelopment. The existing homes will be demolished, and more than 2,000 residents will relocated. The participant, who has lived in this housing project for the past 45 years, is critical of the plan from a practical perspective but also dislikes the idea of splitting up the community:

> They s'posed to be tearin' down and we gonna move. . . . Um-hmm and then they tried to put us way out in the suburbs. Place where we don't have no transportation so I ain't goin' out there. . . . Yeah, you have to have a car 'cause they showed it on there [. . .], they showed it on the TV screen, you know, movie, how you need transportation and everything, back and forth . . . 'cause all us, we know each other . . . so it's kinda hard. . . . And people do look around fo' you and you go right out here and catch the bus or up there and catch the bus. 'Cause all of us don't have cars, 'cause I can't even drive one.

For this woman, 45 years in the same place with the same families creates a community where she feels safe. The displacement, or "root shock,"[31] that she would experience is more stressful than the crime, poverty, or segregation that she currently deals with. The common perception is that people living in the "projects" should be happy to move if they have the chance. Statistics and the media portray African Americans as poor, at risk, prone to violence and drug addiction, and without stability, roots, or connection. Yet the reality is that whole communities are being torn apart and relocated to an inconvenient, foreign area not even in the same city.

Crime. Although women did not always talk outright about the safety of their neighborhoods, I observed incidents that indicated that safety was an issue. One woman always looked out her front window when she was expecting me. She met me on the stoop and took note of where I parked my car. She also met her grandson when he got off the school bus. The school bus driver would honk his horn to let her know the bus was outside, and he would not open the bus door until he saw her standing on the front stoop. This participant is very concerned about the drug dealing that goes on in front of her house (which I also observed), and she has tried to reach out and establish a relationship with the very people that she is afraid of:

> When I first moved over here, the first day I came over here to look at the place, uh, some guys was out, outside the house out there. And I said "What are you all doing," you know? "Oh we just out here." I said "Why?," you know. And I said "What you all doing? You gonna do this all the time?" And

they told me "Yes." . . . And I said "You know what, I'll be friends with you if you be friends with me. If you respect me, give me respect, I'll give you the respect." . . . And so uh after that I got to know them before I moved in. And then they told me, they said "Well you know what, we will try very hard not to give you no problems, and we won't let no one else bother give you problems." That's what they told me. So after I moved in, they did just that. But it got where they would hang around the front, and I didn't like that. And I know what they was doin' . . . and I would see them put all these little nests <baggies of drugs> down side the gate, the fence, out there around the grass.

She did not call the police because she believed that they were in on it:

The police was getting' their kick out of it too. I really feels that way. The policemans are getting money out of it too. Because there was too much stuff goin' on and nobody talked about it.

When I asked why she did not call the police, she explained that if you call them, they know who you are, they will tell someone, and "then they will mess with you." She does not express any sense of personal vulnerability with respect to the drug dealers unless she notifies the police.

Residential Stability. Two participants who live within three blocks of each other had opposing views of the neighborhood. One woman, when asked if she felt safe living there, replied, "There's just so many new faces." In contrast, the other participant describes her neighborhood as being very safe based on her residence there for the past 43 years. No one has ever broken into her house, and the neighbors all watch out for each other. She acknowledges that many people have moved away but feels she knows most people because she has been an election judge for 35 years. "And I see most of the people when they come to vote. Every year, you know, whenever. . . . And I know they children." Although neighborhoods might be low income, or its residents transient, community ties can still survive.

Being a Strong Woman: Sojourner Syndrome

Women often described how they handled life challenges, whether health related, family crises, or just everyday tasks. This persona was articulated by one woman as "being a strong woman." Unfortunately, being a strong woman contributes to stress. In her words, a "strong woman" is

one who is very independent. I never asked anybody for anything. I did it, just like if I was goin' to the grocery store with my girlfriends, instead of waiting on my husband to bring the pop or the beer up, I would do it myself. You know I didn't ever want anybody to do anything for me. . . . But bein' strong is handling all the financial problems. My husband doesn't know what be up, anything. I jus' handle it all. And to me, and then I, I guess because I feel like I'm so strong, I try to help other people. . . . But if people have a problem, they used to all dump it on me. Because I, I'm strong and no one realized that it bothered me. I didn't know how to let it out. . . . I mean it's nothin' to me that I have come in to that I haven't been able to handle. Except for this, well, I'm gonna handle this too, though. That's what I mean by being strong, overcoming any obstacle that comes in my way or whatever.

This participant's comments articulate several aspects of the Sojourner syndrome: the assumption of economic responsibilities, the striving to overcome difficulties, and using one's strength to take care of others.

These same traits of independence, caretaking, and keeping things inside were expressed or demonstrated by several of the other women in the sample. Another woman describes how being unable to work because of her depression has affected her sense of being a strong woman. "I couldn't handle it and to me it was a sign of failure and I couldn't deal with that either. 'Cause I had always been so strong, dealt with everything." She has also suffered a loss of self-esteem now that she is not earning any money. "I never had to ask anyone for anything. . . ." The enforced dependence has been difficult for her, as her husband does not want her to go back to work because of her illness. She discusses how her habit of keeping things inside has caused her physical problems. "They found out that I was having migraines. Due to the stress and the loss of my Mom that I was holdin' inside."

A related feature of keeping things inside is not letting others know that you're sick. One participant told me, "I don't complain a lot about bein' sick. If I'm sick, nobody knows I'm sick. Cause I been in bed and somebody comes, I'm going. I just gotta drag myself outta here and go." Another woman, who suffered two strokes several years ago, does not want to become dependent or unable to do her own housework or bathe and dress herself. She has had to reduce some of her church activities, such as singing in the choir, because she cannot stand for long periods, but she notes that her fellow parishioners tell her, "You don't look like you sick." There's a sense that they do not believe that she is ill. Conversely, she does not want to look sick because of how she perceives that sick people are treated:

> Well, you know, I tell you, it's hard for people to understand. That is the hardest thing, through life, people understandin' you, you know. About your health. They think 'cause you looks well that you well. You understand me? See? And they don't believe I'm on as much medication that they, you know. Like I say, I go to church, "They ain't nuthin' wrong wit you. You don't look like nuthin' wrong wit you." Sometime when I walk up the steps I have to sit down before I can go on down any further. See?

Thus, the very characteristics that allowed these women to endure raising families on their own, handling financial problems, and taking care of others do not serve them once they are ill. Although being a strong woman allows them to have some sense of normalcy, on the other hand, it discredits their assertions that they are sick or in pain.

Discussion

The purpose of this article was to examine older African American women's stories of social and environmental stress in relation to their heart disease through the lens of the weathering conceptual framework. Women reported that stress was a primary cause of, and an ongoing contributor to, their heart disease. They describe stress as a "killer" and believe that it can worsen their heart condition, causing chest pain and heart attacks. An analysis of their descriptions of the stress that they perceive is related to their "bad heart" reveals the daily challenges and chronic stressful situations that these women live with. When their narratives are combined with individual and neighborhood demographic and socioeconomic data, it is evident that these older women's life experiences demonstrate the themes of the weathering framework that lead to accelerated aging, and that they are aware of it. Their stories reveal the depth, detail, and context behind the statistics that point to widening health disparities among blacks and whites in Chicago. This rich contextual background is rarely reported in heart disease research.

Women's stories of chronic stress reflect many of the mechanisms that characterize the weathering conceptual framework.[4] Women described many early incidents in their lives that implied a cumulative stress effect: early loss of a parent, early age at first childbirth, raising children alone, and early onset of chronic illness and disability. Their retrospective stories confirm other studies that associate early childbearing and pregnancy-related hypertension with weathering.[8] However, women also described recent and persistent stressors: living with chronic illness, cultural expectations such as "being a strong woman," caregiving, interactions with social service and other agencies for life's necessities, crime, and persistent financial instability. Their reports confirm other studies[11] in which African American women described a lack of trust in the police, disrespect from social service agencies, and reliance on extended family networks to raise children. These situations and interactions clearly take a toll on their health and well-being.

[. . .]

Most of the women in this sample lived in neighborhoods at the extreme end of the socioeconomic scale in comparison to the statistically average black person residing in Chicago.[21,22] Most women reported incomes that were significantly less than the median for blacks in the city (only the 3 married women reported incomes greater than the median), and women lived in neighborhoods that were much more segregated than the average shown for Chicago. More than 80% of the women lived in the most deadly and violent neighborhoods in Chicago.[24] Only 2 of the participants did not live in one of these violent neighborhoods. Ironically, one of them is the woman whose son was shot.

The resilience and persistence these women portray in their efforts to cope with challenging circumstances is truly inspiring. The cultural description of "being a strong woman" confirms the characteristics of the Sojourner syndrome.[14] These participants also articulated the negative consequence of this coping strategy: They have no one to talk to or listen to their problems. This was stated both directly and indirectly to me. I was told, "You listen like doctors should" and "You're the only one . . . I told *everything* [emphasis added] to." Another woman said, "I'm so glad you came 'cause I just been so full." One woman's doctor referred her to a psychiatrist, and she told him that she did not need one because I was coming to see her. Their need to present themselves as strong women who can cope with anything effectively isolates them from receiving emotional support. Thus, their survival strategy has also had a huge cost to their mental health; they are surviving but not thriving. Evidence of the Sojourner syndrome has important implications for health care clinicians, who need to be sensitive to African American women's emotional isolation. It is likely that black women tell their physicians about what seemingly are nonmedical issues but have great relevance and meaning to them in the context of their stress and its perceived effect on their heart health.

Without understanding the complexity of people's lives, we cannot hope to conquer effectively the health disparities experienced by lower income, underserved, and marginalized populations. [. . .]

References

1. Cohen DA, Farley TA, Mason K. Why is poverty unhealthy? Social and physical mediators. *Social Science and Medicine.* 2003;57(9):1631–1641.

2. American Heart Association. Heart disease and stroke statistics—2004 update. 2005. http://www.heart.org/HEARTORG/General/Heart-and-Stroke -Association-Statistics_UCM_319064_SubHomePage.jsp.

3. Mosca L, Manson JE, Sutherland SE, Langer RD, Manolio T, Barrett-Connor E. Cardiovascular disease in women: A statement for healthcare professionals from the American Heart Association: Writing Group. *Circulation.* 1997;96(7):2468–2482.

4. Geronimus AT. Understanding and eliminating racial inequalities in women's health in the United States: The role of the weathering conceptual framework. *Journal of the American Medical Women's Association.* 2001;56(4): 133–136, 149–150.

5. Geronimus AT, Bound J, Waidmann TA, Colen CG, Steffick D. Inequality in life expectancy, functional status, and active life expectancy across selected black and white populations in the United States. *Demography.* 2001;38(2): 227–251.

6. Geronimus AT. Black/white differences in the relationship of maternal age to birthweight: A population-based test of the weathering hypothesis. *Social Science and Medicine.* 1996;42(4):589–597.

7. Rich-Edwards JW, Buka SL, Brennan RT, Earls F. Diverging associations of maternal age with low birthweight for black and white mothers. *International Journal of Epidemiology.* 2003;32(1):83–90.

8. Wildsmith EM. Testing the weathering hypothesis among Mexican-origin women. *Ethnicity and Disease.* 2002;12(4):470–479.

9. Astone NM, Ensminger M, Juon HS. Early adult characteristics and mortality among inner-city African American women. *American Journal of Public Health.* 2002;92(4):640–645.

10. Sampson RJ, Morenoff JD, Gannon-Rowley T. Assessing "neighborhood effects": Social processes and new directions in research. *Annual Review of Sociology.* 2002;28:443–478.

11. Schulz A, Parker E, Israel DB, Fisher DT. Social context, stressors, and disparities in women's health. *Journal of the American Medical Women's Association.* 2001;56(4):143–149.

12. Schulz AJ, Williams DR, Israel BA, Lempert LB. Racial and spatial relations as fundamental determinants of health in Detroit. *Milbank Quarterly.* 2002;80(4):677–707.

13. Williams DR, Collins C. Racial residential segregation: A fundamental cause of racial disparities in health. *Public Health Reports.* 2001;116(5):404–416.

14. Mullings L, Wali A. *Stress and resilience: The social context of reproduction in central Harlem.* New York: Kluwer Academic/Plenum; 2001.

15. James SA. John Henryism and the health of African Americans. *Culture, Medicine and Psychiatry.* 1994;18(2):163–182.

16. Diez Roux AV. Investigating neighborhood and area effects on health. *American Journal of Public Health.* 2001;91(11):1783–1789.

17. Diez Roux AV, Merkin SS, Arnett D, et al. Neighborhood of residence and incidence of coronary heart disease. *New England Journal of Medicine.* 2001;345(2):99–106.

18. Boardman JD. Stress and physical health: The role of neighborhoods as mediating and moderating mechanisms. *Social Science and Medicine.* 2004; 58(12):2473–2483.

19. LeClere FB, Rogers RG, Peters K. Neighborhood social context and racial differences in women's heart disease mortality. *Journal of Health and Social Behaviour.* 1998;39(2):91–107.

20. Bureau of the Census. *Profile of general demographic characteristics.* Washington, DC: US Government Printing Office; 2000.

21. Logan J, Lewis Mumford Center Research Team. Ethnic diversity grows, neighborhood integration lags behind. Albany: State University of New York at Albany; 2001.

22. Logan J. *Separate and unequal: The neighborhood gap for blacks and Hispanics in metropolitan America.* Albany: Lewis Mumford Center for Comparative Urban and Regional Research, State University of New York at Albany; 2002.

23. Butterfield F. Rise in killings spurs new steps to fight gangs. *New York Times.* January 17, 2004:1.

24. Huppke RW, Heinzmann D. Shoot-first culture stalks streets of murder capital. *Chicago Tribune.* February 1, 2004.

25. Margellos H, Silva A, Whitman S. Comparison of health status indicators in Chicago: Are black-white disparities worsening? *American Journal of Public Health.* 2004;94(1):116–121.

26. Kleinman A. *Patients and healers in the context of culture: An exploration of the borderland between anthropology, medicine, and psychiatry.* Berkeley: University of California Press; 1980.

27. Charmaz K, Mitchell R. Grounded theory in ethnography. In *Handbook of ethnography* (Atkinson P, Coffey A, Delamont S, Lofland J, Lofland L, eds.). London: Sage; 2001:160–174.

28. Strauss A, Corbin J. *Basics of qualitative research: Techniques and procedures for developing grounded theory.* 2nd ed. Thousand Oaks, CA: Sage; 1998.

29. DeVault ML. *Liberating method: Feminism and social research.* Philadelphia: Temple University Press; 1999.

30. Bureau of the Census. American fact finder: Sample data. N.d. http://fact finder.census.gov.

31. Fullilove MT. *Root shock: How tearing up city neighborhoods hurts America, and what we can do about it.* New York: One World/Ballantine; 2004.

CHAPTER TWENTY-FIVE

The Protective Effect of Community Factors on Childhood Asthma

Ruchi S. Gupta, Xingyou Zhang, Lisa K. Sharp, John J. Shannon, and Kevin B. Weiss

Introduction

Asthma is the leading chronic illness of childhood, affecting over 9 million children; however, the burden is not equally distributed in the United States.[1] Racial differences in prevalence have been identified as an important public health concern, as has the problem of increased asthma prevalence in certain U.S. urban populations.[2-5]

Chicago, a city with one of the highest asthma rates in the country, has asthma mortality twice the national average.[6,7] Chicago hospitalization rates have also been shown to be twice as high as suburban Chicago and overall U.S. rates.[8] However, research demonstrates that childhood asthma rates in Chicago vary widely based on the neighborhood in which a child lives.[9]

Researchers exploring the causes of the asthma burden in Chicago and other high-risk urban areas have demonstrated that mortality rates are associated with individual factors such as race and community social economic status.[5-10] Some negative community-level physical environment factors, such as neighborhood violence, air pollution, and housing conditions, have also been implicated in affecting childhood asthma

Originally published in the *Journal of Allergy and Clinical Immunology* 123, no. 6 (June 2009): 1297–304. Copyright © 2009, Elsevier.

prevalence and morbidity.[11–15] To our knowledge, the effect of social and environmental factors thought to enrich a community, i.e., *positive community factors*, has not been fully characterized. In a study limited to a comparison of 3,268 adults in Chicago, it was suggested that collective efficacy, a measure of residents' trust, attachment, and capacity for mutually beneficial action, was protective against asthma and breathing problems.[16]

The Chicago Initiative to Raise Asthma Health Equity (CHIRAH) study was designed to better characterize the factors associated with asthma burden. Initial findings have suggested a wide variation in childhood asthma prevalence.[9] Therefore, the purpose of this study was to determine the effect of positive community factors such as social capital, economic potential, and community amenities on childhood asthma prevalence in Chicago neighborhoods.

Methods

Overview of Study Design

This report is based on a cross-sectional survey screening for asthma that was conducted as part of the CHIRAH study. This study consisted of a large sample of children attending Chicago public and Catholic elementary and middle schools during the 2003 to 2004 and 2004 to 2005 school years. An overview of the study methods follows; for further details on study methods, refer to Shalowitz et al.[17]

School Sample

In 2004, Chicago Public Schools (CPS) had 320,557 students in 486 elementary schools. CPS students were 50% black, 38% Hispanic, and 9% white. Eighty-five percent of CPS students were considered low-income, defined as coming from families who are receiving public aid, living in institutions for neglected or delinquent children, being supported in foster homes with public funds, or being eligible to receive free or reduced-price lunches. In 2004, the Archdiocese of Chicago had 37,333 students in 126 elementary schools. Archdiocese students were 14% black, 17% Hispanic, and 62% white. Twenty-four percent of Archdiocese students were low-income (includes Chicago and suburbs; Chicago-only estimates are higher).

In order to gain a representative sample of students, schools were stratified first by race and then income. Schools were identified by population proportionate and cluster sampling methods within each of the 4 race-income sampling groups (high black/mid-income; high black/low-income; low black/mid-income; low black/low-income), resulting in a final sample of 105 schools. For each school, all children in kindergarten through eighth grade were eligible to be surveyed and asked to participate. A total of 48,917 (79%) completed surveys were returned.

Survey Instrument

The screening survey was distributed at the schools and taken home by the students for an adult caregiver to complete in English or Spanish. It consisted of questions including the child's birth date, height, weight, sex, report of physician-diagnosed or nurse-diagnosed asthma, age at diagnosis, race/ethnicity of the child, current asthma status, relationship to the child of the person completing the survey, names and ages of others living in the same household with asthma, the child's home address, and a short asthma symptom screening tool: the Brief Pediatric Asthma Screen Plus.[18,19] Our analyses included only children with physician-diagnosed or nurse-diagnosed asthma as reported by an adult caregiver. The sampled subjects were geocoded by using ArcGIS US Streetmap and linked with neighborhoods (ESRI GIS and Mapping Software; Redlands, Calif.).

Neighborhood Selection Criteria

To study the possible community-level factors, all children were assigned to a neighborhood. The Chicago neighborhoods used in this analysis represent neighborhoods as defined by the Project on Human Development in Chicago Neighborhoods (PHDCN).[20] The PHDCN Scientific Directors defined *neighborhoods* spatially, as a collection of people and institutions occupying a contiguous subsection of a larger community. The project collapsed 847 census tracts in the city of Chicago to form 343 neighborhoods. The predominant guideline in formation of the neighborhoods was that they should be as ecologically meaningful as possible, composed of geographically contiguous census tracts, and internally homogenous on key census indicators. The project settled on an ecological unit of about 8000 people, which is smaller than the 77 established community areas in Chicago (of which the average size is almost 40,000 people), but large enough to approximate local communities. Geographic boundaries (e.g., railroad tracks, parks, and freeways) and knowledge of Chicago's community areas guided this process. Our sample consisted of children from 287 of the 342 PHDCN neighborhoods; 56 neighborhoods had fewer than 15 children from our sample and were not included in the study.

Community Vitality Index

Community-level socio-environmental characteristics were assigned to each neighborhood and were part of the Community Vitality Index (CVI). The census-tract level CVI was developed by and obtained from the Metro Chicago Information Center (MCIC), an official Census Information Center. The MCIC CVI provides a composite score with 3 components: Social Capital (33.3%), Economic Potential (33.3%) and Community Amenities (33.3%). Each of these components consists of four subindices [table 25A.1]. Subindex scores range from 1 (lowest observed value) to 100 (highest observed value). The values are averaged and then ranked together to produce the overall CVI and CVI component scores for each census tract.

The MCIC CVI generates a score from 1 to 100 for every census tract in the 6-county Chicago metropolitan region. The score is a way to grade each census tract in relation to the region as a whole. For example, if a tract has a CVI score of 87, it means that 87% of the tracts in the region have lower CVI scores. Indicators in this index model were determined through a review of the literature and current practices, small area data availability, and stakeholder input. All data indicators are normalized to account for population density differences. A neighborhood's community indices are the averages of its corresponding census-tract level indices.

Statistical Analysis

Neighborhoods were assigned to a quartile group according to childhood asthma prevalence. The multiple t-test was performed to evaluate the CVI across each quartile group. This method allowed us to test the null hypothesis of no difference in the mean among 3 or more groups simultaneously and produces an accurate assessment of the effects of community factors on asthma prevalence.[20,21] Proc Multtest (Bonferroni option) in SAS was used for this analysis (SAS Institute, Inc., Cary, NC).

In order to accommodate the significant effects of neighborhood racial/ethnic composition on asthma prevalence, we grouped neighborhoods with greater than two-thirds of a specific race: white, black, and Hispanic. We then applied multiple group analysis to evaluate further the effects of community factors on asthma prevalence specific to neighborhoods categorized by race. Mplus3.0 was used to implement the multiple group analysis (Muthén and Muthén, Los Angeles, Calif.).

Multilevel logistic regression analysis was performed for 45,309 individuals nested within 287 neighborhoods to estimate the effect of the 12 CVI subindices on childhood asthma neighborhood variance. A similar analysis was conducted looking at individual and neighborhood factors alongside CVI to assess the impact of each subindex and subindex item on childhood asthma neighborhood variance. SAS GLIMMIX was used for multilevel analysis (SAS Institute, Inc). [. . .]

[. . .]

Results

Study Population

A total of 48,917 children were screened, and 45,177 (92%) were successfully geocoded and resided in one of the 287 Chicago neighborhoods. Among these children, 11% were age 3 to 5 years, 34% were age 6 to 8 years, 33% were age 9 to 11 years, and 22% were 12 years and older. Forty-nine percent were boys, and 29% self-identified as white, 29% as black, and 43% as Hispanic. The asthma prevalence of the overall study population was 13%. White and Hispanic children had a mean asthma prevalence of 10% and 11%, respectively, whereas black children had a mean asthma prevalence of 20% ($P < .0001$). Nine percent of children in the sample had a household member with asthma (table 25.1).

Positive Community Factors and Asthma Prevalence

To assess the effect of positive community factors on asthma prevalence, we categorized the 287 neighborhoods into quartile groups (figure 25.1). Each neighborhood quartile group was characterized by its mean asthma prevalence: 8% in group 1, 12% in group 2, 17% in group 3,

TABLE 25.1 **Demographic characteristics of sample population (n = 45,177)**

Subpopulation	Frequency (n)	Sample prevalence (%)	Cases of asthma in subpopulation (n)	Asthma prevalence in subpopulation (%)
Reported asthma diagnosis				
Yes	5,874	13		
No	39,303	87		
Race/ethnicity				
White	12,915	29	1,227	10
Black	12,998	29	2,534	20
Hispanic	19,264	43	2,113	11
Sex				
Male	22,230	49	3,356	15
Female	22,947	51	2,518	11
Household member with asthma				
Yes	4,114	9	1,493	36
No	41,063	91	4,381	11
Age group (yr.)				
3–5	5,073	11	599	12
6–8	15,273	34	1,907	13
9–11	14,910	33	2,010	14
12 and older	9,921	22	1,358	14

and 25% in group 4. As seen in table 25.2, the mean CVI score differed significantly across each neighborhood quartile group; as asthma prevalence decreased, the mean CVI percentile scores improved significantly ($P < .001$).

There were notable differences seen in the scores for each CVI component and the corresponding subindices. The overall social capital of a neighborhood did not reach statistical significance because the subindices measuring social capital were significant in opposite directions. Neighborhoods with more civic engagement ($P < .0001$) and community diversity ($P < .0001$) had lower childhood asthma rates. In contrast, neighborhoods with more interaction potential ($P < .0001$) and stability ($P < .05$) had higher asthma prevalence (table 25.2).

Neighborhoods with evidence of economic vigor had lower asthma prevalence rates ($P < .0001$), ranging from 64% in the low prevalence neighborhoods to 38% in the high prevalence neighborhoods. Lower asthma rates were also seen in neighborhoods with greater commercial vitality ($P < .0001$), buying power ($P < .0001$), and workforce poten-

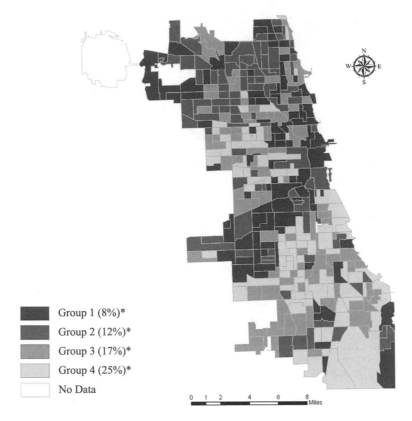

FIGURE 25.1. Asthma prevalence in Chicago arranged in quartile groups by neighborhood asthma prevalence

*Mean asthma prevalence

tial ($P < .0001$). Asthma prevalence was not associated with evidence of confidence and investment in a community (table 25.2).

Neighborhoods with more community amenities also had lower childhood asthma prevalence ($P < .05$). Lower asthma rates were particularly common in neighborhoods with many cultural/entertainment facilities and restaurants ($P < .0001$). However, there were more community institutions (e.g., libraries, universities, and so forth) in neighborhoods with high asthma prevalence ($P < .05$). Health and human service facilities seemed to be distributed equally among all neighborhoods and were not significantly associated with asthma prevalence (table 25.2).

TABLE 25.2 **Asthma prevalence, race/ethnicity distribution, and mean CVI scores arranged in quartile groups by neighborhood asthma prevalence (percentage by neighborhood quartile group)**

Variable	Group 1 ($n = 72$)	Group 2 ($n = 72$)	Group 3 ($n = 72$)	Group 4 ($n = 71$)
Mean asthma prevalence				
Total	8	12	17	25
Race/ethnicity				
White***	59	52	30	15
Black***	14	30	58	75
Hispanic***	32	33	14	12
CVI				
Total	54	55	50	44
Social capital component				
Total	44	53	51	49
Interaction potential***	36	42	59	73
Stability**	40	42	54	53
Community diversity***	52	63	42	31
Civic engagement***	62	61	52	43
Economic potential component				
Total***	64	61	51	38
Commercial vitality***	67	65	54	46
Buying power***	64	63	50	42
Confidence and investment	44	50	52	50
Workforce potential***	60	52	48	33
Community amenities component				
Total**	53	50	48	44
Arts, culture, and leisure***	47	43	34	26
Restaurants***	60	57	47	41
Health and human services	59	56	61	63
Community institutions**	45	45	54	54

**$p < .05$; ***$p < .001$

The Relationship of Race and CVI with Neighborhood Asthma Prevalence

As the black population increased in a community, so did the childhood asthma prevalence ($P < .0001$). To investigate whether CVI indicators were still predictive of asthma prevalence when race/ethnicity was controlled, neighborhoods with ≥ 67% of their population classified as white or black were analyzed individually. Because only 32 neighborhoods had a greater than two-thirds Hispanic population, analyses were not done on this group.

The predominant population in 108 Chicago neighborhoods was black. As asthma prevalence increased in these primarily black neighborhoods, the overall CVI score significantly decreased ($P < .05$). None of the 3 CVI component scores reached statistical significance. However, commercial vitality, an indicator of economic potential, was statistically significant ($P < .05$), with higher commercial vitality predictive of lower asthma prevalence.

The predominant population in 72 Chicago neighborhoods was white. In these neighborhoods, neither the total CVI score nor any of the component scores were significantly related to asthma prevalence. However, community diversity, an indicator of social capital, was nearly significant ($P < .1$), with greater diversity corresponding to higher asthma rates. Economic potential was nearly significant ($P < .1$), with more potential for community development associated with lower asthma prevalence.

Positive Community Factors and Neighborhood Asthma Variance

Eleven of the 12 CVI subindices, with the exception of the degree of confidence and investment in a community, were significantly associated with the neighborhood asthma variation (table 25.3). That being said, each subindex had a small individual impact on the variation seen. Together, indicators of social capital explained 43% of the neighborhood variation seen (from values for neighborhood variance: [Model I – Model VI]/Model I, table 25.3). Indicators of economic potential explained 29% of the variation, whereas indicators of community amenities explained 50%.

In table 25.4, individual characteristics as well as community race and socioeconomic status were added into the models. A child's age, sex, household asthma history, and community racial composition were all significant factors associated with the variation in neighborhood asthma prevalence. A community's socioeconomic status, however, was not significantly associated when modeled with CVI/CVI components and individual characteristics of the child. The CVI continued to contribute significantly when community race was added to the model. The social capital component played a significant role in explaining a degree of the variation seen in asthma prevalence by neighborhood in spite of the inclusion of a community's racial/ethnic composition. Absent race, overall CVI accounted for 50% of the variation in neighborhood asthma; with the inclusion of race, CVI continued to explain 21% of the variance (from values for neighborhood variance: [Model III – Model IV]/ Model I, table 25.4).

TABLE 25.3 **Significance of CVI components on neighborhood asthma prevalence**

Subindex	Model I (null model)	Model II OR (CI)	Model III OR (CI)	Model IV OR (CI)	Model V OR (CI)	Model VI OR (CI)
Analysis of social capital component						
Interaction potential		1.30*** (1.23–1.36)				1.22*** (1.13–1.33)
Stability			1.12*** (1.06–1.18)			1.00 (0.94–1.06)
Community diversity				0.81*** (0.77–0.86)		0.93** (0.86–0.99)
Civic engagement					0.86*** (0.82–0.91)	0.99 (0.93–1.05)
Neighborhood variance (SE)	0.14 (0.02)	0.09 (0.01)	0.13 (0.02)	0.1 (0.01)	0.12 (0.02)	0.08 (0.01)
Median OR (CI)	1.42 (1.35–1.49)	1.32 (1.26–1.38)	1.41 (1.34–1.47)	1.34 (1.28–1.4)	1.38 (1.32–1.44)	1.31 (1.25–1.37)
Analysis of economic potential component						
Commercial vitality		0.83*** (0.78–0.88)				0.89** (0.83–0.96)
Buying power			0.82*** (0.77–0.86)			0.83*** (0.77–0.91)
Confidence and investment				1.03 (0.98–1.09)		1.03 (0.97–1.09)
Workforce potential					0.84*** (0.79–0.88)	1.03 (0.94–1.13)
Neighborhood variance (SE)	0.14 (0.02)	0.12 (0.02)	0.11 (0.02)	0.14 (0.02)	0.12 (0.02)	0.1 (0.02)
Median OR (CI)	1.42 (1.35–1.49)	1.39 (1.32–1.45)	1.36 (1.3–1.42)	1.43 (1.35–1.49)	1.39 (1.32–1.45)	1.35 (1.29–1.41)
Analysis of community amenities component						
Arts, culture, and leisure		0.86*** (0.81–0.91)				0.84*** (0.77–0.93)
Restaurants			0.85*** (0.8–0.9)			0.87** (0.79–0.95)
Health and human services				1.09** (1.03–1.15)		1.13** (1.05–1.21)
Community institutions					1.11*** (1.05–1.18)	1.17*** (1.09–1.26)
Neighborhood variance (SE)	0.14 (0.02)	0.12 (0.02)	0.12 (0.02)	0.13 (0.02)	0.13 (0.02)	0.07 (0.01)
Median OR (CI)	1.42 (1.35–1.49)	1.40 (1.33–1.46)	1.39 (1.32–1.45)	1.40 (1.33–1.47)	1.40 (1.33–1.47)	1.28 (1.22–1.34)

Note: OR = odds ratio. For each CVI component, models II through V incorporate a single subindex for the stated component and show the effect of that subindex on the likelihood of having asthma; model VI incorporates all subindices for the stated component and shows the collective effect of subindices on the likelihood of having asthma.

**p < .05; ***p < .001

TABLE 25.4 **Significance of community and individual characteristics on neighborhood asthma prevalence**

Variable	Model I (null model)	Model II OR (CI)	Model III OR (CI)	Model IV OR (CI)	Model V OR (CI)	Model VI OR (CI)
Individual characteristics						
Age 6–8 vs. age 3–5		1.05 (0.95–1.16)	1.05 (0.95–1.16)	1.05 (0.95–1.16)	1.05 (0.95–1.16)	1.05 (0.95–1.16)
Age 9–11 vs. age 3–5		1.11** (1.00–1.23)	1.11** (1.00–1.22)	1.11** (1.00–1.22)	1.11** (1.00–1.23)	1.11** (1.00–1.23)
Age 12+ vs. age 3–5		1.13** (1.02–1.26)	1.13** (1.01–1.25)	1.12** (1.01–1.25)	1.13** (1.01–1.25)	1.13** (1.01–1.25)
Male vs. female		1.48*** (1.40–1.57)	1.48*** (1.40–1.57)	1.49*** (1.40–1.57)	1.49*** (1.40–1.57)	1.49*** (1.40–1.57)
Household member with asthma vs. without		4.44*** (4.15–4.78)	4.47*** (4.15–4.81)	4.46*** (4.15–4.78)	4.46*** (4.15–4.81)	4.44*** (4.13–4.78)
Community race						
Black vs. white[a]		1.74*** (1.54–1.97)		1.74*** (1.45–2.08)		1.73*** (1.43–2.09)
Hispanic vs. white[b]		1.06 (0.91–1.23)		1.10 (0.91–1.33)		1.11 (0.92–1.35)
Mixed vs. white[c]		1.10* (0.98–1.24)		1.20* (1.03–1.39)		1.25** (1.08–1.46)
Community socioeconomic status						
Low vs. high[d]			1.11 (0.95–1.31)	0.90 (0.76–1.06)	1.06 (0.90–1.25)	0.88 (0.74–1.04)
Moderate vs. high[e]			0.97 (0.87–1.08)	0.89 (0.79–1.00)	0.98 (0.89–1.09)	0.89 (0.79–1.00)
CVI						
Total			0.84*** (0.79–0.90)	0.93** (0.87–0.99)		
Social capital component					0.84*** (0.77–0.91)	0.88** (0.81–0.96)
Economic potential component					1.00 (0.92–1.10)	1.06 (0.98–1.16)
Community amenities component					0.98 (0.93–1.03)	0.96 (0.91–1.01)
Neighborhood variance (SE)	0.14 (0.02)	0.04 (0.01)	0.07 (0.01)	0.04 (0.01)	0.06 (0.01)	0.04 (0.01)
Median OR (CI)	1.42 (1.35–1.49)	1.10 (1.16–1.27)	1.10 (1.23–1.35)	1.10 (1.16–1.27)	1.10 (1.21–1.33)	1.10 (1.16–1.26)

Note: OR = odds ratio. Models II–VI incorporate a collection of variables and show the collective effect of the variables on the likelihood of having asthma.

[a] Where ≥ 2/3 population black vs. ≥ 2/3 population white.

[b] Where ≥ 2/3 population Hispanic vs. ≥ 2/3 population white.

[c] Where < 2/3 population black/Hispanic/white vs. ≥ 2/3 population white.

[d] Where average family income ≤ \$30,638.40 vs. average family income > \$51,632.25.

[e] Where average family income > \$30,638.40 and ≤ \$51,632.25 vs. average family income > \$51,632.25.

$*p < .1; **p < .05; ***p < .001$

Discussion

To our knowledge, this study is the first to show the influence of positive community factors on childhood asthma prevalence. The overall CVI was significantly associated with asthma prevalence, with higher CVI scores in neighborhoods with low asthma rates. Specifically, communities with low childhood asthma rates had greater potential for economic development and, from a social perspective, were more diverse and civically engaged. They also had more restaurants and cultural/entertainment facilities. Neighborhoods with high childhood asthma had more community institutions, such as libraries and universities, and more potential for community interaction; these communities also tended to be more stable. Health and human service agencies, including medical care facilities, were not significantly associated with asthma prevalence. After controlling for individual and community confounders, including race/ethnicity, a community's social capital continued to contribute significantly to neighborhood asthma variation. The overall CVI remained significant but contributed less to neighborhood asthma variation after the addition of community race. Accordingly, race may serve as a proxy for many socio-cultural and environmental risk factors for asthma in our study.

Under the social capital component, neighborhoods with more civic engagement (higher percentage of registered voters) and increased diversity (ethnicity, income, and age) were associated with low asthma prevalence. Interestingly, neighborhoods with high asthma had double the potential for community interaction. However, previous studies have shown that psychosocial factors, including lack of social support networks, led to increased asthma hospitalizations.[22,23] This apparent conflict may be explained by the measure with which interaction was evaluated. In this study, interaction was measured by the percentage of households not linguistically isolated or composed of a single person living alone and having at least 1 household member not in the labor force. Although one can understand how these factors may lead to increased interaction, they may also signify crowding and poverty, which has been associated with increased indoor pollutants and asthma rates.[24,25] Future researchers may wish to question participants about personal social support and interaction networks to measure this variable accurately.

Neighborhoods with high asthma rates were also more stable, indicating that residents in the community were less likely to move. Previous studies have linked more residential stability both with higher and lower asthma rates based on cockroach allergen levels in the home. In the former study, higher asthma rates in more stable communities were attributed to less thorough and frequent maintenance cleaning in homes occupied for a longer period.[26,27] In the latter study, lower asthma rates in more stable communities were suggested to indicate a better built environment in these homes.[27]

If the measures used herein truly capture social support and stability, our findings are encouraging for the development of effective asthma interventions in communities with high asthma rates. Successful interventions are known to require an interactive and stable community in which individuals can develop shared commitments to desired outcomes.[28]

Poverty has been shown to be associated with asthma prevalence, hospitalizations, and mortality in multiple studies.[25,29,30] Likewise, we found a neighborhood's economic potential to be strongly associated with asthma prevalence. Specifically, the greater the number of businesses, number of business loans, aggregate income, degree of educational attainment, number of wage earners, and employment rate were all associated with lower asthma rates. In predominantly black neighborhoods, although the overall potential for economic growth was not associated with asthma prevalence, there *were* significantly more businesses in neighborhoods with lower asthma rates.

Surprisingly, the number of mortgages, home improvement loans, and occupied dwelling units—all representative of the degree of confidence and investment in a community—was not significantly different among neighborhoods. This may be because areas with higher asthma prevalence may also have a higher density of people, resulting in an illusory inflation in the number of mortgages and home improvement loans. Another possible explanation may be the unusually high real estate activity in Chicago in early 2000; many buildings in low income neighborhoods were sold and rehabbed for section 8 rentals, which may have disproportionately increased the number of occupied properties in neighborhoods with high asthma prevalence.

The association of community amenities and asthma rates may be explained by basic supply and demand analysis. Neighborhoods with low asthma rates had more restaurants and cultural/entertainment facilities because they had higher aggregate community income and, accordingly, were able to invest more in these facilities. Neighborhoods with high asthma had more libraries, houses of worship, and institutions of higher education. This too is understandable, because these facilities are typically not-for-profit and are often managed by the local government and religious organizations. Interestingly, the number of health and human services agencies was not related to asthma prevalence. However, previous studies have shown that poor children are less likely to use appropriate health services.[31-33] Although it seems health centers exist equally in neighborhoods regardless of asthma prevalence, a child in a community with high asthma rates may have difficulty accessing services because of insurance, knowledge, and other individual factors.

[...]

Prior studies clearly identify the causes of pediatric asthma to be multifactorial. Negative community factors that have been associated with asthma prevalence include exposure to air pollution; housing problems including sensitization to cockroach, dust mite, mouse, and rat allergens; decreased exposure to endotoxins (the hygiene hypothesis); community income and education; and exposure to violence. Individual factors known to be associated with asthma include age, sex, race, family history, smoking, diet, and stress.[4,15,25,29,34-57] Because asthma is such a complex disease, several of these factors may be related to the positive factors discussed. For example, in neighborhoods with more economic potential, there may be less indoor and outdoor pollutants and less indoor allergen exposure due to a better built environment.

Regardless, with childhood asthma prevalence at a historic high and disparities increasing among low-income and minority populations, further insight is clearly needed to combat this growing problem. Positive community factors have rarely been examined as potential protective factors in childhood asthma even though asthma prevalence has been shown to vary widely by neighborhood.[9,58] Our results suggest that positive community factors are associated with childhood asthma prevalence, and further investigation is warranted. A deeper understanding of positive community factors and the interplay of these factors with individual and negative community factors is an essential step to determining the true causes of neighborhood variation in childhood asthma rates.

Social capital component (33%)

Descriptor of connections between people that allow communities to work together

Subindex	Variable	Definition
Interaction potential (25%)	Neighborhood interaction[1]	% households not linguistically isolated
	Social support[1]	% households not composed of a single person living alone
	Availability[1]	% households with at least 1 adult not in the labor force
Stability (25%)	Mobility[1]	% households that resided in same home 5 yr. earlier
	Immigration[1]	Inversely ranked % foreign-born residents who entered given tract within 5 yr.
Community diversity (25%)	Ethnic diversity[1]	Inversely ranked % tract population of largest single racial/ethnic group
	Age distribution[1]	Inversely ranked % tract population in any single age group (0–24, 25–44, 45+)
	Income mix[1]	% households in any single income group ($0–34,999, $35,000–74,999, $75,000+)
Civic engagement (25%)	Voting rate[2]	% registered voters who voted in Nov. 2002 election

Economic potential component (33%)

Descriptor of features considered important in community development and assets with potential leverage for community change

Subindex	Variable	Definition
Commercial vitality (25%)	Business density[3]	# businesses per square mile
	Small business loans[4]	Aggregate amount of small business loans (< 1 million)
Buying power (25%)	Aggregate income[1]	Total income for all people in given census tract
	Shelter cost burden[1]	Inversely ranked % households spending ≥ 30% monthly income on housing
Neighborhood confidence and investment (25%)	Home investment[5]	# mortgages originated per dwelling unit
	Home improvement[5]	# home improvement loans originated per occupied dwelling unit
	Owner occupancy[1]	% occupied dwelling units
Workforce potential (25%)	Educational attainment[1]	% population > 25 yrs old with at least some college education
	Wage earners[1]	# wage earners age 16–64 per square mile
	Employment rate[1]	% labor force employed

TABLE 25A.1 *(continued)*

Community amenities component (33%)

Descriptor of the impact of cultural and social amenities on the growth of social capital and community development

Subindex	Definition
Arts, culture, and leisure (25%)[6,7]	# of 3-mile buffers around each artistic, cultural, and entertainment facility that include the center of each tract divided by the population density
Restaurants (25%)[6]	# of 1-mile buffers around each restaurant that include the center of each tract divided by the population density
Health and human services (25%)[8]	# of 3-mile buffers around each agency that include the center of each tract divided by the population density
Community institutions (25%)[9]	# of 2-mile buffers around each institution that include the center of each tract divided by the population density

Data sources: [1]2000 U.S. Census. [2]County Board of Elections, Chicago Board of Elections by precinct. [3]2002 commercial listing of all businesses with telephones. [4]1999 Community Reinvestment Act data. [5]1999 Home Mortgage Disclosure Act. [6]Commercial database of businesses with telephones. [7]Database of nonprofit arts/culture organizations. [8]2001 United Way Blue Book. [9]InfoUSA commercial business database.

References

1. Akinbami LJ, Schoendorf KC. Trends in childhood asthma: Prevalence, health care utilization, and mortality. *Pediatrics*. 2002;110(2 pt. 1):315–322.

2. Akinbami L, Centers for Disease Control Prevention National Center for Health Statistics. The state of childhood asthma, United States, 1980–2005. *Advance Data*. 2006;12(381):1–24.

3. Byrd RS, Joad JP. Urban asthma. *Current Opinion in Pulmonary Medicine*. 2006;12(1):68–74.

4. Migliaretti G, Cavallo F. Urban air pollution and asthma in children. *Pediatric Pulmonology*. 2004;38(3):198–203.

5. Grant EN, Malone A, Lyttle CS, Weiss KB. Asthma morbidity and treatment in the Chicago metropolitan area: One decade after national guidelines. *Annals of Allergy, Asthma and Immunology*. 2005;95(1):19–25.

6. Mannino DM, Homa DM, Akinbami LJ, Moorman JE, Gwynn C, Redd SC. Surveillance for asthma—United States, 1980–1999. *MMWR Surveillance Summaries*. 2002;51(1):1–13.

7. Weiss KB, Wagener DK. Changing patterns of asthma mortality—

identifying target populations at high-risk. *Journal of the American Medical Association.* 1990;264(13):1683–1687.

8. Thomas SD, Whitman S. Asthma hospitalizations and mortality in Chicago: An epidemiologic overview. *Chest.* 1999;116(4 suppl. 1):S135–S141.

9. Gupta RS, Zhang X, Sharp LK, Shannon JJ, Weiss KB. Geographic variability in childhood asthma prevalence in Chicago. *Journal of Allergy and Clinical Immunology.* 2008;121(3):639–645 e631.

10. Marder D, Targonski P, Orris P, Persky V, Addington W. Effect of racial and socioeconomic factors on asthma mortality in Chicago. *Chest.* 1992;101(6 suppl.):S426–S429.

11. Crain EF, Walter M, O'Connor GT, et al. Home and allergic characteristics of children with asthma in seven U.S. urban communities and design of an environmental intervention: The Inner-City Asthma Study. *Environmental Health Perspectives.* 2002;110(9):939–945.

12. Schwartz J. Air pollution and children's health. *Pediatrics.* 2004;113 (4 suppl.):1037–1043.

13. Gauderman WJ, Avol E, Lurmann F, et al. Childhood asthma and exposure to traffic and nitrogen dioxide. *Epidemiology.* 2005;16(6):737–743.

14. Swahn MH, Bossarte RM. The associations between victimization, feeling unsafe, and asthma episodes among US high-school students. *American Journal of Public Health.* 2006;96(5):802–804.

15. Wright RJ, Mitchell H, Visness CM, et al. Community violence and asthma morbidity: The Inner-City Asthma Study. *American Journal of Public Health.* 2004;94(4):625–632.

16. Cagney KA, Browning CR. Exploring neighborhood-level variation in asthma and other respiratory diseases: The contribution of neighborhood social context. *Journal of General Internal Medicine.* 2004;19(3):229–236.

17. Shalowitz MU, Sadowski LM, Kumar R, Weiss KB, Shannon JJ. Asthma burden in a citywide, diverse sample of elementary schoolchildren in Chicago. *Ambulatory Pediatrics.* 2007;7(4):271–277.

18. Wolf RL, Berry CA, Quinn K. Development and validation of a brief pediatric screen for asthma and allergies among children. *Annals of Allergy, Asthma and Immunology.* 2003;90(5):500–507.

19. Berry CA, Quinn K, Wolf R, Mosnaim G, Shalowitz M. Validation of the Spanish and English versions of the asthma portion of the Brief Pediatric Asthma Screen Plus among Hispanics. *Annals of Allergy, Asthma and Immunology.* 2005;95(1):53–60.

20. Ottenbacher KJ. Quantitative evaluation of multiplicity in epidemiology and public health research. *American Journal of Epidemiology.* 1998;147(7): 615–619.

21. Farcomeni A. A review of modern multiple hypothesis testing, with par-

ticular attention to the false discovery proportion. *Statistical Methods in Medical Research.* 2008;17(4):347–388.

22. Wainwright NW, Surtees PG, Wareham NJ, Harrison BD. Psychosocial factors and incident asthma hospital admissions in the EPIC-Norfolk cohort study. *Allergy.* 2007;62(5):554–560.

23. Weil CM, Wade SL, Bauman LJ, Lynn H, Mitchell H, Lavigne J. The relationship between psychosocial factors and asthma morbidity in inner-city children with asthma. *Pediatrics.* 1999;104(6):1274–1280.

24. Baxter LK, Clougherty JE, Laden F, Levy JI. Predictors of concentrations of nitrogen dioxide, fine particulate matter, and particle constituents inside of lower socioeconomic status urban homes. *Journal of Exposure Science and Environmental Epidemiology.* 2007;17(5):433–444.

25. Almqvist C, Pershagen G, Wickman M. Low socioeconomic status as a risk factor for asthma, rhinitis and sensitization at 4 years in a birth cohort. *Clinical and Experimental Allergy.* 2005;35(5):612–618.

26. Peters JL, Levy JI, Rogers CA, Burge HA, Spengler JD. Determinants of allergen concentrations in apartments of asthmatic children living in public housing. *Journal of Urban Health.* 2007;84(2):185–197.

27. Rauh VA, Chew GR, Garfinkel RS. Deteriorated housing contributes to high cockroach allergen levels in inner-city households. *Environmental Health Perspectives.* 2002;110(suppl. 2):323–327.

28. Peterson JW, Lachance LL, Butterfoss FD, et al. Engaging the community in coalition efforts to address childhood asthma. *Health Promotion Practice.* 2006;7(2 suppl.):S56–S65.

29. Miller JE. The effects of race/ethnicity and income on early childhood asthma prevalence and health care use. *American Journal of Public Health.* 2000;90(3):428–430.

30. Grant EN, Lyttle CS, Weiss KB. The relation of socioeconomic factors and racial/ethnic differences in US asthma mortality. *American Journal of Public Health.* 2000;90(12):1923–1925.

31. Halfon N, Newacheck PW. Childhood asthma and poverty: Differential impacts and utilization of health services. *Pediatrics.* 1993;91(1):56–61.

32. Davidson AE, Klein DE, Settipane GA, Alario AJ. Access to care among children visiting the emergency room with acute exacerbations of asthma. *Annals of Allergy, Asthma and Immunology.* 1994;72(5):469–473.

33. Crain EF, Kercsmar C, Weiss KB, Mitchell H, Lynn H. Reported difficulties in access to quality care for children with asthma in the inner city. *Archives of Pediatrics and Adolescent Medicine.* 1998;152(4):333–339.

34. Tatum AJ, Shapiro GG. The effects of outdoor air pollution and tobacco smoke on asthma. *Immunology and Allergy Clinics of North America.* 2005;25(1):15–30.

35. Gauderman WJ, Avol E, Gilliland F, et al. The effect of air pollution on lung development from 10 to 18 years of age. *New England Journal of Medicine.* 2004;351(11):1057–1067.

36. Gruchalla RS, Pongracic J, Plaut M, et al. Inner City Asthma Study: Relationships among sensitivity, allergen exposure, and asthma morbidity. *Journal of Allergy and Clinical Immunology.* 2005;115(3):478–485.

37. Litonjua AA, Carey VJ, Burge HA, Weiss ST, Gold DR. Exposure to cockroach allergen in the home is associated with incident doctor-diagnosed asthma and recurrent wheezing. *Journal of Allergy and Clinical Immunology.* 2001;107(1):41–47.

38. Morgan WJ, Crain EF, Gruchalla RS, et al. Results of a home-based environmental intervention among urban children with asthma. *New England Journal of Medicine.* 2004;351(11):1068–1080.

39. Lau S, Illi S, Sommerfeld C, et al. Early exposure to house-dust mite and cat allergens and development of childhood asthma: A cohort study: Multicentre Allergy Study Group. *Lancet.* 2000;356(9239):1392–1397.

40. Eder W, Ege MJ, von Mutius E. The asthma epidemic. *New England Journal of Medicine.* 2006;355(21):2226–2235.

41. Matsui EC, Krop EJ, Diette GB, Aalberse RC, Smith AL, Eggleston PA. Mouse allergen exposure and immunologic responses: IgE-mediated mouse sensitization and mouse specific IgG and IgG4 levels. *Annals of Allergy, Asthma and Immunology.* 2004;93(2):171–178.

42. Perry T, Matsui E, Merriman B, Duong T, Eggleston P. The prevalence of rat allergen in inner-city homes and its relationship to sensitization and asthma morbidity. *Journal of Allergy and Clinical Immunology.* 2003;112(2):346–352.

43. Braun-Fahrlander C, Riedler J, Herz U, et al. Environmental exposure to endotoxin and its relation to asthma in school-age children. *New England Journal of Medicine.* 2002;347(12):869–877.

44. Weiss ST. Eat dirt—the hygiene hypothesis and allergic diseases. *New England Journal of Medicine.* 2002;347(12):930–931.

45. Strachan DP. Family size, infection and atopy: The first decade of the "hygiene hypothesis." *Thorax.* 2000;55(suppl. 1):S2–S10.

46. Cesaroni G, Farchi S, Davoli M, Forastiere F, Perucci CA. Individual and area-based indicators of socioeconomic status and childhood asthma. *European Respiratory Journal.* 2003;22(4):619–624.

47. Wright RJ, Steinbach SF. Violence: An unrecognized environmental exposure that may contribute to greater asthma morbidity in high risk inner-city populations. *Environmental Health Perspectives.* 2001;109(10):1085–1089.

48. Debley JS, Redding GJ, Critchlow CW. Impact of adolescence and gender on asthma hospitalization: A population-based birth cohort study. *Pediatric Pulmonology.* 2004;38(6):443–450.

49. Fagan JK, Scheff PA, Hryhorczuk D, Ramakrishnan V, Ross M, Persky V. Prevalence of asthma and other allergic diseases in an adolescent population: Association with gender and race. *Annals of Allergy, Asthma and Immunology.* 2001;86(2):177–184.

50. Slezak JA, Persky VW, Kviz FJ, Ramakrishnan V, Byers C. Asthma prevalence and risk factors in selected Head Start sites in Chicago. *Journal of Asthma.* 1998;35(2):203–212.

51. Bener A, Janahi IA, Sabbah A. Genetics and environmental risk factors associated with asthma in schoolchildren. *European Annals of Allergy and Clinical Immunology.* 2005;37(5):163–168.

52. Gilmour MI, Jaakkola MS, London SJ, Nel AE, Rogers CA. How exposure to environmental tobacco smoke, outdoor air pollutants, and increased pollen burdens influences the incidence of asthma. *Environmental Health Perspectives.* 2006;114(4):627–633.

53. Cook DG, Strachan DP. Health effects of passive smoking: 3. Parental smoking and prevalence of respiratory symptoms and asthma in school age children. *Thorax.* 1997;52(12):1081–1094.

54. Black PN, Sharpe S. Dietary fat and asthma: Is there a connection? *European Respiratory Journal.* 1997;10(1):6–12.

55. Mihrshahi S, Peat JK, Marks GB, et al. Eighteen-month outcomes of house dust mite avoidance and dietary fatty acid modification in the Childhood Asthma Prevention Study (CAPS). *Journal of Allergy and Clinical Immunology.* 2003;111(1):162–168.

56. Wright RJ, Cohen S, Carey V, Weiss ST, Gold DR. Parental stress as a predictor of wheezing in infancy: A prospective birth-cohort study. *American Journal of Respiratory and Critical Care Medicine.* 2002;165(3):358–365.

57. Wright RJ, Rodriguez M, Cohen S. Review of psychosocial stress and asthma: An integrated biopsychosocial approach. *Thorax.* 1998;53(12):1066–1074.

58. Gupta RS, Carrion-Carire V, Weiss KB. The widening black/white gap in asthma hospitalizations and mortality. *Journal of Allergy and Clinical Immunology.* 2006;117(2):351–358.

PART V

Taking Action

It can never be enough simply to write about health inequities without identifying ways to reduce or eliminate them. In this part are articles from Chicago that address the idea of taking action against health inequities. If structural violence is a cause of health inequities, then the solutions must necessarily address the structural causes as well. In this *Reader*, there are many more articles that point out the problems with health inequity than ones that point to solutions. Sadly, in our review of over one thousand articles on health inequity in Chicago since the early twentieth century, there were few that delivered solutions to addressing these disparities. Yet there are inspiring accounts of collective action and social change (see figure 6).

The photograph shows protestors calling for the opening of an adult trauma center on the city's South Side. This protest was directly connected to the empirical work published by Marie Crandall et al., seen earlier in this book, which showed that suffering from a gunshot wound more than five miles from a trauma center was associated with an increase in the mortality rate. But, above all, it was an action taken in response to the death of eighteen-year-old Damian Turner, as chronicled in this part in an article by Claire Bushey and Kristen Schorsch (originally published in a business magazine, *not* an academic journal).

The selections describe important examples of the type of actions that can be taken to improve community health. John McKnight outlines what one Chicago community did when they were given data from their local hospitals and acted on it. His article attempts to address the question, "What is the relationship between a community's political and economic self-determination and its health status?" He strives to free people from "medical clienthood" and move them to political action that

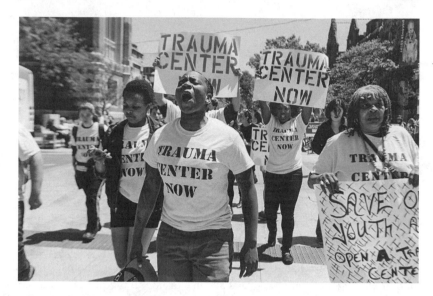

FIGURE 6. Protest for a South Side trauma center, June 2015
Source: http://loveandstrugglephotos.com.

improves health. He observed that a close inspection of hospitalization data suggests that "modern medical systems are usually dealing with maladies—social problems—rather than disease." For McKnight and his community partners, this powerful realization activated citizens and community organizations for social change.

Also in this part is a document detailing the groundbreaking work of CeaseFire—an innovative violence reduction program that has now been replicated in other cities in the United States. Nancy Ritter's account of CeaseFire's prevention, intervention and community-mobilization strategies offers important lessons in taking action against one of the most visible manifestations of inequity in Chicago today.

Later in this part, we present the work of David Ansell et al., who led a community effort to reduce the black/white breast cancer mortality disparity in Chicago. Ansell et al. outline the creation of a social entrepreneurial not-for-profit organization designed to tackle racial inequity in breast cancer mortality in Chicago, the Metropolitan Chicago Breast Cancer Task Force. Their position is clear: "solutions must be pursued with all available energy," and these solutions necessarily call for collaboration across institutions and sectors.

Finally, the last article in this part outlines an action plan created by the Chicago Department of Public Health in collaboration with hundreds of community partners, including academic researchers, health providers, and community members. Called Healthy Chicago 2.0, this plan for public health improvement sets almost sixty measurable health improvement goals across many health categories from access to care, community development, education, behavioral health, child and adolescent health, chronic diseases, infectious diseases, and violence as well as overarching health goals. Ambitious in scope, it includes targets for addressing the structural drivers of health inequity such as reducing hardship and perceived discrimination. It includes traditional public health targets aimed at "modifiable risk factors" like tobacco use and unhealthy diet, but it also sets specific targets for far more structural and deep-rooted drivers of health in Chicago, from strengthening social cohesion ("shared values and trust among neighbors") to reducing discrimination in the criminal justice system ("percentage of adults who report ever experiencing discrimination, been prevented from doing something or been hassled or made to feel inferior from the police or in the courts because of their race, ethnicity or color").

The goal, of course, is to overcome inequities, not just to write about them. With such deep health inequities in Chicago, why has relatively little attention been given to evaluating systematic solutions? We think the answer may lie in the structural nature of the inequities. Racism, poverty, housing and school segregation, and doctor and hospital gaps in black neighborhoods all contribute to Chicago's health inequities. Tackling these entrenched inequities requires major systematic, structural investments from national, state, and city resources into the marginalized poor and minority neighborhoods that suffer the most.

This part of the *Reader* is frustratingly brief. Clearly, much of the literature has focused on describing health inequities and testing hypotheses about associations and causal factors, and relatively less attention has been given to implementing and testing solutions, an idea that we will return to in the conclusion of the *Reader*.

CHAPTER TWENTY-SIX

Community Health in a Chicago Slum

John L. McKnight

Is it possible that out of the contradictions of medicine one can develop the possibilities of politics? The example I want to describe is not going to create a new social order. It is, however, the beginning of an effort to free people from medical clienthood, so that they can perceive the possibility of being citizens engaged in political action.

The example involves a community of about 60,000 people on the West Side of Chicago. The people are poor and black, and the majority are dependent on welfare payments. They have a community organization which is voluntary, not part of the government. The community organization encompasses an area in which there are two hospitals.

The neighborhood was originally all white. During the 1960s it went through a racial transition. Over a period of a few years, it became largely populated with black people.

The two hospitals continued (analogous to colonial situations) to serve the white people who had lived in the neighborhood before the transition. The black people, therefore, struggled to gain access to the hospitals' services.

This became a political struggle, and the community organization finally "captured" the two hospitals. The boards of directors of the hospitals then accepted people from the neighborhood, employed black peo-

Originally published in *Health/PAC Bulletin* 11, no. 6 (July–August 1980): 13–18.

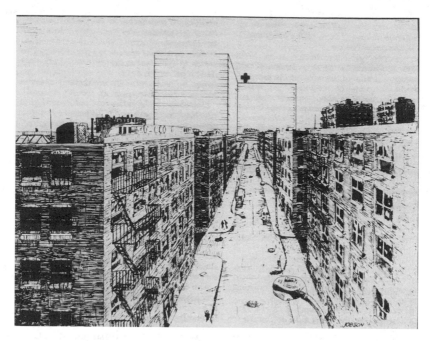

ple on their staffs and treated members of the neighborhood rather than
the previous white clients.

After several years, the community organization felt that it was time
to stand back and look at the health status of their community. As a result of their analysis, they found that, although they had "captured" the
hospitals, there was no significant evidence that the health of the people
had changed since they had gained control of the medical services.

The organization then contacted the Center for Urban Affairs, where
I work. They asked us to assist in finding out why, if the people controlled the two hospitals, their health was not any better.

The Causes of Hospitalization

It was agreed that we would do a study of the hospitals' medical records
to see why people were receiving medical care. We also took a sample of
the emergency room medical records to determine the frequency of the
various problems that brought the people into the hospitals.

We found that the seven most common reasons for hospitalizations, in order of frequency, were:

1. Automobile accidents
2. Interpersonal attacks
3. Accidents (non-auto)
4. Bronchial ailments
5. Alcoholism
6. Drug-related problems (medically administered and non-medically administered)
7. Dog bites

The people from the organization were startled by these findings. The language of medicine is focused upon disease—yet the problems we identified have very little to do with disease. The medicalization of health had led them to believe that "disease" was the problem which hospitals were addressing, but they discovered instead that the hospitals were dealing with many problems which were not "diseases." It was an important step in conscientization to recognize that modern medical systems are usually dealing with maladies—social problems—rather than disease. Maladies and social problems are the domain of citizens and their community organizations.

Community Action

Having seen the list of maladies and problems, the people from the organization considered what they ought to do, or could do, about them. I want to describe the first three things that they decided to do because each makes a different point.

First of all, as good political strategists, they decided to tackle a problem where they felt they could win. They didn't want to start out and immediately lose. So they went down the list and picked dog bites, which cause about 4% of the emergency room visits at an average hospital cost of $185.

How could this problem best be approached? It interested me to see the people in the organization thinking about that problem. The city government has employees who are paid to be "dog catchers," but the organization did not choose to contact the city. Instead, they said: "Let us see what we can do ourselves." They decided to take a small part of their money and use it for "dog bounties"! Through their block clubs they let it be known that for a period of one month, in an area of about a square mile, they would pay a bounty of five dollars for every stray dog (not house dog) that was brought in to the organization or had its location identified so that they could go capture it.

There were packs of wild dogs in the neighborhood that had frightened many people. The children of the neighborhood, on the other hand, thought that catching dogs was a wonderful idea—so they helped to identify them. In one month, 160 of these dogs were captured, and cases of dog bites in the hospitals decreased.

Two things happened as a result of this success. The people began to learn that their action, rather than the hospital, determines their health. They were also building their organization by involving the children as community activists.

The second course of action was to deal with something more difficult—automobile accidents. "How can we do anything if we don't understand where these accidents are taking place?" the people said. They asked us to try to get information which would help to deal with the accident problem, but we found it extremely difficult to find information regarding "when," "where," and "how" an accident took place.

We considered going back to the hospital and looking at the medical records to determine the nature of the accident that brought each injured person to the hospital. If medicine were a system that was related to the possibilities of community action, it should have been possible. It was not. The medical record did not say, "This person has a malady because she was hit by an automobile at six o'clock in the evening on January 3rd at the corner of Madison and Kedzie." Sometimes the record did not even say that the cause was an automobile accident. Instead, the record simply tells you that the person has a "broken tibia." It is a record system that obscures the community nature of the problem, by focusing on the therapeutic to the exclusion of the primary cause.

We began, therefore, a search of the data systems of macro-planners. Finally we found one macro-planning group that had data regarding the nature of auto accidents in the city. It was data on a complex, computerized system, to be used in macro-planning to facilitate automobile traffic! We persuaded the planners to do a "print-out" that could be used by the neighborhood people for their own action purposes. This had never occurred to them as a use for "their" information.

The print-outs were so complex, however, that the organization could not comprehend them. So we took the numbers and translated them on to a neighborhood map showing where the accidents took place. Where people were injured, we put a blue X. Where people were killed, we put a red X.

We did this for accidents for a period of three months. There are 60,000 residents living in the neighborhood. In that area, in three months, there were more than 1,000 accidents. From the map the people could see, for example, that within three months six people had been injured, and one person killed, in an area 60 feet wide. They immediately identified this place as the entrance to a parking lot for a department store. They were then ready to act rather than be treated by dealing with the storeowner because information had been "liberated" from its medical and macro-planning captivity.

The experience with the map had two consequences. First, the opportunity was offered to invent several different ways to deal with a health problem that the community could understand. The community organization could negotiate with the department store owner and force a change in its entrance.

The second consequence was that it became very clear that there were accident problems that the community organization could not handle directly. For example, one of the main reasons for many of the accidents was the fact that higher authorities had decided to make several of the streets through the neighborhood major throughways for automobiles going from the heart of the city out to the affluent suburbs. Those who made this trip were a primary cause of injury to the local people. Dealing with this problem is not within the control of people at the neighborhood level—but they understand the necessity of getting other community organizations involved in a similar process, so that together they can assemble enough power to force the authorities to change the policies that serve the interests of those who use the neighborhoods as their freeway.

The third community action activity developed when the people focused on "bronchial problems." They learned that good nutrition was a factor in these problems, and concluded that they did not have enough fresh fruit and vegetables for good nutrition. In the city, particularly in the winter, these foods were too expensive. So could they grow fresh fruit and vegetables themselves? They looked around, but it seemed difficult in the heart of the city. Then several people pointed out that most of their houses are two story apartments with flat roofs: "Supposing we could build a greenhouse on the roof, couldn't we grow our own fruit and vegetables?" So they built a greenhouse on one of the roofs as an experiment. Then, a fascinating thing began to happen.

Originally, the greenhouse was built to deal with a *health* problem— adequate nutrition. The greenhouse was a tool, appropriate to the environment, that people could make and use to improve health. Quickly, however, people began to see that the greenhouse was also an *economic development* tool. It increased their income because they now produced a commodity to use and also to sell.

Then, another use for the greenhouse appeared. In the United States, energy costs are extremely high and are a great burden for poor people. One of the main places where people lose (waste) energy is from the rooftops of their houses—so the greenhouse on top of the roof converted energy loss into an asset. The energy that did escape from the house went into the greenhouse, where heat was needed. The greenhouse, therefore, was an *energy* conservation tool.

Another use for the greenhouse developed by chance. The community organization owned a retirement home for elderly people, and one day one of the elderly people discovered the greenhouse. She went to work there and told the other old people, and they started coming to the greenhouse every day to help care for the plants. The administrator of the old people's home noticed that the attitude of the older people changed. They were excited. They had found a function. The greenhouse became a tool to *empower older people*—to allow discarded people to be productive.

The people began to see something about technology that they had not realized before. Here was a simple tool—a greenhouse. It could be built locally, used locally, and its "outputs" were, at least, *health, economic development, energy conservation and enabling older people to be productive*. A simple tool requiring minimum "inputs" produced multiple "outputs" with few negative side effects. We called the greenhouse a "multility."

Most tools in a modernized consumer-oriented society are the reverse of the greenhouse. They are systems requiring a complex organization with multiple inputs that produce only a single output. Let me give you an example. If you get bauxite from Jamaica, copper from Chile, rubber from Indonesia, oil from Saudi Arabia, lumber from Canada, and labor from all these countries, and process these resources in an American corporation that uses American labor and professional skills to manufacture a commodity, you can produce an electric toothbrush! This tool is what we call "unitility." It has multiple inputs and one output. This is a unique tool, this toothbrush. If a tool is basically a labor-saving device, this toothbrush is an anti-tool. If you added up all the labor put into producing this electric toothbrush, its sum is infinitely more than the labor saved by its use.

The electric toothbrush and the systems for its production are the essence of the technological mistake. The greenhouse is the essence of the technological possibility. The toothbrush (unitility) is a tool that disables capacity and maximizes exploitation. The greenhouse (multility) is a tool that minimizes exploitation and enables community action.

Similarly, the greenhouse is a health tool that creates citizen action and improves health. The hospitalized focus on health disables community capacity by concentrating on therapeutic tools and techniques requiring tremendous inputs, with limited outputs in terms of standard health measures.

Conclusions

Let me draw several conclusions from the health work of the community organization.

First, out of all this activity, it is most important that the health action process has strengthened a community organization. Health is a political issue. To convert a medical problem into a political issue is central to health improvement. Therefore, as our action has developed the organization's vitality and power, we have begun the critical health development. Health action must lead away from dependence on professional tools and techniques, towards community building and citizen action. Effective health action must convert a professional-technical problem into a political, communal issue.

Second, effective health action identifies what you can do at the local level with local resources. It must also identify those external authorities and structures that control the limits of the community to act in the interest of its health.

Third, health action develops tools for the people's use, under their own control. To develop these tools may require us to *diminish* the resources consumed by the medical system. As the community organization's health activity becomes more effective, the swollen balloon of medicine should shrink. For example, after the dogs were captured, the hospital lost clients. Nonetheless, we cannot expect that this action will stop the medical balloon from growing. The medical system will make new claims for resources and power, but our action *will* intensify the contradictions of medicalized definitions of health. We can now see people saying: "Look, we may have saved 185 dollars in hospital care for many of the 160 dogs that will not now bite people. That's a lot of money! But it still stays with that hospital. We want our 185 dollars! We want to begin to trade in an economy in which you don't exchange our action for more medical service. We need income, not therapy. If we are to act in our health interest, we will need the resources medicine claims for its therapeutic purposes in order to diminish our therapeutic need."

The three principles of community health action suggest that "Another Development in Health" is basically moving *away* from being "medical consumers" with the central goal being full access to medical care. Rather, the experience I have described suggests that the sickness which we face is the captivity of tools, resources, power and consciousness by medical "unitilities" that create consumers.

Health is a political question. It requires citizens and communities. The health action process can enable "another health development" by translating medically defined problems and resources into politically actionable community problems.

CHAPTER TWENTY-SEVEN

CeaseFire

A Public Health Approach to Reduce Shootings and Killings

Nancy Ritter

The bloodshed in some of the Windy City's toughest neighborhoods declined substantially with the advent of the CeaseFire violence reduction program.

A rigorous evaluation of the program, sponsored by the National Institute of Justice, confirmed anecdotal evidence that had already led officials in other cities to adopt Chicago's CeaseFire model. Researchers found that CeaseFire had a significant positive impact on many of the neighborhoods in which the program was implemented, including a decline of 16–28% in the number of shootings in four of the seven sites studied.

"Overall, the program areas grew noticeably safer in six of the seven sites, and we concluded that there was evidence that decreases in the size and intensity of shooting hot spots were linked to the introduction of CeaseFire in four of those areas. In two other areas shooting hot spots waned, but evidence that this decline could be linked to CeaseFire was inconclusive," the researchers reported.

Led by Wesley Skogan, a political science professor at Northwestern University, the evaluation team meticulously measured CeaseFire's im-

Originally published in the *National Institute of Justice Journal*, no. 264 (November 2009): 20–25.

pact on shootings and killings in Chicago.[a] The researchers spent three years evaluating the program. The findings are encouraging.

What Is CeaseFire?

CeaseFire uses prevention, intervention and community-mobilization strategies to reduce shootings and killings. The program was launched in Chicago in 1999 by the Chicago Project for Violence Prevention at the University of Illinois at Chicago School of Public Health. By 2004, 25 CeaseFire sites existed in Chicago and a few other Illinois cities. Some of the program's strategies were adapted from the public health field, which has had notable success in changing dangerous behaviors. For example, public health campaigns have helped to decrease smoking and increase childhood immunizations. In fact, the program's executive director, Gary Slutkin, is an epidemiologist who views shootings as a public health issue.

As the researchers note in their report, a significant amount of street violence is "surprisingly casual in character." Men shoot one another in disputes over women, or because they feel they have been "dissed." Simply driving through rival gang territory can be fatal. In the gang world, one shooting can lead to another, starting a cycle of violence that can send neighborhoods careening.

CeaseFire uses various tools to target this violence:

- Community mobilization.
- A major public education campaign.
- Services, such as GED programs, anger-management counseling, drug or alcohol treatment, and help finding child care or looking for a job that can improve the lives of at-risk youth, including gang members.

In their evaluation, the researchers detail the program's approaches to building collaborations in the CeaseFire sites. The successes and pitfalls were many, as could be expected in a complex program that required law enforcement agencies, businesses, service providers, schools, community groups, political leaders and one of CeaseFire's most important partners, churches, to work together.

Of all of the program's facets, the most notable involves hiring "violence interrupters." CeaseFire's violence interrupters establish a rapport with gang leaders and other at-risk youth, just as outreach workers in a public health campaign contact a target community. Working alone or in pairs, the violence interrupters cruise the streets at night, mediating conflicts between gangs. After a shooting, they immediately offer nonviolent alternatives to gang leaders and a shooting victim's friends and relatives to try to interrupt the cycle of retaliatory violence. Violence interrupters differ from community organizers or social workers. Many are former gang members who have served time in prison, which gives them greater credibility among current gang members.

CeaseFire's message travels from violence interrupters to gang members, from clergy to parishioners, and from community leaders to the neighborhood through conversations, sermons, marches and prayer vigils. The message appears on banners at postshooting rallies, which are a major part of the program. The message is simple: "The killing must stop!"

Measuring Results

The evaluation included two parts: process and outcomes.

In the process evaluation, the researchers looked at how the program worked in the field. They interviewed CeaseFire staff, police, social service workers, and business, religious and community leaders at 17 sites. The researchers also interviewed 297 gang members and street youth to get their assessment of the program.

The evaluation of outcomes was challenging because the researchers had to find comparable areas without the program to make valid comparisons to CeaseFire neighborhoods. They found seven such sites within the city of Chicago.

Statistical Analysis

Analysis based on 17 years of data showed that, as a direct result of CeaseFire, shootings decreased 16–28% in four of the seven sites studied. The researchers called this decrease in gun violence "immediate and permanent" in three of the sites and "gradual and permanent" in the fourth site.

Hot Spots Analysis

Using crime mapping techniques, the researchers compared shooting patterns before and after CeaseFire started to those in areas that had no CeaseFire program. Six of the sites grew noticeably safer overall, but the researchers could credit this to CeaseFire in only four of those areas. In two sites, shooting hot spots waned, but there was not enough evidence to link this to CeaseFire.

Gang Social Network Analysis

Gang killings declined in two CeaseFire sites. The researchers also looked at the proportion of gang homicides that were sparked by an earlier shooting. This violence was a special focus of the violence interrupters. In four sites, retaliatory killings decreased more than in the comparison areas.

Impact on Young People

The researchers also looked at CeaseFire's impact on gang members and other at-risk street youth ("clients") that the program targeted. More than 80% of CeaseFire's clients had past arrests, 56% had spent more than a day in jail, 20% had been to prison, and about 40% had been on probation or parole. Most CeaseFire clients had been involved in a gang. Nearly 60% had only a grade school education.

Many clients said in interviews that they had received significant help from CeaseFire. More than three-fourths of the clients said they needed a job; 87% of that group received significant help. Of the 37% who said they wanted to get back into school or a GED program, 85% said they had received help through the program. Nearly every one of the 34% who told the researchers that they wanted help in leaving a gang reported that they had received such guidance. However, although two-thirds of the clients became active in CeaseFire after they had formed a relationship with a violence interrupter—and indeed, half of them took part in marches and vigils after a shooting occurred in their neighborhood—70% of the clients were still in a gang when they were interviewed.

That said, the researchers found that CeaseFire had a positive influence on these at-risk youth.

"A striking finding was how important CeaseFire loomed in their lives," the researchers stated in the report. "Clients noted the importance of being able to reach their outreach worker at critical moments— when they were tempted to resume taking drugs, were involved in illegal activities, or when they felt that violence was imminent."

CeaseFire also had a positive influence on the violence interrupters themselves. The program employed 150, many of whom had been in a gang and served time in prison. CeaseFire gave them a job in an environment where ex-offenders have limited opportunities, and the researchers note, "Working for CeaseFire also offered them an opportunity for personal redemption and a positive role to play in the communities where many had once been active in gangs."

Challenges and Cautions

Evaluating Chicago CeaseFire was not a neat laboratory experiment. Because the program runs in the real world, boundaries were not always clear between CeaseFire neighborhoods and other neighborhoods. For example, the violence interrupters had to go where gang members and other potential perpetrators of gun crime (and their potential victims) lived or hung out. "Spillover" between targeted areas and other areas was inevitable, although the researchers pointed out that this could have resulted in underestimating the program's impact.

Other programs, such as Project Safe Neighborhoods, were running in and around some of the CeaseFire sites during part of the time the researchers evaluated the program. Despite their best efforts to avoid such areas when selecting comparison sites, it was not always possible to do so. When this occurred, the researchers stated they were unable to determine empirically that CeaseFire alone was responsible for the decrease in violence.

Other issues made it difficult to discover the exact effect of CeaseFire in as straightforward and precise a way as policymakers and citizens might like. For example, in looking at the statistical data about violence, the researchers had to pick a month as the pre- and post-CeaseFire demarcation. However, pinpointing a precise date for the start of a program as large and multifaceted as CeaseFire is not easy. Community-mobilization and public education efforts got under way at different times in different areas, and the hiring of violence interrupters came a few years after the program started.

Another issue to consider when looking at the findings is that the researchers were able to examine only events that were reported to and recorded by police.

Finally, one overarching caveat to keep in mind is that Chicago experienced a huge drop in violence beginning in 1992.[b] As the researchers state in their report, "The reasons for this decline are, as elsewhere in the nation, ill-understood, and we could not account for possible remaining differences between the target and comparison areas in terms of those obviously important factors."

Still, It Worked

Despite these caveats, the evaluation showed that the program made neighborhoods safer. CeaseFire decreased shootings and killings (including retaliatory murders in some of the sites), making shooting hot spots cooler and helping the highest-risk youth.

The full report contains an extensive discussion of many topics, including:

- How sites were selected and organized, and how the central CeaseFire management worked.
- Challenges in areas with notably weak community bases.
- The crucial role of local police in providing immediate information about a shooting. This cooperation was not automatic, and readers may want to learn more about how this evolved.

Like other criminal justice programs, CeaseFire was vulnerable to the vagaries of funding fluctuations. Policymakers in particular will want to read sections of the evaluation to understand how the program was funded and the role that fluctuations played throughout the years. Also, CeaseFire was a small-scale program. Although it varied among the sites, the typical CeaseFire site's annual budget during the period covered in the evaluation was about $240,000. In the summer of 2007, the program was dramatically downsized because of budget cuts. The researchers found that they did not have enough data to do a rigorous statistical analysis of this cutback's impact. They did state, however, that "[a] detailed examination of the existing data did not reveal any dramatic shifts in crime following the closures [of CeaseFire sites], when compared to trends in the comparison areas."

CeaseFire is still running in 16 Chicago communities and six other Illinois cities. The CeaseFire model is going national. Recently, CeaseFire has collaborated with the Baltimore City Health Department to set up the model in four sites. Parts of the model are being implemented in Kansas City, Mo., and officials are considering implementing it in Columbus, Ohio; Detroit; Jacksonville, Fla.; and New Orleans. Other programs modeled on CeaseFire are being launched in eight New York cities, including Albany, Buffalo, New York City, Rochester and Syracuse.

The NIJ evaluation was supported by the Bureau of Justice Assistance and the Office of Juvenile Justice and Delinquency Prevention.

Notes

a. Skogan was the lead investigator on the NIJ-funded evaluation. Other researchers who participated in the evaluation include So Yung Kim (Korea Advanced Institute of Science and Technology); Richard Block (Loyola University Chicago); Andrew Papachristos (University of Massachusetts Amherst); and Susan Hartnett and Jill DuBois (Northwestern University).

b. Crime and violence decreased throughout Chicago in both the target and the comparison sites during the time that the researchers considered data, so they used fairly complex analyses to examine whether crime dropped significantly, hot spots visibly moved or cooled, and gang homicide weakened more in the CeaseFire sites than in the comparison areas.

CHAPTER TWENTY-EIGHT

A Community Effort to Reduce the Black/White Breast Cancer Mortality Disparity in Chicago

David Ansell, Paula Grabler, Steven Whitman, Carol Ferrans, Jacqueline Burgess-Bishop, Linda Rae Murray, Ruta Rao, and Elizabeth Marcus

Background

In October 2006, a group of Chicago breast cancer researchers released a report entitled "Breast Cancer in Chicago: Eliminating Disparities and Improving Mammography Quality" and called for a metropolitan Chicago summit to address the issue.[1] The major objective of the report was to present new data looking at breast cancer epidemiology in Chicago from 1980 to 2003. Trends in black/white female breast cancer incidence, mortality, stage of diagnosis and mammography screening rates in Chicago were analyzed. This was the first comprehensive study of breast cancer mortality disparity in Chicago and showed a substantial and growing disparity in Chicago black/white breast cancer mortality, a disparity that was greater than that reported for the United States as a whole.[1,2] The authors of the report concluded that there were three possible hypotheses to explain the differences in breast cancer mortality: black women receive fewer mammograms, black women receive mammograms of inferior quality, and black women receive different quality

Originally published in *Cancer Causes and Control* 20 (2009): 1681–88. Copyright © 2009, Springer Science+Business Media B.V.

of treatment for breast cancer, once diagnosed. In March 2007, a Breast Cancer Summit was held with researchers, providers, government, advocacy groups, survivors, and community groups to discuss the problem and propose solutions. The outcome of the Breast Cancer Summit was the Metropolitan Chicago Breast Cancer Task Force that organized action workgroups around the three major hypotheses. Each workgroup was charged with reviewing the literature and data, conducting interviews and focus groups with providers, and holding Town Hall meetings with the public. The goal of the Task Force was to reach conclusions regarding the reasons for the mortality disparity, propose evidence-based recommendations for reducing the breast cancer mortality disparity in Chicago, and set forth strategies for successfully implementing them. The report, "Improving Quality and Reducing Disparities in Breast Cancer Mortality in Metropolitan Chicago,"[3] was released on 16 October 2007. This paper describes the process that was employed to create plans to eliminate the disparities, presents some of the data that guided the decision-making process, and discusses the key findings and recommendations of the Task Force.

Methods

A total of 102 individuals from 74 Chicago area organizations were involved in the Task Force and participated in the three Action workgroups addressing each of the three hypotheses. The Action workgroups met bi-weekly from March to September 2007 with additional meetings of workgroup subcommittees. The workgroups reviewed the literature, assembled the data, and proposed recommendations.

Breast cancer mortality rates for non-Hispanic black and non-Hispanic white women were assembled for Chicago using a methodology described elsewhere.[2] Breast cancer mortality rates from New York City for black and white women were calculated (from vital records) using the same methodology. Breast cancer mortality from SEER was utilized to calculate the non-Hispanic black and non-Hispanic breast cancer mortality rates in the United States from 1980 to 2005.[3,4]

Town Hall meetings, designed to elicit community input, were held in four low income, predominantly African American Chicago neighborhoods and were facilitated by community leaders. The opinions and perspectives of 184 African American women were obtained regarding their perceptions of the causes of breast cancer disparity in Chicago, their ability to access screening and treatment, financial limitations, and other barriers. In addition, focus groups and interviews were held with safety net primary care providers, mammography technicians, and general radiologists who read mammograms in community hospital settings to identify their perspectives on breast cancer care in Chicago. A general solicitation to primary care physicians in private practice, those in community health centers, and those working in the County Health system produced a group of eight diverse physicians and physician assistants who provided care to underrepresented minorities in Chicago. They participated in a focus group on the mammography process as it impacted their patients and practices. In addition, eight mammography technologists representing six Chicago area institutions were also participants in a separate focus group. Phone surveys of eight individuals involved with breast cancer treatment across the metropolitan area including medical oncologists, surgeons, and health advocates were also conducted to elicit ideas regarding barriers to treatment. The focus groups used a structured questionnaire and were facilitated. The phone surveys of eight radiologists from eight Chicago institutions were conducted by research assistants. The detailed accounts of these focus groups and surveys are included in the Task Force report.[3]

A mammography capacity survey in Chicago was conducted. All 87 providers of mammography services in metropolitan Chicago were identified from the Food and Drug Administration Web site of accredited facilities[5] and were mailed surveys. Eighty-two percent of Chicago area mammography providers returned these surveys (86% from Chicago facilities and 76% from suburban facilities), many after being individually contacted by Task Force members.[3] Mammography capacity was calculated using the Government Accountability Office methodology.[3,6] For the 18% nonreporting facilities, an estimate of capacity was derived by using the average number of mammograms provided at the reporting facilities as the imputed baseline for capacity calculations.

Of 49 mammography screening facilities within the city of Chicago, 42 facilities completed the 35 question surveys and 40 facilities including all major academic facilities provided data on patient race/ethnicity. In order to examine potential differences in the quality of mammography services by race, facilities were surveyed about quality-related issues including the availability of digital mammography and ultrasound, the qualifications of those reading the mammograms, whether the facility was an academic, private nonacademic, or public facility, and whether abnormal results were delivered face-to-face. A facility was considered predominately minority if greater than 75% of the clientele were reported to be either African American or Hispanic. A facility was considered predominately white if > 75% of their clientele were reported to be white. *p* values were calculated with chi-squared test for contingency tables or by Fischer Exact test based on weighted cell count rounded to the nearest integer. The lower of the two *p* values is reported.

Finally, all 25 Chicago area acute care healthcare institutions were surveyed by phone to ascertain the extent of the breast cancer treatment facilities available and whether these treatment services had received approval from the American College of Surgeons Commission on Cancer.[7] There are 77 distinct community areas in Chicago of which 31 are predominately black, 20 predominately white, 12 Hispanic, and 14 mixed. Maps depicting the 25 communities in Chicago with the highest breast cancer mortality were assembled and overlaid with the locations of the fourteen Chicago institutions that had American College of Surgeons Commission on Cancer approved cancer programs.

Results

Figure 28.1 presents the main findings that stimulated the work of the Task Force, including two more recently acquired years' data. The breast cancer mortality rates for black and white women in Chicago were the same in 1980 (38 per 100,000, age adjusted). Rates remained similar until the early 1990s, when they began to diverge. By the late 1990s, a substantial disparity was present. By 2005, the mortality gap had widened to 116% with the age-adjusted black mortality rate of 41.3 more than twice that of the age-adjusted white rate of 19.2. Thus, from a position of equity in 1980, a large gap in black/white breast cancer mortality emerged and continued to widen through 2005. This occurred because the black rate remained constant over this period, while the white rate declined by almost one-half (49%).

Figure 28.2 presents the black/white breast cancer mortality disparity in Chicago, the United States, and New York City for the years 2000–2005. While there are black/white breast cancer mortality disparities for all three locations, the disparity has been smaller in the United States and New York City over the same time period, while the gap in Chicago

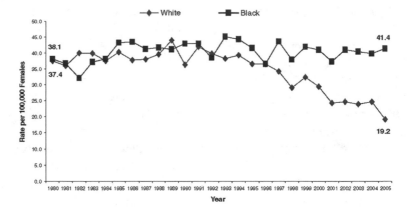

FIGURE 28.1. Black and white age-adjusted breast cancer mortality, Chicago, 1980–2005

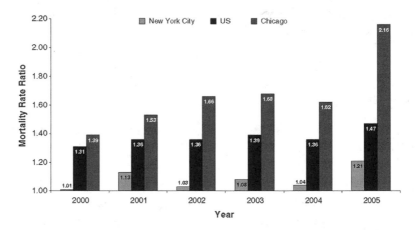

FIGURE 28.2. Black/white breast cancer mortality disparity, New York City, United States, and Chicago, 2000–2005

has continued to grow. From 2002 through 2005, the breast cancer mortality disparity in Chicago has on average been twice that of the United States and five times that of New York City.

Based on the response to the mammography survey, 206,000 screening mammograms were performed for women living in Chicago in 2007, far short of the 588,000 women in the 40–69 age range in Chicago according to the 2000 Census. According to the mammography centers' responses, there is potential for 254,000 screening mammograms in Chicago. Using the Government Accountability Office methodology for determining mammography capacity, Chicago has the maximum potential to perform 371,000 mammograms.[3,6] Both of these estimates are far short of the numbers needed to provide annual screening for the 588,000 women.

Predominantly minority populations were more likely to have their mammograms performed at public institutions (31 vs. 0%), less likely to be screened at academic (27 vs. 71%) and private nonacademic institutions (43 vs. 29%), and $p < .03$ than predominately white populations. Predominately minority populations were also less likely than predominately white populations to receive care at facilities where digital mammography was used (18 vs. 71%, $p < .003$) and less likely to have all their mammograms read by a trained specialist (23% compared to 87%), $p < .003$.

Figure 28.3 presents the geographic distribution of the 25 community areas in Chicago with the highest breast cancer mortality rates and juxtaposes the locations of hospitals with American College of Surgeons Commission on Cancer approved cancer programs.[7] Of the 25 Chicago community areas (out of a total of 77) with the highest breast cancer mortality rates, 24 are predominately black, and most are located on the

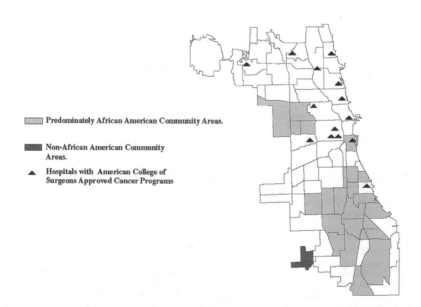

FIGURE 28.3. Chicago community areas with the highest 2000–2005 average annual breast cancer mortality rates

south side of the city. Only one community area with a high breast cancer mortality rate has a hospital with an approved cancer program residing within it, and there are only two hospitals with approved cancer programs on the south side of Chicago.

Results from the Town Hall meetings, focus groups of primary care physicians, mammography technicians, and oncologists and radiologists identified a number of recurring themes. First, there was agreement that there needed to be more breast cancer education and outreach programs for black women and other minorities. Secondly, the mammography process was broken in Chicago, and both patients and providers could identify quality differences in the manner in which the centers provided care and reported back. Finally, there were a number of reported barriers to

TABLE 28.1 **Proposed quality measures recommended by the Task Force**

Measure	Goal
Evaluating access	
Proportion of patients referred for screening mammography	100%
Proportion of patients actually receiving mammograms (annually)	80%
Evaluating mammography performance (ACR)[a]	
Positive predictive value of an abnormal mammogram (PPV$_1$)	5%–10%
Positive predictive value of a recommended biopsy (PPV$_2$)	25%–40%
Tumors found—stage 0 or 1	> 50%
Tumors found—minimal (invasive ≤ 1 cm or DCIS)	> 30%
Node positivity rate	< 25%
Cancer detection rate per 1,000 screened	2–10
Percent patients recalled from screening for additional imaging	< 10%
Evaluating follow-up	
Proportion not returning for follow-up within 60 days of screening overall and by BI-RADS	< 10%
Proportion never returning for treatment (overall and by stage)	< 10%
Evaluating timeliness	
Number of days from abnormal screening to initial diagnostic workup	< 30 days
Number of days from screening to final diagnosis (all diagnostic tests complete)	< 30 days
Number of days from diagnosis to treatment	< 30 days
Evaluating breast cancer treatment quality (ASCO)[b]	
Radiation therapy administered to the breast within 1 year of diagnosis for women under age 70 receiving breast conservation therapy	90%
Combination chemotherapy considered or administered within 4 months of diagnosis for women under 70 with AJCC T1c, II, III and hormone receptive negative breast cancer	90%
Tamoxifen or 3rd generation aromatase inhibitor (whichever appropriate) is considered or administered within 1 year of diagnosis for women with AJCC T1c, II, III and hormone receptor positive breast cancer	90%

[a]American College of Radiology (ACR). *Breast imaging reporting and data systems (BI-RADS).* 4th ed. Reston, VA: American College of Radiology; 2003. Rosenberg RD, Yankaskas BC, Abraham LA, et al. Performance benchmarks for screening mammography. *Radiology.* 2006;241(1):55–66.

[b]https://www.asco.org/ASCO/Downloads/Cancer.

diagnosis and treatment identified including fear, the lack of primary care, the burden of insurance co-pays and deductibles, providers who refused to treat patients on Medicaid, and noncompletion of treatment for social or economic reasons.

Table 28.1 presents a series of quality measures for the breast cancer screening, diagnosis, and treatment process proposed by national organizations and the Task Force.[3,8–10] The Task Force has recommended that these quality measures be systematically measured in institutions across Metropolitan Chicago and used to drive improvement in breast care for all women. In table 28.2, the key findings of the Task Force are summarized.[3]

TABLE 28.2 **Metropolitan Chicago Breast Cancer Task Force recommendations**

1. Access to and cost of mammography and breast cancer treatment
    Fully fund the Illinois breast and cervical cancer screening program
    Increase Medicaid payment rates for mammograms and breast cancer treatment
    Eliminate insurance co-pays and deductibles for mammograms
    Fully fund and staff Chicago public health and hospital breast cancer screening and
        treatment facilities
2. Breast cancer education and outreach
    Create culturally relevant grassroots community education and outreach efforts to improve
        screening rates
    Create one metropolitan Chicago phone number that women can call to access screening and
        treatment services
3. Capacity and the safety net
    Assemble a blue ribbon committee to address screening and treatment capacity deficiencies
        in metropolitan Chicago
    Identify solutions to geographic gaps for breast cancer screening, diagnosis, and treatment
    Create a public-private collaboration to coordinate screening, diagnosis, and treatment of
        breast cancer across metropolitan Chicago
    Expand use of digital mammograms to facilitate electronic transfer of images to central sites
        for reading
    Expand the use of breast cancer navigators to facilitate increased screening and completion
        of treatment
4. Quality improvement for mammography and treatment
    Create a Chicago breast cancer quality consortium
    Develop quality measures across the continuum of care from screening, diagnosis through
        treatment
    Share institutional quality outcomes among the institutions and with the community
5. Diagnostic and follow-up communication
    Women should be able to self-refer for breast cancer diagnostic tests
    Breast cancer diagnostic testing results should be communicated verbally with women in
        addition to referring physicians
    Patients with breast abnormalities should be directly referred for treatment by breast cancer
        screening facilities rather than relying only on the primary care physician
6. Mammography specialist workforce
    Expand the training of breast imagers at Chicago academic health centers
    Develop a community fellowship to train community-based radiologists to improve their
        breast cancer screening and diagnostic skills

Discussion

The Task Force concluded that the problem of breast cancer disparity in Chicago had many components but was primarily caused by gaps in education and access to screening and gaps in the quality of breast care across the continuum of care. Recommendations by the Task Force on remedies to the problem of black/white breast cancer mortality disparity address two overarching principles. The first was that no single entity in Chicago could "fix what was broken" and that this effort would thus require the participation of all institutions. Secondly, simply fixing one part of the breast health "system" would not be enough; all aspects had to be fixed together. What good would it be to expand outreach activities if the facilities do not have capacity? What good would it be to assure access to mammography if the mammograms and the reading of the mammograms were of poor quality such that small cancers were missed? What good would be served by finding cancers but not having access to quality treatment?

The fact that black breast cancer mortality in Chicago has not decreased among black women since 1980 (it has actually increased by a small amount) suggests that the major advances in breast cancer diagnosis and treatment in the past 25 years have not benefited black women in Chicago, while white women have experienced a large decrease in mortality. The disparity in Chicago is larger than that seen in New York City and the United States, which suggests something uniquely different and of great concern is occurring in Chicago with regard to breast cancer outcomes for black women. We believe that similar poor breast cancer outcomes may be present in other minority populations in Chicago, but do not have the data to corroborate the veracity of this hypothesis.

The growing black/white breast cancer mortality disparity in Chicago cannot be easily attributed to biological or co-morbid differences between blacks and whites but suggests that differential screening and treatment are contributors.[3,11–14] The comparisons with the United States and New York City disparity ratios shown in figure 28.2 make this clear, as one would not expect that the biological changes or co-morbidities that are alleged to drive breast cancer mortality could appear since 1980 or affect black women differentially in New York compared to Chicago. Rather, the reasons must involve breakdowns in the access to and the quality of breast care for black women across Chicago.

The communities with the highest mortality for breast cancer in Chicago are also those communities without hospitals with American College of Surgeons approved cancer treatment facilities, as shown in figure 28.3. These communities can be viewed as "health care deserts," as one participant in the Town Hall meetings described them, abandoned over the years by health care providers. Feedback from women in these communities as well as interviews with providers of breast cancer care revealed major problems women face trying to access services often miles from their homes and requiring long bus and train rides. Added to this geographic problem is the likelihood that the quality of breast care for black women in Chicago is different from that received by white women. White women in Chicago are more likely than black women to attend academic and private facilities, and their mammograms more likely to be read by specially trained radiologists.[3] Research has demonstrated that specialists are more likely to detect early breast cancers than general radiologists, and that diagnostic mammograms performed by academic facilities are associated with higher diagnostic accuracy.[15,16] Finally, white women are more likely than minority women to attend facilities with digital mammography, which research has demonstrated to be more effective in detecting breast cancer in women aged 40–50.[17]

The solutions to this disparity are neither straightforward nor simple. The literature suggests that the racial disparities in breast cancer outcomes can be reduced or eliminated by adequate screening and equivalent treatment.[13,18] Racial disparity in health outcomes has been described as a significant quality of care problem that can be addressed by tracking race specific outcomes.[19] A number of studies have demonstrated that for diseases other than breast cancer, when the quality of care is measured, made transparent, and improved, the black/white disparity in various health care processes can be reduced or even eliminated.[20,21] We believe the same is true for the processes of care that contribute to breast cancer mortality disparity in Chicago.

There are obvious challenges ahead. We are not aware of any community that has attempted to use quality improvement methodology to address racial disparity in breast cancer mortality across the continuum of care. While many institutions in Chicago have expressed an interest in joining such an effort, it will require developing new measurement tools and an unprecedented inter-institutional collaboration. Cost has also been shown to be a major barrier to the receipt of mammography services and should be eliminated as a barrier.[22] This will certainly be facilitated by a new state of Illinois rule, stimulated by the work of the Task Force, which makes Illinois the first state to pay for mammograms and treatment for all uninsured women, under the Illinois Breast and Cervical Cancer Screening Program.[23] However, while the coverage of all uninsured women is significant, there is an absolute annual capacity deficit for screening mammography in Chicago of at least 200,000 screening mammograms.[3] Capacity building is necessary but probably not sufficient as we heard from women, providers, and community organizations that issues of public transportation, childcare, work, and insurance copays are significant barriers even for insured women.[3] Navigation programs have been shown to provide some reduction in delay time to treatment and reduce anxiety in women and have been recommended by the Task Force.[24,25] While improving mortality is a daunting task, if we proceed in Chicago as we have been doing for the past 25 years, the outcomes for black women will likely fail to improve.

This is, of course, not a viable option. The Metropolitan Chicago Breast Cancer Task Force has documented the problem and proposed solutions. Now the solutions must be pursued with all available energy. Philosophers have noted that it is not enough to identify a problem and then do nothing to fix it. As Martin Luther King Jr. noted, "All that is necessary for evil to triumph is for good men to do nothing."[26]

References

1. Hirschman J, Whitman S, Ansell D, Grabler P, Allgood K. *Breast cancer in Chicago: Eliminating disparities and improving mammography quality.* Chicago: Sinai Urban Health Institute; 2006.

2. Hirschman J, Whitman S, Ansell D. The black:white disparity in breast cancer mortality: The example of Chicago. *Cancer Causes and Control.* 2007; 18(3):323–333.

3. Metropolitan Chicago Breast Cancer Task Force. *Improving quality and reducing disparities in metropolitan Chicago.* Chicago; 2007.

4. National Bureau of Economic Research. Mortality data—Vital Statistics NCHS' multiple cause of death data, 1959–2015. Cambridge, MA; 2009.

5. US Department of Health and Human Services. *Mammography facilities.* Washington, DC: US Food and Drug Administration. https://www.accessdata .fda.gov/scripts/cdrh/cfdocs/cfMQSA/mqsa.cfm.

6. Government Accounting Office (GAO). *Mammography capacity generally exists to deliver services.* Report no. GAO-02-5322002. Washington, DC; 2002.

7. http://web.facs.org/cpm/CPMApprovedHospitals_Result.cfm [link inactive].

8. American College of Radiology (ACR). *Breast imaging reporting and data systems (BI-RADS)*. 4th ed. Reston, VA: American College of Radiology; 2003.

9. Rosenberg RD, Yankaskas BC, Abraham LA, et al. Performance benchmarks for screening mammography. *Radiology*. 2006;241(1):55–66.

10. https://www.asco.org/ASCO/Downloads/Cancer.

11. Li CI, Malone KE, Daling JR. Differences in breast cancer stage, treatment, and survival by race and ethnicity. *Archives of Internal Medicine*. 2003; 163(1):49–56.

12. Newman LA. Breast carcinoma in African-American and white women: Application of molecular biology to understand outcome disparities. *Cancer*. 2004;101(6):1261–1263.

13. Smith-Bindman R, Miglioretti DL, Lurie N, Abraham L, Barbash RB, Stzelczyk J, et al. Does utilization of screening mammography explain racial and ethnic differences in breast cancer? *Annals of Internal Medicine*. 2006;144(8): 541–553.

14. Tammemagi CM, Nerenz D, Neslund-Dudas C, Feldkamp C, Nathanson D. Comorbidity and survival disparities among black and white patients with breast cancer. *Journal of the American Medical Association*. 2005;294(14): 1765–1772.

15. Sickles EA, Wolverton DE, Dee KE. Performance parameters for screening and diagnostic mammography: Specialist and general radiologists. *Radiology*. 2002;224(3):861–869.

16. Miglioretti DL, Smith-Bindman R, Abraham L, et al. Radiologist characteristics associated with interpretive performance of diagnostic mammography. *Journal of the National Cancer Institute*. 2007;99(24):1854–1863.

17. Pisano E, Gatsonis C, Hendrick E, et al. Diagnostic performance of digital versus film mammography for breast cancer screening. *New England Journal of Medicine*. 2007;353:1773–1783.

18. Dignam JJ. Differences in breast cancer prognosis among African-American and Caucasian women. *CA: A Cancer Journal for Clinicians*. 2000; 50(1):50–64.

19. Fiscella K, Franks P, Gold MR, Clancy CM. Inequality in quality: Addressing socioeconomic, racial, and ethnic disparities in health care. *Journal of the American Medical Association*. 2000;283(19):2579–2584.

20. Sehgal AR. Impact of quality improvement efforts on race and sex disparities in hemodialysis. *Journal of the American Medical Association*. 2003;289(8): 996–1000.

21. Trivedi AN, Zaslavsky AM, Schneider EC, Ayanian JZ. Trends in the quality of care and racial disparities in Medicare managed care. *New England Journal of Medicine*. 2005;353(7):692–700.

22. Trivedi AN, Rakowski W, Ayanian JZ. Effect of cost sharing on screening mammography in Medicare health plans. *New England Journal of Medicine.* 2008;358(4):375–383.

23. http://dph.illinois.gov/topics-services/life-stages-populations/womens-health-services/ibccp.

24. Ferrante JM, Chen PH, Kim S. The effect of patient navigation on time to diagnosis, anxiety, and satisfaction in urban minority women with abnormal mammograms: A randomized controlled trial. *Journal of Urban Health.* 2008; 85(1):114–124.

25. Battaglia TA, Roloff K, Posner MA, Freund KM. Improving follow-up to abnormal breast cancer screening in an urban population: A patient navigation intervention. *Cancer.* 2007;109(2 suppl.):359–367.

26. http://charactercounts.org/pdf/speech_MLK.pdf [link inactive].

CHAPTER TWENTY-NINE

The Fight for a University of Chicago Adult Trauma Center

The Rumble and the Reversal

Claire Bushey and Kristen Schorsch

The Rumble

From 61st and Cottage Grove, above still-leafless trees, you can see the complex where University of Chicago Medicine will house its future trauma center. It didn't exist when Damian Turner was shot at the corner almost six years ago.

The random victim of someone else's vendetta, the 18-year-old was hit shortly after midnight on Aug. 15, 2010, just three blocks south of U of C's medical campus. He struggled to his sister's apartment, his back bleeding, and collapsed in front of his young nieces and nephews. A neighbor called 911.

Despite a national reputation for excellence, U of C Medicine hadn't operated an adult trauma care center in more than 20 years. So the paramedics chose the nearest option, driving 10 miles north to Northwestern Memorial Hospital. Turner died at 1:23 a.m., leaving friends and family haunted by a question: Could treatment at a closer facility have saved his life?

Two weeks later, about 30 members of Fearless Leading by the Youth,

Originally published in *Crain's Chicago Business*, April 11, 2016. Reprinted with permission, Crain's Chicago Business 2016. © Crain Communications, Inc.

a community organization Turner helped found in 2007, clustered in the community room of a Woodlawn apartment complex to rage and grieve. That's where group leader Brittany Blaney spoke up: FLY should campaign for a new trauma center, to help prevent other deaths and spare others the pain they felt.

"That hit home," says Darrius Lightfoot, Turner's best friend. That was the beginning.

It would take five years, but the three-hospital health system eventually would reverse course and announce plans to offer the highest-level trauma care at its Hyde Park campus. The racial dynamics of Chicago would shift over that stretch, with the national Black Lives Matter movement drawing attention to polices shootings, and activists here opposing closures of mental health clinics and neighborhood schools located predominantly in poor, minority neighborhoods. After last November, when a judge released a video showing a Chicago police officer firing 16 bullets into teenager Laquan McDonald, the trauma center organizers would be joined by other protesters in the streets.

That a group of young, black community organizers built enough power to reckon with one of Chicago's most formidable institutions is "significant and unprecedented," says Elizabeth Todd-Breland, an assistant history professor at the University of Illinois at Chicago who has studied black political organizing in the city. While the campaign echoes earlier town-gown struggles, its youthful leadership and strategic nimbleness makes it an example—not just here in Chicago but nationally—that activists can emerge victorious.

"One of the chants you constantly hear among young black people is, 'I believe that we will win,'" Todd-Breland says. "When you actually have wins like the one that happened with the trauma center, you have every right to believe that you can."

Lingering Rift

The University of Chicago, which sits between 55th and 61st streets, and Woodlawn, the community that borders it to the south, have never been comfortable neighbors. In the 1960s, the university clashed with Bishop Arthur Brazier and the Rev. Leon Finney Jr., community leaders trained by legendary Chicago organizer Saul Alinsky, as it sought to expand its territory. Eventually the two men secured a written promise from U of C that it would never extend south of 61st Street.

Today, Hyde Park, the university's home, is a racially mixed community of 27,000. Forty percent of households earn $25,000 to $75,000 annually; 30% earn more. Meanwhile, the population of its southern neighbor has shrunk from more than 81,000 in 1960 to just under 22,000. Nearly three-quarters of Woodlawn's residents are unemployed or have stopped looking for work, and half of families there make less than $25,000, according to data from the 2013 American Community Survey. Of Chicago's 77 community areas, Woodlawn ranks in the top third for deaths caused by firearms or kidney disease, and near the top third for diabetes.

To understand why Turner's death was such a catalyzing event, it helps to know more about him. He grew up in Woodlawn's Grove Parc Plaza with his mother, three sisters and a brother; his father visited the family every week. In 2007, the summer he was 15, he and Lightfoot got jobs through an inaugural youth program at the community organization Southside Together Organizing for Power. The 12 junior organizers were determined "to make this into something real," recalls Lightfoot, now 24. They chose their own name, FLY, and their first campaign: improving conditions at the Cook County Juvenile Temporary Detention Center, historically called the Audy Home.

With Turner at 6-foot-4 and Lightfoot nearly a foot shorter, they were a mismatched pair but tight as brothers. When teenagers at the Audy Home said they had no clean underwear, the duo—who had collaborated

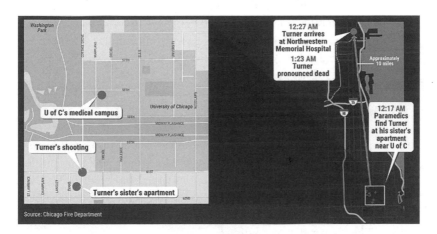

FIGURE 29.1. The gunshot heard around Chicago

Before Laquan McDonald was killed by police, the death of a Woodlawn activist named Damian Turner became a catalyst for one of the biggest movements in recent Chicago history.

on a rap about the conditions at the center—delivered underwear to the office of Todd Stroger, then Cook County Board president. They helped form a tenants association at Grove Parc Plaza. Turner even considered a campaign for a trauma center, says his mother, Sheila Rush, after a friend was shot and killed.

"Damian was a leader," Lightfoot says. Though young, he "moved with the heart of a full-grown soldier. He stood his ground."

But it wasn't all organizing. Turner was a neighborhood fixture who played basketball in a league run by Dr. Byron Brazier's Apostolic Church of God and danced with a hip-hop troupe. After attending three high schools, he struggled to graduate. He was applying to Job Corps when he died.

Building Momentum

On Sept. 28, 2010, which would have been Turner's 19th birthday, about 250 members of FLY and their allies marched from the site of the crime to a point near Duchossois Center for Advanced Medicine on campus. They carried a 4-foot-high white cardboard cake with red trim covered with photos of the teen, whose killing remains unsolved.

From that day, it would take seven months to get a meeting with anyone in management at U of C Medicine. When they did, Lightfoot recalls one of the vice presidents saying the health system's brief foray into running a trauma center, from 1986 until 1988, "did not work out" and that a new one on the South Side would "not save lives."

In all, it would take five years to force a meeting with Dr. Kenneth Polonsky, the executive vice president for medical affairs who reports directly to U of C President Robert Zimmer.

The activists' strategy: become a problem the university couldn't ignore. FLY organizers recruited students, religious leaders and other nonprofits to unify under an umbrella, Trauma Care Coalition. They chose strategic moments for civil disobedience—signing up, for example, for a public tour in January 2013 of U of C Medicine's new $700 million Center for Care and Discovery. "The optics were kind of absurd," given the university had argued it lacked the funds to operate a trauma center, says Alex Goldenberg, executive director of STOP, FLY's parent organization. "They never saw us coming."

Four activists were arrested that day, including a U of C graduate student. University police used batons to sweep the demonstrators out of the lobby. Overnight, a petition asking the university to drop charges against the protesters had 600 signatures. Three days later, administrators called for a "faculty-led dialogue" that culminated in a May 28 open meeting where, for the first time, Polonsky publicly supported a "regional solution" to the South Side's lack of trauma care.

The comment registered as progress. The campaign advanced, with organizers occupying a construction site in 2014 until police dragged them from it. They prayed in a hospital lobby, and when police kicked them out, they returned weekly to pray on the sidewalk. When Dr. Paul Farmer, an expert on medicine for the poor, came to speak on campus, they won his support by slipping a briefing paper into the car collecting him from the airport. They blocked traffic on Michigan Avenue.

In an interview with *Crain's*, U of C Medicine officials downplay the effect the organizers had on the institution's decision. "This isn't an issue that can be looked at in a silo," says Cristal Thomas, the community liaison for the health system. "We are engaged with our community, we assess their health needs, we listen to what they want and need from our hospital. We heard the voice of the trauma coalition; we heard the voice of many of our stakeholders."

But no other stakeholders staged die-ins on the medical campus or carried coffins through the streets.

A significant shift in the campaign came in spring 2014, when the organizers zeroed in on a particular weakness: the U of C's bid for Barack Obama's presidential library. "No trauma, no 'bama," they said, making national headlines.

Their first tangible victory came soon after, on Dec. 9, 2014, when U of C Medicine agreed to raise the age for admission to the trauma center at Comer Children's Hospital from 15 to 17.

Incremental Progress

One of the leaders to emerge from the campaign was Veronica Morris-Moore, 23, a Hyde Park Academy High School graduate who had been drawn to activism through a friend at FLY. After writing a senior English paper on young, black revolutionaries, she adopted the motto of Fred Hampton, a Black Panther activist killed by police in 1969: "Living for other people, struggling for other people and dying for other people."

In the runup to alumni weekend last June, Morris-Moore, now a staff organizer at FLY, was among nine who used U-locks and plywood to barricade themselves in Edward H. Levi Hall, the Ellis Avenue building housing the president, other administrators and, ironically, the Office of Civic Engagement.

"I honestly thought they would give us what we wanted," Morris-Moore says. "That's not what happened. About two hours into it, we started hearing banging on the walls."

Firefighters were hacking a hole in the wall. When that failed, they broke in through a window. Morris-Moore and the others were arrested and banned from campus. Police took them to lockup, where they waited 46 hours in the gloomy chill. The sound of slamming bars, she says, is a noise "that you don't ever forget."

Two months after the sit-in, Morris-Moore and Goldenberg, of STOP, finally got what they wanted: a meeting with Polonsky, brokered by the Rev. Julian DeShazier, a socially active senior pastor at University Church in Hyde Park.

A month later, the university announced that it would partner with Sinai Health System to open a trauma center at Holy Cross Hospital in Marquette Park. University officials hadn't mentioned the deal in their two meetings with the organizers—Morris-Moore found out the night before the Sept. 11 announcement. When she and other organizers tried to attend the news conference, Sinai representatives stopped them at the front desk. She's still banned from U of C's campus.

It looked like victory, albeit a bittersweet one, since the surprise of the Sinai announcement had deepened the organizers' distrust of the university. Almost a year had passed since administrators agreed to raise the age for admitting patients to the children's trauma center. And while paperwork was filed with the Illinois Department of Public Health, the health system still hasn't fulfilled the promise.

On the one-year anniversary of that announcement, the organizers held a news conference calling on the university to keep its promise. Another message, unspoken, was broadcast, too: We're not going away.

The Reversal

The activists had put up a long, hard fight. But they weren't running a hospital in the brutal, expensive reality of today's health care environment. Trauma is a money-loser, a service that even administrators at the richest hospitals avoid so they don't have to sacrifice other critical programs.

Adding to the complexity, it wasn't clear even to researchers who study trauma that another center was actually needed. Perhaps the problem, some say, is that Chicago has an appropriate number of trauma centers, but they're in the wrong places.

To be sure, University of Chicago Medicine is one of the most affluent health systems in the Chicago area, with $1.54 billion in 2015 revenue and a reputation for top-notch specialists. The activists, who grew up in the poor, violent neighborhoods around the university, and the U of C students who joined the cause, knew the system had deep enough pockets to take on trauma, if it wanted to.

After the surprise announcement last September that U of C Medicine would partner with Sinai Health System to build a trauma center 6 miles west at its Holy Cross Hospital in Marquette Park, the deal fell apart. Just before Christmas, U of C Medicine announced it would house the center on its Hyde Park campus after all and later revealed a massive $270 million expansion, a plan set to go before state regulators in May. The proposal also has to get the nod from rival Chicago trauma directors and the Illinois Department of Public Health.

In a recent interview, the Rev. Julian DeShazier, who helped broker discussions between activists and top U of C Medicine and university officials, asks the question on everyone's mind: What really triggered the health system's change of heart?

"Why was it right for them now?" he asks. "It's always been right for the community."

Two compelling reasons: the university's campaign to snag the prestigious Obama presidential library and a lucrative cancer institute. Activists could have derailed these projects if a trauma center didn't happen.

Long and Labored Process

U of C Medicine operates a three-hospital campus where about 1,800 doctors treat around 180,000 patients a year—the biggest, most well-resourced health complex on the South Side in a sea of modest community hospitals that mainly treat the poor and uninsured. Even combined, eight surrounding hospitals report just over half as much revenue. Most of these facilities send their sickest patients to U of C Medicine, which also is a feeder system for its growing network of suburban hospital partners.

In an interview, Sharon O'Keefe, a former nurse who has been president of the system since 2011, and Cristal Thomas, the former Illinois deputy governor to Democrat Pat Quinn, who now is a community liaison for the health system, say the long and labored decision-making process was about more than plugging a trauma gap on the South Side. Rather, it was about addressing community needs holistically. (Dr. Kenneth Polonsky, executive vice president for medical affairs, who oversees the health system, and Derek Douglas, university vice president of civic engagement and a former Obama aide who also attended the meetings with activists, declined interview requests.)

"People could argue that it might have been a convoluted trail that we followed," O'Keefe says. "But getting to the right decision is more important than anything else."

The emotional and political reasons to establish a center were obvious. But the evidence behind one—not so much.

"There's plenty of evidence to say there's a need, and there's plenty of evidence to say there's not a need," says Lee Friedman, an associate professor at the University of Illinois at Chicago who has studied the issue. "You're in the land of gray."

The argument for a center looks like this: There are no adult trauma centers on the city's South Side—a cruel irony for patients given that it has some of the most violent neighborhoods in the city. Of the nearly 19,000 total patients who were transported by Chicago paramedics from late 2012 to 2015, 3,900 suffered from gunshot wounds, the most common trauma injury today.

There are, however, four of these highly specialized centers elsewhere in Chicago: Mount Sinai Hospital in Lawndale on the West Side; Northwestern Memorial Hospital downtown in Streeterville; John H. Stroger Jr. Hospital on the Near West Side; and Advocate Illinois Masonic Medical Center in Lakeview. Last year, 26% of all trauma victims in Chicago were shuttled down the Dan Ryan Expressway to Advocate Christ Medical Center in suburban Oak Lawn, about 13 miles southwest of Hyde Park, a trip that takes a typical driver at least 30 minutes.

The most compelling case for U of C Medicine to reopen such a center is a 2013 study of nearly 12,000 area gunshot victims led by Dr. Marie Crandall, then a Northwestern trauma surgeon. "What we found was that being more than 5 miles away (from a trauma center), you're more

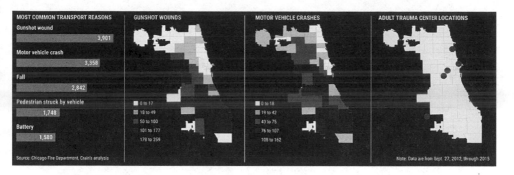

FIGURE 29.2. The void a South Side trauma center could fill

While gunshot victims are the most common patients transported by Chicago paramedics, emergency personnel are also busy with cases such as car crashes and falls.

likely to die," says Crandall, now a research director at the University of Florida, supporting a long-held belief among trauma surgeons that there is a "golden hour" to transport the seriously injured to a center and have them survive.

Activists, politicians and state regulators have seized on Crandall's study to bolster their argument that U of C Medicine needs to open such a center. But other research doesn't support that view.

A 2010 study led by Dr. Craig Newgard at Oregon Health and Science University analyzed nearly 3,700 trauma patients who were transported to 51 trauma centers nationwide. It found no significant link between transport times and death.

In Cook County, a regional 2011 study led by UIC's Friedman, corroborates this finding. After Franciscan St. James Hospital in Olympia Fields closed its trauma center in 2008, Friedman analyzed patient outcomes at nearby hospitals and found no increase in deaths or complications because patients had to travel farther.

Crain's attempted its own analysis, but each city or state agency we requested records from (Chicago Fire Department, Chicago Office of Emergency Management and Communications, Illinois Department of Public Health) either denied portions of the request or provided data that was missing key pieces. For example, the Fire Department doesn't track whether patients live or die once they reach trauma centers. The state does, but it cited an Illinois law in not identifying trauma centers by name.

Advocate Christ trauma director Dr. James Doherty hasn't found evidence that his trauma patients who travel longer distances suffer more in comparison. And he says there's no consensus among local trauma surgeons that another one is needed. "We certainly don't want to have a trauma center come in and cripple another," Doherty says. But he supports U of C Medicine's efforts, he says, because there's an obvious gap in trauma care around it.

White House Ties

The activists had armed themselves with data and steadily linked research supporting their case to a university pressure point: its desire to host a presidential library and museum for Barack Obama, a project estimated to cost at least $500 million. It would be a sorely needed tourist destination and South Side place-maker for a president whose regional roots run deep. Obama got his start as a community organizer and later taught constitutional law at the esteemed university. First Lady Michelle Obama was an executive at the medical center.

The Rev. Michael Pfleger, the prominent St. Sabina pastor who is a powerful figure in the South Side black community, says he told university officials who sought his support, including Susan Sher, the former chief of staff to Michelle Obama and now senior adviser to University of Chicago President Robert Zimmer, that he was "100 percent" for the library—but only if a trauma center was opening, too. "If not, I had every intention of stopping the building of the Obama presidential library," he says. Sher listened and said, "I hear you," Pfleger recalls.

Sher remembers her in-person meeting with Pfleger but emphasizes that while activists and others have tied the library to the trauma center, "from the university's perspective, one had nothing to do with the other." O'Keefe and Thomas also say no outside factors played into the trauma decision. But others clearly connected the dots.

Timuel Black Jr., a community stalwart and a civil rights activist who lives in Bronzeville, was on the university's 12-person advisory committee for the library. "I said if you want me to be here, a trauma center is very important," Black says.

Emails obtained by *Crain's* through Freedom of Information Act requests show that Sher and top-level aides to Mayor Rahm Emanuel kept in communication about the trauma center and exchanged details before they were made public. This despite the fact that Sher worked for the university, not the health system, which have two separate boards. Sher says she had a working relationship with both Sinai—she used to be on that health system's board before working at the White House—and

Emanuel's top aide, David Spielfogel, so she kept him and others in the loop.

Spielfogel says that the mayor has been "pretty vocal for the past few years about expanding health options throughout the city, and particularly on the South Side. But he obviously deferred to [U of C] in terms of how that would happen."

Spielfogel left the mayor's office recently to launch a tech startup. O'Keefe says the mayor's office had no influence in the system's decision.

Cash and Cachet

O'Keefe was close to ending years of angst when she and Sinai CEO Karen Teitelbaum announced in September that they planned to open a Level I trauma center, the highest state designation, at Holy Cross. It was a strategic deal that included a one-time $40 million payment from U of C Medicine, not to mention the cachet of bringing the system's surgeons to an aging community hospital.

The deal wasn't what the activists wanted: Holy Cross was on the other side of the Dan Ryan Expressway. While that Southwest Side facility also is surrounded by neighborhoods racked with violence, according to a *Crain's* analysis of Chicago Fire Department data, trauma patients there are closer to existing trauma centers than those near Hyde Park.

But the marriage didn't last. O'Keefe says that while they were hammering out the details, it became clear that the health system should house trauma on its own campus, which already has a burn center and a pediatric trauma center. Why have a satellite team of surgeons toiling

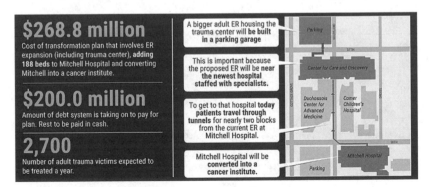

FIGURE 29.3. U of C Medicine's grand overhaul
Four trauma bays are a small part of a much bigger vision for the Hyde Park campus.

away elsewhere when they could stay at U of C Medicine's complex and assist with other patients between trauma cases?

She says she could better sustain the exorbitant costs of a trauma center by having it on her campus. "Those nuances only became clear to us during planning," she says. Even though most trauma patients are typically poor or uninsured, the system wouldn't have to share reimbursement payments from private and government insurers with Holy Cross.

Teitelbaum declined an interview request. But people familiar with the collapse of the deal say Sinai was caught by surprise. It had been in the midst of gathering data to present to regulators. Then its Hyde Park partner pulled the plug.

Five months after dropping Sinai, U of C Medicine produced a bold $270 million plan—a proposal that likely would have drawn heat from the community and local lawmakers if it didn't include trauma. The plan includes expanding the system's cramped adult emergency room, which fed-up patients frequently leave before seeing a doctor, and adding four trauma bays. Nearly 200 more patient beds will be added to aging Mitchell Hospital, which will be transformed into a new cancer institute. That would help showcase its specialty, ranked 34th out of roughly 900 hospitals nationwide by *U.S. News and World Report.*

This facility could become a branding booster for the health system and a moneymaker to offset giant losses U of C Medicine expects from adding emergency services. In 2015, the adult ER alone lost more than $30 million.

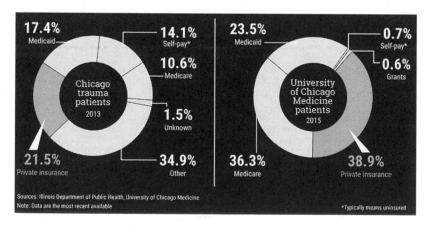

FIGURE 29.4. Why trauma is a money loser

Trauma patients tend to be poor and uninsured. In Chicago in 2013, only 1 in 5 had private insurance.

The move could prompt academic rivals like Northwestern Medicine and Rush University Medical Center to beef up their cancer programs as they vie for patients, says Dan Marino, Chicago-based executive vice president at consultancy GE Healthcare Camden Group. "I think [U of C Medicine] is trying to brand themselves even more—not just as a metropolitan center but as a regional and national destination" for cancer care, Marino says.

O'Keefe says the big plans help lay the groundwork for the future. Not only are the system's specialists in high demand, especially as baby boomers live longer, but cancer is among the most lucrative services, along with orthopedics and cardiology. The money it brings in is needed to cover the ER expansion and new trauma service.

An Olive Branch

For all the heightened emotion behind it, the deal likely wouldn't have happened if U of C Medicine didn't balance out losing so much money on trauma. The cancer institute is a key piece of that puzzle.

Time will tell what effect the trauma center will have on repairing the health system's—and the university's—relationship with the community that surrounds it.

"The politics of it. The community demand for it. The economic impact of these health care facilities. All of that ultimately factors into if one is built or kept open," says local health care consultant Duane Fitch. "It's well beyond the more simplistic, 'Does this marketplace support one: yes or no?'"

The question of need is not as simple as one trauma center, says a voice from inside the walls of U of C Medicine. Dr. Philip Verhoef works in the intensive care unit and treats adults and children with severe injuries. He has been on both sides of the issue, also serving as an adviser to the activists. Sure, these services will likely lose money, but, quite simply, he says, it's the right thing to do. He recalls a recent conversation he had with a trauma leader at a health system in Philadelphia that faced a similar town-gown clash two decades earlier. Opening a trauma center helped heal their fractured relationship.

"I'd love to see that be an outcome here, too," Verhoef says, "that this starts to mend the divide."

CHAPTER THIRTY

Selections from *Healthy Chicago 2.0: Partnering to Improve Health Equity, 2016–2020*

Chicago Department of Public Health

Dear Partners,

Chicago is my home. My parents came to Chicago after being relocated from the west coast during World War II. With the support of community organizations, churches and extended family, they were able to create a safe, stable and supportive environment for my brothers and me. As a result, we have been able to lead healthy and productive lives and my husband and I have been able to do the same for our two children. My vision is for all Chicago residents to have the same opportunities that have allowed my family and me to thrive. As Commissioner for the Chicago Department of Public Health (CDPH), I have the unique opportunity to lead a department that has the responsibility to do just that.

CDPH is responsible for maximizing the health and well-being of every Chicago resident, but our department alone can't accomplish that goal. We know that good health depends on numerous factors, including many that are outside of the traditional public health sphere. The availability of economic resources, the conditions of the homes in which we live, our educational opportunities and the degree to which we feel safe and connected in our neighborhoods play critical roles in improving our health. That is why the development of Healthy Chicago 2.0 is an important milestone for Chicago.

Reprinted courtesy of the Chicago Department of Public Health.

Healthy Chicago 2.0 is a plan for the entire city. As part of the planning process, we convened representatives from more than 130 organizations across a broad range of sectors to review data and then identify actionable strategies to address our city's most pressing health issues and their root causes.

The plan is a result of a collaborative effort. Its implementation, similar to its development, is dependent on partners across the city working together to make the changes necessary to improve health. I am grateful for the businesses, non-profit organizations, philanthropic agencies, faith-based networks, advocacy groups, other government agencies and residents who devoted a great deal of time and energy to create this plan and who have committed resources and human capital to see that the goals in this plan are realized.

Achieving health equity will take time, resources and dedication. I look forward to working together to create a Chicago where every resident has the opportunities, resources and information necessary to live a healthy life.

Julie Morita, M.D.
Commissioner, Chicago Department of Public Health

TABLE 30.1 **Healthy Chicago 2.0 indicators: Baseline data and 2020 targets**

Indicator	Description	Citywide baseline & year	Priority population	Priority population baseline & year	2020 target & percentage change from baseline
		Overarching			
Overall health status	Percentage of adults who report their health as "good," "very good," or "excellent"[1]	81.6% (2014)	Citywide	81.6% (2014)	85.7% (5% increase)
Life expectancy	Life expectancy at birth in years[2]	77.8 (2012)	Citywide	77.8 (2012)	79.4 (2% increase)
Preventable hospitalization	Age-adjusted rate of potentially preventable hospitalizations, which includes certain acute illnesses (e.g., dehydration) and worsening chronic conditions (e.g., hypertension) that might not have required hospitalization had these conditions been managed successfully by primary care providers in outpatient settings[3]	172.3 per 10,000 (2011)	Citywide	172.3 per 10,000 (2011)	163.7 per 10,000 (5% decrease)
Obesity	Percentage of Chicago Public School kindergartners who are obese[4]	19.1% (2012–2013)	Citywide	19.1% (2012–2013)	18.2% (5% decrease)
	Percentage of adults who are obese[2]	28.8% (2014)	Citywide	28.8% (2014)	27.4% (5% decrease)
Discrimination	Percentage of adults who report ever experiencing discrimination, been prevented from doing something, or been hassled or made to feel inferior because of their race, ethnicity or color[1]	Data available 2016			
Economic hardship	Population living in communities experiencing high economic hardship[5]	835,249 (2014)	Citywide	835,249 (2014)	793,487 (5% decrease)
Child opportunity	Number of children (0–17 years) living in communities with low or very low child opportunity[6]	297,352 (2014)	Citywide	297,352 (2014)	282,484 (5% decrease)
Trauma-informed city	City agencies and community-based organizations are trained and understand the impact that violence and trauma has on individuals and communities		Data and metric forthcoming		

		Access			
Primary care provider	Percentage of adults who have a personal doctor or health[1] care provider	80.8% (2014)	Hispanic	68.4% (2014)	75.2% (10% increase)
No health insurance	Percentage of population without health insurance[5]	18.7% (2014)	Hispanic	28.1% (2014)	22.5% (20% decrease)
Dental care emergencies	Age-adjusted rate of dental-related emergency department visits[3]	39.0 per 10,000 (2011)	High hardship communities	53.8 per 10,000 (2011)	51.1 per 10,000 (5% decrease)
Health care satisfaction	Percentage of adults who were satisfied with the health care they received[1]		Data available 2016		
Routine checkup	Percentage of adults who visited a doctor or health care[1] provider for a routine checkup in the past year[1]	76.8% (2014)	Citywide	76.8% (2014)	80.6% (5% increase)
Received needed care	Percentage of adults who report it is "usually" or "always"[1] easy to get the care, tests, or treatment they needed through their health plan		Data available 2016		
Annual dental cleanings	Percentage of adults who report having had their teeth cleaned by a dentist or dental hygienist in the past year[1]		Data available 2016		
		Built environment, economic development, housing			
Housing cost burden	Percentage of households whose housing costs are at least 35% of household income[5]	38.7% (2014)	Citywide	38.7% (2014)	36.8% (5% decrease)
Permanent supportive housing	Number of permanent supportive housing units[7]	6,946 (2014)	Citywide	6,946 (2014)	7,293 (5% increase)
Healthy homes	Adoption of model of healthy homes codes		Data and metric forthcoming		
Lead poisoning	Percentage of children less than 3 years of age with elevated blood lead levels (> 6 mcg/dL)[8]	3.4% (2014)	Very low child opportunity communities	5.7% (2014)	3.7% (35% decrease)
Unemployment	Percentage of civilian labor force who are unemployed[9]	8.4% (2014)	Citywide	8.4% (2014)	7.6% (10% decrease)
Savings and assets	Asset development through capital, such as savings, financial securities (stocks and bonds), property ownership, as well as education, job training, and access to credit.		Data and metric forthcoming		

(continued)

TABLE 30.1 (continued)

Indicator	Description	Citywide baseline & year	Priority population	Priority population baseline & year	2020 target & percentage change from baseline
Active transportation	Percentage of workers who walk, bike, or take public transportation as their primary mode of getting to work[1]	37.0% (2014)	Citywide	37.0% (2014)	40.7% (10% increase)
Neighborhood safety	Percentage of adults who feel safe in their neighborhood "all" or "most" of the time[1]			Data available 2016	
Traffic crash injuries	Number of serious injuries resulting from traffic crashes (all roadway users)[10]	2,213 (2014)	Citywide	2,213 (2014)	1,452 (34% decrease)
Education					
Early childhood education	Percentage of eligible 3- and 4-year-olds in early childhood education[11]	73.0% (2014)	Citywide	73.0% (2014)	80.0% (10% increase)
School attendance	Percentage of school days attended by Chicago Public School students[4]	93.0% (2013–2014)	Homeless students	77.0% (2013–2014)	93.0% (21% increase)
Postsecondary programs	Percentage of Chicago Public School students who enroll in postsecondary programs (e.g., college, community college, vocational training)[4]			Data available 2016	
Behavioral health					
Serious psychological distress	Percentage of adults who reported serious psychological distress based on how often they felt nervous, hopeless, restless or fidgety, depressed, worthless, or that everything was an effort in the past 30 days[1]	5.2% (2014)	High poverty communities	10.3% (2014)	9.8% (5% decrease)
Behavioral health treatment	Percentage of adults who experience serious psychological distress and who are currently taking medicine or receiving treatment from a doctor or other health professional for any type of mental health condition or emotional problem[1]	50.3% (2014)	Adults with serious psychological distress	50.3% (2014)	55.3% (10% increase)
Suicide attempts	Percentage of high school students who attempted suicide that resulted in an injury, poisoning, or overdose that had to be treated by a doctor or nurse in the past 12 months[12]	3.5% (2013)	LGBTQ youth	11.3% (2013)	10.2% (10% decrease)

Depression	Percentage of high school students who reported feeling sad or hopeless almost every day for 2 or more weeks in a row so that they stopped doing some usual activities during the past 12 months[2]	32.5% (2013)	Female adolescents	40.7% (2013)	38.7% (5% decrease)
Prescription opiate abuse	Percentage of adults who report in the past 12 months either ever taking prescription pain relievers, such as oxycodone or hydrocodone, at a higher dosage or taking it more often than directed in the prescription or ever taking a prescription pain reliever that was not prescribed to them[1]	Data available 2016			
Opiate overdose	Number of ambulance runs in response to suspected opiate overdose[13]	2,506 (2014)	Citywide	2,506 (2014)	2,005 (20% decrease)
Binge drinking	Percentage of adults who report binge drinking in the past month[14]	29.0% (2011)	Non-Hispanic white males	45.8% (2011)	43.5% (5% decrease)
Behavioral health hospitalizations	Age-adjusted rate of hospitalizations due to behavioral health disorders[3]	226.8 per 10,000 (2011)	Citywide	226.8 per 10,000 (2011)	204.1 per 10,000 (10% decrease)
Primary care utilization	Percentage of adults who visited a doctor or health care provider for a routine checkup in the past year[1]	76.8% (2014)	Adults with serious psychological distress	78.9% (2014)	86.8% (10% increase)

Child & adolescent health

Infant mortality	Rate of deaths before age 1[15]	7.8 per 1,000 births (2013)	High hardship communities	9.7 per 1,000 births (2013)	8.7 per 1,000 births (10% decrease)
Early intervention services	Number of children with developmental delays less than 4 years of age who have a plan for special services[16]	Data available 2016			
School-based health services	Number of Chicago Public School students who receive a school-based vision exam[17]	43,878 (2014–2015)	Citywide	43,878 (2014–2015)	48,753 (10% increase)
	Number of Chicago Public School students who receive a school-based dental exam[17]	115,238 (2014–2015)	Citywide	115,238 (2014–2015)	144,048 (20% increase)
	Number of Chicago Public School students who receive a school-based screening for sexually transmitted infections[17]	6,399 (2014–2015)	Citywide	6,399 (2014–2015)	7,039 (10% increase)

(continued)

TABLE 30.1 (continued)

Indicator	Description	Citywide baseline & year	Priority population	Priority population baseline & year	2020 target & percentage change from baseline
Teen birth rate	Rate of births to mothers aged 15–19 years[18]	35.5 per 1,000 (2013)	Very low child opportunity communities	57.3 per 1,000 (2013)	51.6 per 1,000 (10% decrease)
	Chronic disease				
Fruits and vegetable servings	Percentage of high school students who reported consuming five or more fruit and vegetable servings daily in the past week[12]	18.3% (2013)	Citywide	18.3% (2013)	20.3% (10% increase)
	Percentage of adults who reported consuming five or more fruit and vegetable servings yesterday[1]	29.2% (2014)	African Americans	18.9% (2014)	20.8% (10% increase)
Soda consumption	Percentage of high school students who reported consuming one or more can/bottle/glass of soda daily in the past week[12]	23.1% (2013)	Citywide	23.1% (2013)	21.9% (5% decrease)
	Percentage of adults who drank soda or pop at least once per day in the past month[1]			Data available 2016	
Physical activity	Percentage of high school students who were physically active at least 60 minutes per day during the last week[12]	19.6% (2013)	Citywide	19.6% (2013)	20.6% (5% increase)
	Percentage of adults with no leisure time physical activity in the past month[1]	18.3% (2014)	High poverty communities	22.7% (2014)	21.6% (5% decrease)
Smoking	Percentage of high school students who currently smoke cigarettes[12]	10.7% (2013)	Citywide	10.7% (2013)	9.6% (10% decrease)
	Percentage of adults who currently smoke cigarettes[1]	18.4% (2014)	Citywide	18.4% (2014)	16.6% (10% decrease)
	Percentage of adults who currently use electronic cigarettes[1]	3.9% (2014)	Adults aged 18–29 years	6.3% (2014)	5.7% (10% decrease)
Cancer screenings	Percentage of women aged 50–74 years reporting having a mammogram in the past 2 years[1]	75.6% (2014)	Citywide	75.6% (2014)	79.4% (5% increase)
	Percentage of women aged 21–65 years reporting having a Pap test within the past 3 years[1]	82.9% (2014)	Citywide	82.9% (2014)	87.0% (5% increase)

	Percent of adults aged 50–75 years reporting having a sigmoidoscopy/colonoscopy in the past 10 years, having a sigmoidoscopy/colonoscopy in the past 5 years and a blood stool test in the past 3 years, or having a blood stool test in the past year[1]	60.4% (2014)	High poverty communities	47.9% (2014)	52.7% (10% increase)
HPV vaccination	Percentage of female adolescents aged 13–17 years who received three or more doses of HPV vaccine[19]	52.6% (2014)	Citywide	52.6% (2014)	80.0% (52% increase)
Breast cancer mortality	Age-adjusted rate of female breast cancer deaths[2]	24.9 per 100,000 (2013)	African American women	33.3 per 100,000 (2013)	30.0 per 100,000 (10% decrease)
Asthma emergency department visits	Age-adjusted emergency department visit rate due to asthma for the population less than 18 years of age[3]	147.7 per 10,000 (2011)	African Americans	280.0 per 10,000 (2011)	252.0 per 10,000 (10% decrease)
Diabetes-related hospitalizations	Age-adjusted hospitalization rate due to diabetes-related lower extremity amputations[3]	2.0 per 10,000 (2011)	High hardship communities	3.0 per 10,000 (2011)	2.7 per 10,000 (10% decrease)

Infectious disease

Hepatitis C treatment	Access and availability to treatment for persons diagnosed with Hepatitis C		Data and metric forthcoming		
HIV incidence	Number of new HIV infections[20]	973 (2014)	African American men who have sex with men	355 (2014)	320 (10% decrease)
Linkage to HIV care	Percentage of persons with newly diagnosed HIV infections that are linked to HIV medical care within 90 days of diagnosis[20]	81.5% (2014)	African Americans	78.6% (2014)	90.0% (15% increase)
Engagement in HIV care	Percentage of persons living with HIV that are engaged in HIV medical care[20]	55.0% (2012)	Citywide	55.0% (2012)	74.3% (35% increase)
HIV viral suppressions	Percentage of persons living with HIV who have an undetectable viral load[20]	45.0% (2012)	Citywide	45.0% (2012)	90.0% (100% increase)
Chlamydia	Rate of reported chlamydia cases[21]	1,013 per 100,000 (2013)	African American females under 25 years	4,567 per 100,000 (2013)	3,425 per 100,000 (25% decrease)

(continued)

TABLE 30.1 (continued)

Indicator	Description	Citywide baseline & year	Priority population	Priority population baseline & year	2020 target & percentage change from baseline
		Violence			
Gun-related homicides	Age-adjusted homicide rate as the result of firearm use[2]	10.8 per 100,000 (2013)	African American males	55.4 per 100,000 (2013)	44.3 per 100,000 (20% decrease)
Nonfatal shootings	Number of nonfatal shootings reported[22]	2,435 (2014)	Citywide	2,435 (2014)	1,948 (20% decrease)
Sexual assault	Number of sexual assault crimes reported[22]	2,395 (2014)	Citywide	2,395 (2014)	2,156 (10% decrease)
Violent crime in public spaces	Number of gun-related violent crimes reported that occurred in public spaces (e.g., street, sidewalk, park, etc.)[22]	9,577 (2014)	Citywide	9,577 (2014)	7,662 (20% decrease)
Suspensions	Percentage of Chicago Public School students who received out-of-school suspensions[4]	2.6% (2014–15)	Citywide	2.6% (2014–2015)	1.3% (50% decrease)
School fights	Percentage of high school students who were in a physical fight on school property one or more times during the past 12 months[12]	16.9% (2013)	Citywide	16.9% (2013)	12.7% (25% decrease)
Bullying	Percentage of high school students who report being bullied on school property[12]	13.0% (2013)	LGBTQ youth	30.4% (2013)	27.4% (10% decrease)
School safety	Percentage of high school students who reported missing school due to safety concerns	12.9% (2013)	Citywide	12.9% (2013)	10.3% (20% decrease)
Social cohesion	Shared values and trust among neighbors[12]	Data and metric forthcoming			
Discrimination from criminal justice system	Percentage of adults who report ever experiencing discrimination, been prevented from doing something or been hassled or made to feel inferior from the police or in the courts because of their race, ethnicity or color	Data available 2016			

Data sources: [1]Healthy Chicago Survey, Chicago Department of Public Health (CDPH). [2]Death Data, Division of Vital Records, Illinois Department of Public Health (IDPH). [3]Discharge Data, Division of Patient Safety and Quality, IDPH. [4]Chicago Public Schools (CPS). [5]American Community Survey 2010–2014, US Census Bureau. [6]diversitydatakids.org, Kirwan Institute for the Study of Race and Ethnicity. [7]Department of Family and Support Services, City of Chicago. [8]Lead Poisoning Prevention, CDPH. [9]US Department of Labor, Bureau of Labor Statistics. [10]Illinois Department of Transportation. [11]CPS, Department of Family and Support Services, City of Chicago. [12]Youth Risk Behavioral Surveillance System, CPS. [13]Chicago Fire Department. [14]Behavioral Risk Factor Surveillance System, Illinois Center for Health Statistics, IDPH. [15]Birth and Death Data, Division of Vital Records, IDPH. [16]Illinois Department of Human Services. [17]Adolescent & School Health, CDPH. [18]Birth Data, Division of Vital Records, IDPH. [19]National Immunization Survey—Teen, National Center for Immunization and Respiratory Diseases, Centers for Disease Control and Prevention. [20]HIV Surveillance, CDPH. [21]STI Surveillance, CDPH. [22]Chicago Police Department.

Conclusion

Researchers have grappled for over a century with the social divisions that characterize Chicago, a city that has been described as one of "sumptuous wealth and profound indifference."[1] Chicago is not a poor city; it is an unequal city, one with significant health inequities. And, although these inequities have persisted over generations—documented by the wide range of methodologies seen in the selections in this *Reader*—this does not imply that health inequities are natural or inevitable. On the contrary. Chicago's patterns of health inequities are the result of *structural violence*; our social divisions *produce* unnecessary, unfair, and avoidable inequities in health.

We prepared this *Reader* to bring together seemingly disparate literatures to show, with some level of detail, the ways in which structural violence operates in Chicago. We are not aware of any other book that has attempted to create such a compilation. We hope that viewing health equity through the lens of Chicago may serve as an example for other cities. Taking stock of what has been experienced, what has been debated, and what have been offered as solutions is important, though not always prioritized in the pursuit of the new. In our minds, there are significant strengths in this Chicago literature—in the value it places on local community data, the development and refinement of concepts to describe observed patterns, the integration of quantitative and qualitative research methods, the search for structural causes, the identification of community-level processes such as collective efficacy, and the recognition that inequities in health are, indeed, avoidable, unnecessary, and unfair. At its best, this Chicago literature provides models for meaningful action based on data, blurring the traditional lines between researchers, advocates, and the community.

There are significant gaps in this literature, and many challenges remain. Much of Chicago's research attention has been devoted to identifying a community's deficits rather than naming and investing in its strengths. Compounding this issue is the well-known publication bias in scholarly journals toward statistically significant findings, resulting in a lopsided empirical record with more studies finding differences rather than null results. And, while there are important examples of research involving community partnerships, the research process as a whole remains an unequal relationship, with research institutions wielding the most power to define questions and methods. However, despite these limitations, health equity researchers have created a valuable empirical record, now collectively documented in this *Reader*.

Our Challenge

We chose to write a historical book, one that looks backward into our collective efforts to understand and address Chicago's marked inequities. We chose to do this because we know that history matters and because we believe that there is insight to be gained from bringing these works together into one collection. Yet, while our book looks backward, our preoccupation is, of course, with the present and the future.

We live in a time when all the parts of the book—"A Divided City," "The Health Gap," "Separate and Unequal Health Care," "Communities Matter," and "Taking Action"—are alive. The city's social divisions are entrenched but dynamic—and surely the Chicago of twenty or thirty years from now will be different than the city it is today. Will it be more equal? What will the data tell us about the health gap? It could change, we believe it must change, and Healthy Chicago 2.0 has set some important targets— but will it work? *How are we living, and how are we going to live?* Will large segments of the city continue to be systematically excluded from the full benefits of the health care system? What of collective efficacy, social capital, and other aspects of communities that were documented in this book as central to our well-being? Will they be recognized and strengthened or eroded? What kinds of collective action will we see in the coming decades? What will mobilize us to work for the common good?

In *I Call It Murder*, a 1979 British documentary about the famed Chicago public hospital, County, Quentin Young argued:

Our patients represent the crystallized oppressions of our society as expressed in illness. . . . What we are seeing here are the most oppressed of our society, the most vulnerable, those least equipped by education, by birth, by economic resources to resist the numerous oppressions of our society, from the air we breathe to the nasty housing that the poor are condemned to, and it ends up in all variety of diseases. . . . The conclusion you draw from that analysis is that you're dealing with a total societal failure, and working with the health question you can begin that transformation that will make us more civilized than we are.[1]

Nearly four decades later, we continue to grapple with Young's analysis, which, in turn, echoed arguments offered in different places by Rudolph Virchow and Friedrich Engels in the 1840s.[2] The idea that social conditions influence community health is not new. But what this collection of Chicago health equity work teaches us, above all, is that we cannot assume that things will get better over time, that health disparities will diminish on their own through scientific, technical, or economic advancements in society. To be sure, there have been significant improvements in population health over time—across the city, people live longer lives than ever before. Yet the fundamental patterns of inequity have not changed substantially over the time frame of the studies in this book, and structural violence—particularly racism—continues to exert a deadly toll. So our collective challenge remains much the same as it was for Young—to work with the "health question" (now framed in the language of health equity) to "make us more civilized than we are."

Moving Forward

To continue with business as usual would be unethical.[3] We know that health inequities exist, that they are substantial, and that they systematically deprive people (and communities) of the capacity to lead long and healthy lives. And we know that our current approaches to dealing with disease will almost certainly *not* alter that fundamental picture unless we put equity in health at the center of our actions. In that spirit, we offer several suggestions for reorienting the health equity agenda so that the health profile of Chicago ten, twenty, or thirty years ahead will not remain trapped by its past.

1. *Raise public awareness to view health equity as an achievable goal.* Other cities have prioritized health for all residents and have diminished, or even eliminated, some patterns of inequity. In the case of low birth weight (seen in this book as a sensitive indicator used to explore the health effects of racism and discrimination), two cities in Canada show what can be accomplished. In Vancouver, the social gradient in low birth weight births is flat, meaning that low-income residents have the same risk of having low birth weight babies as high-income residents.[4] And, in Toronto, there appears to be no relationship between a community's racial/ethnic makeup and the prevalence of low birth weight births in that community.[5] While neither Vancouver nor Toronto is a utopian city without inequality or social problems, at least some of the health effects of social inequality have been blunted, and more of their residents have the capacity to lead full and long lives. And this is possible not only in relatively rich places like Vancouver and Toronto but also in relatively poor places like Cuba—which now reports a low birth weight prevalence and infant mortality rate on par with those of Canada and the United Kingdom.[6] What would Chicago be like if health equity was recognized as a realistic vision and all its residents saw themselves as valued by society? To recognize health equity as a realistic vision requires that we acknowledge that our current patterns of health inequities are manmade—the result of the unequal distribution of power and resources in our society and of policies that do not value all lives equally.

2. *Understand and teach health inequities in the context of time and place.* For the most part, public health and its associated fields are taught ahistorically, without recognition of the deep roots of contemporary problems. Our collective attention is often devoted to the latest idea—be it a new data set, a new intervention, a new program, or a new policy— and we are often quick to support new initiatives without fully considering what has been tried and perhaps has failed in the past. Yet as the social epidemiologist Nancy Krieger reminds us: "History is vital. . . . We live our history."[7] Chicago is a testament to that idea; the collective history of its communities shapes the health and well-being of its residents today. The challenge is clear: to address health inequities, we need to understand a community's history (and thus its memory) *and* the history of how our respective disciplines have engaged with that community.

3. *Challenge our disciplines to think and act holistically, recognizing disease in its social/structural and political context.* We need to continue the movement in epidemiology away from individual-level risk factor

studies and toward a critical *social* epidemiology focused on structural violence. We need fewer studies of race and more studies of racism, especially studies that document the health effects of institutionalized racism and lead to the design of interventions to eliminate it.[8–10] As Camara Jones has explained through her American Public Health Association initiative on racism and health, we need to (a) put racism on the agenda, naming it as a critical social determinant of health, (b) ask, "How is racism operating here?," identifying the processes through which racism disadvantages some *and* advantages others, and (c) organize to act, promoting work that addresses racism and its negative effects on community health. We need to continue to challenge the disciplinary silos that restrict our capacity to see structural violence—particularly its manifestation as racism—as a determinant of health. We need the next generations of professionals to engage in health equity throughout their professional and civic lives. This training will require a more refined language to describe the patterns of structural forces shaping health equity, better evidence to support or alter the theoretical mechanisms outlined in the current social, economic, and structural determinant models of health, enhanced methods of inquiry to address multicausal chains, and efficient dissemination mechanisms to give people the right knowledge at the right time to take action.

4. *Contribute to and organize social movements that fight to protect health as a human right, both locally and globally.* This *Reader* includes works that demonstrate the power of collective action—from the Committee to End Discrimination in Chicago Medical Institutions in the 1950s to the Medical Committee for Human Rights in the 1960s to the more recent efforts of the Metropolitan Chicago Breast Cancer Task Force and Fearless Leading by the Youth. It is through these moments of collective action that health equity research becomes most meaningful and shifts from describing the world to changing it.

5. *Promote solution-focused research.* The actions proposed above will not matter if we lack the will to design and implement solutions. Much of our research infrastructure is devoted to problem-focused activities—describing the magnitude of problems, identifying risk factors and establishing connections between risk factors and health outcomes, and sometimes comparing how these connections vary from place to place or over time. And, while there is a strong need for continued surveillance and monitoring of how health inequities change over time, we know full well that health inequities *exist*—the challenge, of

course, is to do something about them. Pointing out this limitation, Pat O'Campo and others at Toronto's Centre for Urban Health Solutions argue for investments in solution-focused research geared toward generating evidence needed for the design of equity-based interventions.[11] This could involve, for example, developing more opportunities for true collaboration and resource sharing between communities and research institutions.[12,13]

In the relatively short but historically significant arc of Chicago's experience, structural violence can be traced as the root cause of health inequities. If we do not do so, we run the risk of seeing health as only a personal trouble—something that can be explained by the beliefs, behavior, or biology of individuals. If health is seen solely as a personal trouble, our attention is devoted to seeing the cause of poor health as individuals themselves—a classic case of blaming the victim. But, if we recognize health to be a public rather than a personal issue, and if we recognize that health inequities result from structural violence, our attention is shifted to *structural solutions*.

Structural solutions target unjust systems and practices that benefit some at the expense of others. They necessitate addressing racial/ethnic segregation, discrimination, economic inequality (not just poverty), and other forms of oppression as the root cause of unnecessary morbidity and mortality in our city. The lesson for all of us is that we must challenge ourselves, our respective professions, disciplines, and institutions, to act decisively to mitigate these historical injustices that lead to poor health or risk perpetuating them by our passivity.

References

1. BBC. *I call it murder* [documentary]. 1979.

2. De Maio FG. *Health and social theory*. Basingstoke: Palgrave Macmillan; 2010.

3. Muntaner C, Sridharan S, Solar O, Benach J. Against unjust global distribution of power and money: The report of the WHO Commission on the Social Determinants of Health: Global inequality and the future of public health policy. *Journal of Public Health Policy*. 2009;30(2):163–175.

4. Direction de Santé Publique. *Social inequalities in health in Montréal*. Montréal: Agence de la Santé et des Services Sciaux de Montréal; 2011.

5. De Maio F, Shah RC, Schipper K, Gurdiel R, Ansell D. Racial/ethnic mi-

nority segregation and low birth weight: A comparative study of Chicago and Toronto community-level indicators. *Critical Public Health*. 2017;27(5):541–553.

6. Bonet Lopez N, Choonara I. Can we reduce the number of low-birth-weight babies? The Cuban experience. *Neonatology*. 2009;95:193–197.

7. Krieger N. Public health, embodied history, and social justice: Looking forward. *International Journal of Health Services*. 2015;45(4):587–600.

8. Jones CP. Levels of racism: A theoretic framework and a gardener's tale. *American Journal of Public Health*. 2000;90(8):1212–1215.

9. Jee-Lyn Garcia J, Sharif MZ. Black Lives Matter: A commentary on racism and public health. *American Journal of Public Health*. 2015;105(8):e27–e30.

10. Paradies Y. A systematic review of empirical research on self-reported racism and health. *International Journal of Epidemiology*. 2006;35(4):888–901.

11. O'Campo O, Dunn J, eds. *Rethinking social epidemiology: Towards a science of change*. Berlin: Springer; 2011.

12. Hernandez SG, Genkova A, Castaneda Y, Alexander S, Hebert-Beirne J. Oral histories as critical qualitative inquiry in community health assessment. *Health Education and Behavior*. 2017;44(5):705–715.

13. Peek ME, Wilkes AE, Roberson TS, et al. Early lessons from an initiative on Chicago's South Side to reduce disparities in diabetes care and outcomes. *Health Affairs (Millwood)*. 2012;31(1):177–186.

Suggestions for Further Reading

Choosing which documents to include and which to exclude from this book was a daunting task. We know that our collection is only a small snapshot of the rich literature that has developed around health equity in Chicago. For readers interested in more empirical studies, we recommend browsing through the *American Journal of Public Health*, *Social Science and Medicine*, and related journals. On our Center for Community Health Equity Web site (https://www.healthequitychicago .org), we offer an extended list of relevant articles that we considered but could ultimately not include in this book as well as a "Voices of Health Equity" interview series that features many of the authors of these studies. At the same time, we encourage readers to branch out from traditional public health and medical journals—there is valuable insight to be gained from reading reports from community-based nonprofits and advocacy organizations as well as academic institutions.

There are also many excellent books in this area. We highlight a few:

Everybody in, Nobody Out: Memoirs of a Rebel without a Pause (Friday Harbor, WA: Copernicus Healthcare, 2013), the biography of Quentin Young, is an inspiring book, required reading for anyone interested in engaging with Chicago health equity work. *Urban Health: Combating Disparities with Local Data*, ed. S. Whitman, A. M. Shah, M. R. Benjamins (New York: Oxford University Press, 2011) is an edited collection of some of the work of the Sinai Urban Health Institute (SUHI). SUHI has set the example of how to collect and leverage data for community health programs. *Heat Wave: A Social Autopsy of Disaster in Chicago*, by Eric Klinenberg (Chicago: University of Chicago Press, 2002), is a sociological analysis of a landmark public health crisis. Along with Robert Sampson's *Great American City: Chicago and the Enduring Neighbor-*

hood Effect (Chicago: University of Chicago Press; 2012), *Heat Wave* represents some of the best analysis of the social divisions of Chicago and how these divisions manifest in unequal life chances for its residents.

Moving further away from health research, we would encourage readers to examine *Black Picket Fences: Privilege and Peril among the Black Middle Class* (Chicago: University of Chicago Press, 1999), by the sociologist Mary Pattillo-McCoy, an important analysis of how life in the city remains separate and unequal for many people. Similarly, *Family Properties: How the Struggle over Race and Real Estate Transformed Chicago and Urban America* (New York: Picador, 2010), by Beryl Satter, details the institutionalized system of legal and financial exploitation (institutionalized racism) that has shaped Chicago's communities. Satter's book informed Ta-Nehisi Coates's essay "The Case for Reparations" in the *Atlantic* (June 2014), which has quickly become a classic. *Neoliberal Chicago*, edited by Larry Bennett, Roberta Garner, and Euan Hague (Champaign: University of Illinois Press, 2017), explores how a philosophy of fiscal austerity and regulation reduction has transformed the city. And *Gentrifier*, by John Joe Schlichtman, Jason Patch, and Marc Lamont Hill (Toronto: University of Toronto Press, 2017), examines the process of gentrification—one of the most important challenges we face in community development.

Some of the best descriptions of the structural determinants that drive health disparities in Chicago are found in narrative fiction and nonfiction. In the narrative nonfiction category, *The Warmth of Other Suns: The Epic Story of America's Great Migration*, by Isabel Wilkerson (New York: Random House, 2010), offers the experiences of a family making the great African American migration from the South to Chicago. In the narrative fiction category, Upton Sinclair's *The Jungle* (1906) provides a portrait of immigrants and working conditions in the stockyards of Chicago, while Richard Wright's *Native Son* (1940) provides a portrait of growing up in Chicago's African American community in the 1930s.

Author Index

Subject Index